NURSING PROCESS
Application of
Conceptual Models

NURSING PROCESS
Application of Conceptual Models

EDITED BY

Paula J. Christensen, RN, PhD

Clinical Assistant Professor,
The University of Illinois at Chicago,
College of Nursing,
Rockford, Illinois

Janet W. Kenney, RN, PhD

Professor,
Arizona State University,
College of Nursing,
Tempe, Arizona

Fourth Edition
with 25 illustrations

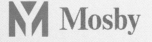 Mosby

St. Louis Baltimore Boston Carlsbad Chicago Naples New York Philadelphia Portland
London Madrid Mexico City Singapore Sydney Tokyo Toronto Wiesbaden

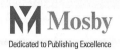
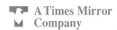

Publisher: Nancy Coon
Managing Editor: Loren Stevenson Wilson
Associate Development Editor: Brian Dennison
Project Manager: Dana Peick
Production Editor: Cindy Deichmann
Interior Design: Elizabeth Fett
Cover Design: Amy Buxton
Manufacturing Supervisor: Theresa Fuchs

Fourth Edition

Printed in the United States of America
Composition by University Graphics, Inc.
Printing/binding by Wm. C. Brown Publishers

Mosby-Year Book, Inc.
11830 Westline Industrial Drive
St. Louis, Missouri 63146

International Standard Book Number 0-8151-1401-X

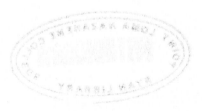

95 96 97 98 99 / 9 8 7 6 5 4 3 2 1

CONTRIBUTORS

Judith A. Barton, RN, PhD
Associate Professor,
University of Colorado,
School of Nursing,
Denver, Colorado

Joanne R. Cross, RN, PhD, NCC
Faculty Emeritus,
Wright State University,
School of Nursing,
Dayton, Ohio

Linda J. Dries, RN, MS, CDE
Clinical Nurse Specialist,
Swedish American Hospital,
Rockford, Illinois

Elizabeth S. Fayram, RN, MSN
Associate Professor,
Edgewood College,
Department of Nursing,
Madison, Wisconsin

Wealtha Yoder Helland, RN, MS
Associate Professor,
Rockford College,
Department of Nursing,
Rockford, Illinois

Karen Saucier Lundy, RN, PhD
Associate Professor,
University of Southern Mississippi,
School of Nursing,
Hattiesburg, Mississippi

Cynthia Makielski Martz, RNC, MSN
Assistant Professor,
Research College of Nursing,
Kansas City, Missouri

Cathy D. Meade, RN, PhD
Associate Professor,
University of Wisconsin-Milwaukee,
School of Nursing,
Milwaukee, Wisconsin

To all professional nurses and nursing students
who aspire to integrate theories in the nursing process
within contemporary nursing practice

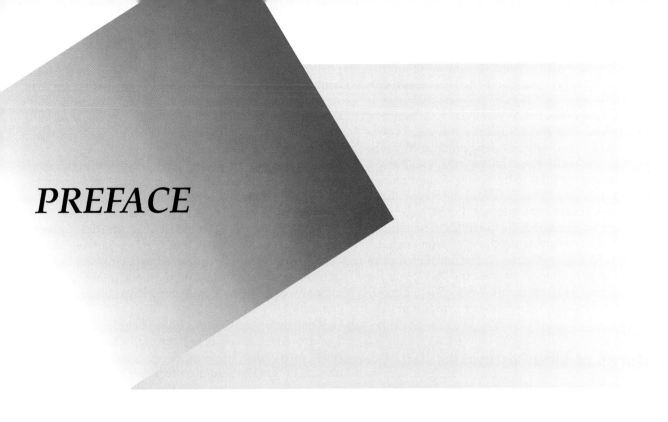

PREFACE

Today nursing is considered a professional discipline that includes the *art* of applying *scientific knowledge* to practice. The body of nursing knowledge encompasses four areas—empirical, ethical, esthetic, and personal knowledge—that are consistently used in making nursing decisions. Critical thinking skills are also required in nursing decisions to determine what information is relevant and how the information should be interpreted to arrive at sound judgments. The nursing process provides the structure for decision-making to assist clients in meeting their health care needs. Nursing models complement the use of the nursing process by guiding what information is relevant to the clients' situation and how to interpret that information. The nursing process ensures consistency in using a scientific approach, while theories and nursing models provide a unique perspective to frame the client's health concern. Together they ensure *theory-based nursing practice*, the basis for demonstrating accountability and responsibility of nurses' decisions.

Over the last two decades nurses have gradually shifted from a reliance on traditional empirical knowledge within the biomedical model to a more holistic, humanistic model based on applying all four forms of knowledge. As nursing leaders recognized the limitations in using mainly objective, empirical knowledge to make clinical decisions, humanistic nursing science evolved. This approach considers clients from a holistic perspective and explores the meaning of their life patterns and experiences in relation to their past, present, and future. It relies on the use of all four types of nursing knowledge, including personal knowledge, which develops with experience and trust in one's own judgment. Thus nursing decisions are currently based on empirical or scientific knowledge, ethical and esthetic knowledge, and personal knowledge, which includes self-awareness and intuition. The nurse's possession of a wealth of knowledge in all four areas is essential to clinical practice. All types of nursing knowledge are applied throughout the nursing process to enhance the quality of decision-making, nursing judgments, and, ultimately, client care.

Twelve years ago the editors and contributors wrote the first edition of *Nursing Process: Application of Theories, Frameworks, and Models*. At that time we could not foresee subsequent editions. However, theory-based practice remains an important aspect of professional nursing. Thus we decided to write the ensuing editions, including this fourth edition. This book was written primarily to provide nursing students, practitioners, and educators with a foundation for understanding how to apply theoretical approaches used in the nursing process. The way in which nurses use the nursing process and theories or models depends on their level of proficiency in practice. Novice practitioners follow a more structured approach. As expertise develops, nurses rely more on their own experience. They internalize the nursing process and theories as part of their broad knowledge base. Patricia Benner researched and delineated levels of nurses' proficiency. Her work is introduced in the first chapter and is integrated throughout the chapters on the nursing process.

Theory-based nursing practice will continuously evolve and change in response to major societal, economic, and professional trends. Some of these trends include changes in the health care system, consumers' needs, medical and technological advances, professional nursing organizations' viewpoints, and educational preparation for advanced practice nurses. Nursing models continue to be developed and refined as nursing practice changes. These models will address how nurses strive to enhance clients' well-being and how nursing responds to society's ever-changing health care needs. Nursing practice based on the nursing process facilitates clients in meeting their health care needs. Application of theories and models in the nursing process ensures theory-based nursing practice, which is responsive to changing trends and optimal client care.

Features of This Edition

This fourth edition of *Nursing Process: Application of Conceptual Models* incorporates major recent developments in the nursing profession. The essential skills of critical thinking in applying models to each component of the nursing process are described and integrated throughout. We also have added *critical thinking exercises* that apply the nursing process to the first 12 chapters of the book. The use of empirical knowledge, as well as ethical, esthetic, and personal knowledge, is explored in chapters describing the components of the nursing process.

In addition to some theoretical and philosophical changes, the fourth edition offers some new practical features. Section I discusses the importance of theory-based nursing practice and the use of critical thinking skills. The evolution of the nursing process and theory development in nursing are described. An overview of theories, models, and frameworks currently used in nursing and other disciplines is presented. These theoretical approaches serve both as an introduction to different models and as a reference for understanding their application in subsequent chapters.

Section II describes the nursing process in detail. The basic components—assessment, analysis and diagnosis, planning, implementation, and evaluation—are illustrated with different frameworks and models. Guidelines for applying each component and exam-

ples of using them with the individual, family, and community client are also given. The chapter on assessment of the community client may be applied to the client as a geographical population or an aggregate group with similar interests or needs. The chapters on nursing diagnosis have been significantly revised to enhance clarity in understanding the complex process of making nursing judgments and writing nursing diagnoses. The planning chapters now address identification of expected outcomes, which reflect the most recent standards of practice by the American Nurses Association. Various nursing intervention strategies are presented to facilitate selection of those that are appropriate for the specific client situation, whether the client is an individual, family, or community.

We recommend that the reader begin with Chapter 1 and proceed in sequence through Chapter 12, because each chapter builds on previous chapters. It is important that the reader understand the rationale for a theoretical approach and the interrelationships of the components before implementing the nursing process. The 10 chapters in Section II provide the foundation for understanding the case studies in Section III. The Appendixes contain a glossary of important terms, the complete list of guidelines for each component of the nursing process, and, selected examples of individual and family nursing assessment tools based on nursing models.

•••

We have been challenged and excited about the revisions in this edition as we strengthened several chapters and incorporated the critical thinking process within them. We believe the addition of critical thinking exercises will enhance the reader's ability to make judgments based on various ways of knowing. Our goal is to illuminate how the nursing process can guide nursing practice while recognizing that nurses are individuals with different talents and abilities. Nurses' unique experiences, levels of proficiency, and ways of knowing contribute to the richness of our profession and to the quality of care provided to our many clients.

Paula J. Christensen
Janet W. Kenney

CONTENTS

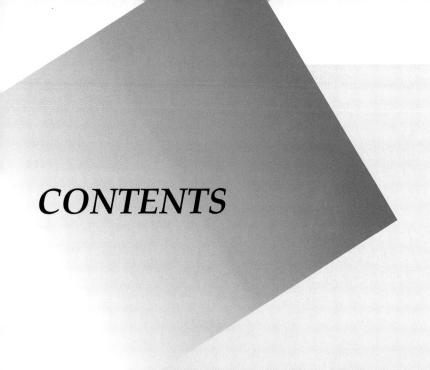

APPENDIXES

NURSING PROCESS
Application of
Conceptual Models

Theory-Based Nursing Practice

CHAPTER 1

RELEVANCE OF THEORY-BASED NURSING PRACTICE

Janet W. Kenney

Nursing is a professional discipline that applies many forms of knowledge and critical thinking skills to each client situation through the use of nursing models in the nursing process. We believe that nurses must exercise critical thinking skills and apply nursing models in each component of the nursing process. The nursing models in existence today vary in their degrees of specification; however, each can be used in nursing practice. In the literature, theorists' works are referred to as theories, frameworks, and models; we collectively call these works *models* unless otherwise specified. Also, because the models present different perspectives, they are considered complementary rather than competitive. Throughout this book the term *client* refers to the individual, family, or community, unless specifically identified.

This chapter begins with an overview of the nursing discipline and forms of knowledge. Historical perspectives of nursing and nursing practice are discussed, including Benner's (1984) levels of nursing proficiency. Next, critical thinking skills are described and related to the nursing process. The purposes and characteristics of the nursing process are also presented. A brief history of theory development in nursing is discussed, followed by current trends in nursing theory. The structural and functional components of theory follow. Terms such as *assumptions, concepts, propositions, conceptual model, theoretical framework,* and *theory* are explained. General perspectives of nursing models are addressed, including the purposes and characteristics of nursing models. The chapter con-

cludes with a discussion on how nurses can implement theory-based nursing practice.

Nursing as a Discipline

A professional discipline is identified by a specific field of inquiry and the shared values and beliefs of its members about its social commitment and the nature of its service. Nursing is recognized as an emerging professional discipline with a unique perspective developed over the past four decades. This perspective is based on an evolving philosophy, past history, and nursing's expanding scope of practice. In addition, new ideas of nurse scholars, theory development, and nursing research have all contributed to the discipline. The consensus is that nursing's unique focus is on persons, health, the environment, and the role of the nurse. As each discipline develops it directs the way that its domain, or field of knowledge, will develop. In the development of nursing knowledge, Meleis (1985) identified four major areas that are addressed:

- Major concepts and problems of nursing
- Assessment, diagnosis, and intervention processes
- Tools to assess, diagnose, and intervene
- Research designs and methods congruent with nursing

Nursing has made tremendous progress in each of these areas. The major concepts identified by the discipline are *client, health, environment,* and *nursing.*

Determining the nurse's role in facilitating the client's health in the environment is the complex problem on which nursing focuses. As an applied discipline, nurses use their broad knowledge base within the nursing process to gather and analyze data, interpret their meanings, and determine the most effective nursing action. There is a growing consensus that theory-based nursing practice provides an effective framework to deliver holistic, comprehensive nursing care and to evaluate the outcomes of nursing practice. Use of a broad knowledge base and nursing models within the nursing process requires critical thinking skills to apply knowledge and general principles, make decisions, and solve problems in specific client situations. Thus nurses must be well-educated, critical thinkers.

Forms of Nursing Knowledge

During the 1960s the nursing discipline sought to define itself as a true profession with a scientific base for its practice and emerging theories. Empirical knowledge became the dominant pattern, and traditional nursing followed the medical model, which embodied the empirical scientific approach. The empirical method focuses on observable, objective, logical hard data, and an analytical, verbal, and linear line of reasoning. Other ways of knowing, especially personal knowledge, which includes subjectivity, sensing, feeling, intuition, emotion, and experience, were devalued or discredited. Science, or "true" knowledge, was based on the superiority of empirical validation; all other forms of knowledge were considered mere speculation.

Since the 1980s there has been a growing awareness that too much reliance on empirical knowledge has led to a distorted view of the world. Each discipline's body of knowledge would be incomplete if it were based only on empirical, observable evidence. In 1978 Carper described four "patterns of knowing" within nursing: empirical, ethical, esthetic, and personal knowledge. Each pattern requires a specific process of discovery and has its own method for determining credibility of knowledge in each field. While some disciplines rely more heavily on one pattern of knowing, other disciplines, especially nursing, integrate all four patterns of knowing for a more complete picture of reality. All are valid ways of knowing and are useful for certain purposes. Each of these patterns is described and its application in nursing is identified here.

Empirical or *scientific knowledge* is based on objective evidence obtained by the senses; it requires validation and verification by others. Within the nursing discipline, scientific knowledge consists of principles, theories, and conceptual models, as well as research findings from nursing and related disciplines. This knowledge is used to relate concepts, order knowledge, and describe, explain, and predict nursing actions and outcomes. Knowledge of interpersonal relationships guides nurses' communication and interaction with clients. Knowledge of technical skills guides performance of procedures. Knowledge of nursing models and theories guides thinking, observations, interpretation of client information, and nursing interventions.

Ethical knowledge examines philosophical premises of justice and seeks credibility through logical justification. Nursing practice is based on accepted Standards of Clinical Nursing Practice established by the American Nurses Association (1991) and defined by each specialty, the scope of nursing practice within each state, and the institutional guidelines for procedures in the nurse's employment setting. Ethical knowledge also includes application of the Code for Nurses (ANA), which explicates nurses' values and how to treat clients. Codes of conduct specify nurses' accountability to clients and each other, along with basic moral principles of obligation to clients and processes for determining right and wrong nursing actions.

Esthetic knowledge is used for creativity, form, structure, and beauty through criticism of the meaning of the creative process and product. The creative way in which nurses structure and apply their knowledge in caring for clients is considered the *art of nursing* and requires esthetic knowledge. This knowledge encompasses sensitivity, empathy, and sincere caring for clients and is acquired through experience in practice.

Personal knowledge integrates and analyzes current interpersonal situations with past experience and knowledge. With increasing experience nurses acquire a growing knowledge about themselves, their client's health patterns, and their ability to interpret selected information and take action. This growing knowledge occurs through encounters with clients and others, thoughtful introspection, reflection, and analysis. Some consider personal knowledge to be the same as intuition, which may reflect a synthesis of knowing based on past experiences. *Intuition* is an awareness of meanings, relationships, and possibilities by way of insight, without conscious knowledge. It can be a sudden perception of a pattern in a seemingly unrelated series of events or a creative discovery. Personal knowledge includes a process of reaching accurate conclusions with limited information or perceiving a gestalt or "whole" of a situation rather than "bits and pieces" of information. As they gain experience, nurses rely more on their personal knowledge to recognize client problems and make decisions.

While each of the four patterns of knowing provide

a unique perspective and contribution to nursing, these patterns are also interrelated in nursing practice. Nurses apply all forms of knowledge in each component of the nursing process. As nurses analyze client information and make clinical judgments, they use a combination of scientific, ethical, esthetic, and personal knowledge to make decisions upon which nursing actions are based. These forms of knowledge are also used to select and apply models for care of clients.

Historical Perspectives

Before the 1960s nursing practice was generally based on apprenticeship learning, the performance of technical skills, and application of isolated acts and principles, such as aseptic technique and principles of mobility. Nurses depended on the physician's diagnosis and orders, which usually consisted of vital signs and simple treatments. Hygienic and comfort measures were initiated by nurses. The medical model, which views body and mind separately and focuses on cure and treatment of pathological problems, was adopted by nurses. Also, nurses, like physicians, believed they knew what was best for the patient. Only ill patients—those under a physician's care—were considered the passive recipients of nursing care.

The need for knowledge specific to nursing was identified by Florence Nightingale, who was the first nurse to systematically collect, record, and analyze data related to disease during the Crimean war. A century later, in the 1960s, the scientific era stimulated development of the nursing profession and the aim of creating a science of nursing. The interpersonal, intellectual, and scientific aspects of nursing were emphasized by the profession. Early nurse theorists viewed nursing as an interaction process and focused on the process and methods of assessment. Orlando (1961) addressed the interpersonal aspects of the nurse-client relationship. She also emphasized the need to deliberate and to validate client needs rather than the use of an intuitive approach. Knowles (1967) applied the scientific approach to her definition of nursing, which included discovery, delving, doing, and discrimination. With continued focus on the scientific approach, nursing leaders explained how to apply this approach in the nursing process. In 1966 Kelly described available data for nursing assessment as the client's physical signs and symptoms, the medical history and diagnosis, the social history and cultural background, and the physical or psychological factors in the environment. Johnson (1967) stressed the importance of systematically collecting data and rigorously analyzing it. Nursing diagnosis was defined at that time as determining the etiology of a symptom and its alleviation.

In 1967 Yura and Walsh wrote the first comprehensive book describing four components of the nursing process. These authors emphasized the intellectual, interpersonal, and technical skills of nursing practice. Since the nursing process has been developed and refined, it has become the primary method and focus of nursing practice; however, the number and definition of components are not completely agreed upon by nurses. In 1973 the American Nurses Association adopted and legitimized the components of the nursing process in *Standards of Nursing Practice.* The manual of the Joint Commission on Accreditation of Hospitals requires documentation of the nursing process. Since 1975 most states have revised their nurse practice acts to reflect this broader scope of nursing practice. State board NCLEX examinations currently test knowledge of all five major components of the nursing process.

By the 1970s the nursing profession viewed itself as a scientific discipline evolving toward a theoretically based practice that focused on the client. Many nursing theorists, such as Abdellah, Hall, Henderson, Johnson, King, Levine, Neuman, Orlando, Orem, Rogers, and Roy, had published their beliefs and ideas about nursing, and some had developed conceptual models. These theorists' views of nursing often were more idealistic than practical and realistic. Thus nurses had difficulty applying them to practice.

In the 1980s most graduate nursing education programs and some undergraduate programs offered required courses in nursing theories. As nurses became familiar with nursing models, they began to apply them to clients in various clinical settings. Gradually nursing practice included the application of theories and models in the nursing process. Many nurses are familiar with some models, such as Maslow's (1970) hierarchy of needs and Erikson's (1963) developmental stages. Other nurses are familiar with nursing models, such as Orem's (1980) self-care model and Roy's (1984) adaptation model. Increasingly, health care agencies are adapting nursing models as a framework for practice. Studies are being conducted to identify the benefits of using nursing models to determine direct client outcomes, along with staff and organizational outcomes.

Nursing Practice

Nursing is an applied science and an art, which uses all four forms of knowledge. A *science* is an organized body of knowledge, composed of specialized concepts and terminology, interrelated beliefs, facts, principles, laws, theories, and research methods that are used in education, research, and practice. Nursing science incorporates the synthesis and application of knowledge from the biophysical, behavioral, and humanistic sciences, along with the study of relationships between nurses and their clients and the environment within the context of health. This knowledge base rapidly changes and expands as research and new theories provide additional information. Nurses apply this broad knowledge base through critical thinking, psychomotor skills, and interpersonal actions to assist clients to achieve their optimum health potential. The *art* of nursing is the interpersonal relationship and interaction process between the person and the nurse within a social environment during delivery of nursing care. The science and art of nursing are creatively applied within the nursing process by critical thinking.

Levels of Nurse Proficiency

In 1984 Benner described five different ways that nurses think and act, based on their learning and experience. Benner found that nurses' levels of practice are directly related to their levels of knowledge, experience, and expertise. The five levels of nursing proficiency that Benner identified were novice, advanced beginner, competent, proficient, and expert. These proficiency levels were explicated in the Dreyfus Model of Skill Acquisition, which assumes that with increasing experience, nurses:

1. Rely less on rules and principles, making greater use of knowledge acquired in previous experiences
2. Rely less on analytic, rule-based thinking and more on intuition
3. Change their perception of situations from analyzing numerous equally relevant bits of information to visualizing an increasingly complex whole in which certain parts are more relevant
4. Move from being a detached observer to becoming fully involved in a situation. (Benner, Tanner, and Chesla, 1992).

The first level, *novice* or student, operates from a set of rules in a context-free situation. Guidelines and principles are used to determine the course of actions. *Advanced beginners* use learned procedures to determine immediate requirements for action. They are aware of the client's current status and immediate multiple, competing tasks to be accomplished to maintain the status, but cannot anticipate changes in the client's situation or adapt rapidly to changing situations. *Competent* nurses have more experience from which they have gained confidence in their ability to recognize impending problems and take appropriate nursing actions. They rely less on the certitude of others' judgments and rely more on their background of knowledge acquired with practice. Competent nurses establish goals for their clients and plans for their work, rather than tasks to be accomplished. They se-

lect nursing actions that fit their goals and organize their work with consistency, predictability, and time management. However, their focus on goals and organization may hinder their recognition of subtle changes in clients that need their attention.

With increasing experience, *proficient* nurses have the ability to recognize relevant changes in their clients. They perceive subtle contextual and situational changes in the client's status and initiate actions other than planned, based on their personal knowledge and experience. Proficient nurses notice when the client's condition has changed sufficiently to call for a redefinition of the situation, although they may need to think further about appropriate actions to take in response to the client's new patterns. They analyze and interpret new situations faster and understand the meanings of subtle changes in the client's patterns better.

Expert nurses quickly understand important aspects of a client situation, and can identify salient changes. Their understanding is not based on set expectations or formal knowledge, although this remains in their background. They have confidence in their ability to intuitively recognize subtle interacting factors, identify those which are relevant, and take appropriate actions. The thinking process is internalized because these practitioners use a holistic approach and see possibilities for their clients. However, experts do not overlook important facts, nor do they rely solely on their intuition to make decisions. After years of practice, they have developed trust in their intuition, and thus make accurate decisions.

As nurses' clinical experience increases, they integrate and synthesize their experiences from using different nursing models in the nursing process. The models and nursing process become basic, internalized frameworks for practice. Thus expert nurses who have developed proficiency may not think about each model or component in the nursing process, but intuitively apply them in their practice.

Roles of Nurses

While practicing the art and science of nursing, nurses also assume responsibility and accountability to the client, team members, other health care providers, the agency, and the state. The nurse is a team member in the health care system and assumes a variety of roles and responsibilities. Some of these roles are practitioner, educator, researcher, collaborator, advocate, case manager, and administrator. Two of these roles, advocate and collaborator, are discussed here. Other roles are integrated in the chapters or addressed in other books.

As *advocates*, nurses encourage clients to provide information about themselves and their views of health and illness and to participate in all decisions.

Client advocacy means the client and family are adequately informed about all relevant health or illness areas so that they can make knowledgeable decisions and that nurses support their decisions. Most clients do not want to be passive recipients of care; they prefer to receive sufficient accurate information so that they can make decisions that affect their lives. Supporting a client's decisions means assuring the client's right to choose and respecting the client's decision without giving approval or disapproval. The Patient's Bill of Rights is an example of the shift of the decision-making power to clients, along with the explanation and signing of "informed consent" for all treatments and operations.

Most nurses are members of a health care team and collaborate with other members to provide comprehensive client care and long-term planning. *Collaboration* with other health care providers assumes an interdependent relationship in a complementary role. Nurses rely on the expertise of specialists, such as respiratory therapists, geriatric practitioners, nutritionists, or neonatologists to perform services or offer assistance in the treatment and care of clients. Health team members also rely on nurses for their expertise in understanding the multiple factors influencing the client's health and in coordinating multiple services to meet the client's health care needs.

Critical Thinking in Nursing

Nurses practice in situations in which the client's conditions, treatments, procedures, and medications are constantly changing. Therefore nurses are constantly required to make numerous decisions based on up-to-date information and critical thinking skills. Critical thinking skills are needed to accurately collect and interpret relevant information, and to make sound judgments that contribute to good decisions within complex health care environments.

Critical thinking involves an attitude of honest inquiry and intellectual skills used in the reasoning process (Wilkinson, 1992). A skeptical attitude of inquiry is necessary to examine whether statements, observations, and facts are valid and relevant to a decision, rather than blindly accepting information. According to Paul (1988), critical thinkers hold the following attitudes:

1. *Intellectual humility*—an awareness of the limits of one's knowledge and sensitivity to one's possible biases and prejudice. Nurses and health providers should not claim to know more than they do.
2. *Intellectual courage*—the willingness and openness to listen and honestly examine others' ideas, although one may be strongly opposed to

those ideas. It requires courage to consider and examine others' viewpoints and to honestly weigh the strengths and shortcomings of one's own views.
3. *Intellectual empathy*—the ability to imagine oneself in someone else's place so that one can understand their views and line of reasoning.
4. *Intellectual integrity*—the willingness to apply the same rigorous intellectual standards of proof to one's own knowledge that one applies to others' knowledge. This requires the honesty to examine and acknowledge errors or inconsistencies in one's own thoughts, judgments, and actions.
5. *Intellectual perseverance*—the willingness to seek further insights and truths despite difficulty and frustrations. Considerable time and energy may be required to obtain and consider new information and form new insights.
6. *Faith in reason*—confidence in oneself and the willingness to pursue rational thinking and to believe that others are capable of the same.
7. *Intellectual sense of justice*—the willingness to examine others' viewpoints with the same intellectual standards, and not be influenced by one's own or others' interests or advantages.

Critical thinking also requires several active intellectual processes that are essential in collecting data, making decisions, setting priorities, solving problems, and planning nursing care. These processes are:

1. *Rational, logical and reasonable thinking*—Based on linking solid evidence, observations, and facts to draw conclusions, rather than making decisions based on ignorance, preferences, prejudice, or self-interest.
2. *Reflective thinking*—Taking time to examine and analyze data accurately identify client problems and desired health outcomes. Possible actions to achieve the outcomes are considered and compared with the benefits, harms, and costs of each action. The nurse does not jump to conclusions, but weighs the information in a disciplined manner.
3. *Autonomous thinking*—Thinking for oneself, not just accepting or being manipulated by others' views. Autonomous thinkers analyze information and decide what has the most evidence and credibility.
4. *Creative thinking*—A purposeful, goal-directed way to relate or synthesize information so that it is seen in a new way or provides a unique conclusion. It is the ability to establish relationships, transfer information to new situations, design alternative options, and find new solutions to problems. Creative thinkers consider the contex-

tual relevance and frame of reference of information and recognize that usually many factors affect each situation.

5. *Deciding conclusions and actions*—Includes analyzing and evaluating the evidence, comparing the options, weighing the costs, risks, and benefits, and estimating the success of achieving desired outcomes.

Nurses, as educated practitioners, are expected to have an *attitude* of skeptical inquiry and the *intellectual ability* to use rational, logical, and reflective thinking as they consider observations and information about each client. Throughout each component of the nurs-

ing process, nurses use critical thinking attitudes and abilities to determine the relevancy, meaning, and interrelationship of client data and to select and implement appropriate nursing models. The quality of nursing care is based on the use of critical thinking to make good judgments. Nurses' decisions determine which actions are taken that ultimately affect the client's care and health.

The Nursing Process

The nursing process provides a systematic guide or method to assist students and novices develop a style of

Table 1-1	Application of Critical Thinking Skills to Components of the Nursing Process
Components & definitions	**Critical thinking skills & activities**
Assessment	
An ongoing process of data collection to determine the client's strengths and health concerns	Collect relevant client data by observation, examination, interview and history, and reviewing the records
	Distinguish relevant data from irrelevant
	Distinguish important data from unimportant
	Validate data with others
Diagnosis	
The analysis/synthesis of data to identify patterns and compare with norms and models	Organize and categorize data into patterns
	Identify data gaps
	Recognize patterns and relationships in data
	Compare patterns with norms and theories
	Examine own assumptions regarding client's situation
A clear, concise statement of the client's health status and concerns appropriate for nursing intervention	Make inferences and judgments of client's health concerns
	Define the health concern and validate with the client and health team members
	Describe actual and potential concerns and the etiology of each diagnosis
	Propose alternative explanations of concerns
Planning	
Determination of how to assist the client in resolving concerns related to restoration, maintenance, or promotion of health	Identify priority of client's concerns
	Determine client's desired health outcomes
	Select appropriate nursing interventions by generalizing principles and theories
	Transfer knowledge from other sciences
	Design plan of care with scientific rationale
Implementation	
The carrying out the plan of care by the client and nurse	Apply knowledge to perform interventions
	Compare baseline data with changing status
	Test hypotheses of nursing inteventions
	Update and revise the care plan
	Collaborate with health team members
Evaluation	
A systematic, continuous process of comparing the client's response with the desired health outcomes	Compare client's responses with desired health outcomes
	Use criterion-based tools to evaluate
	Determine the client's level of progress
	Revise the plan of care

thinking that leads to appropriate clinical judgments. Nurse educators originally developed the nursing process as a teaching tool to guide students in learning critical thinking skills for nursing practice. Nurse leaders believed that the scientific approach of the nursing process would raise nursing to a recognized profession in the 1960s. However, Benner's research (1984) implied that too much reliance on the nursing process may reduce the proficient and expert nurse's intuitive and creative approach to nursing practice.

The nursing process and various nursing models can be considered the "training wheels" of practice. They guide and direct the student and novice practitioner in applying knowledge bases to practice. Nursing models provide a viewpoint for the components of the nursing process that assist beginners in defining nursing and directing the goals of nursing care. Expert nurses have internalized the nursing process and various models; therefore, they combine their experience with theoretical knowledge to analyze and identify the rationale underlying their apparently intuitive decisions. Models help expert nurses to consider the interrelationship of data and to explain the basis for their judgments.

Use of Nursing Models

Some nurses consistently use nursing models in their practice. Many unique nursing and developmental models are applicable in nursing practice. These models provide a frame of reference that can be applied to each component of the nursing process. The use of critical thinking skills in each component of the nursing process is shown in Table 1-1. Nursing models are used in the nursing process to:

- Collect, organize, and classify data
- Understand, analyze, and interpret client's health situations

- Guide formulation of nursing diagnoses
- Plan, implement, and evaluate nursing care
- Explain nursing actions and interactions with clients
- Describe, explain, and possibly predict clients' responses
- Demonstrate responsibility and accountability
- Achieve desired outcomes for clients

The nursing process is a deliberate activity whereby the practice of nursing is performed in a systematic manner. Throughout the nursing process the nurse uses a comprehensive knowledge base to assess the client's health status, to make judicious judgments and diagnoses, to identify the client's desired health outcomes, and to plan, implement, and evaluate appropriate nursing actions to achieve these outcomes. Critical thinking skills are continuously used to effectively carry out each component of the nursing process and to implement high quality nursing care, as shown in Table 1-1.

Components

The nursing process has five components, each with several phases, that are interactive and sequential. A nursing model is selected to guide the process; other models may supplement the primary nursing model. The nursing process can be represented in a schematic form as shown in Figure 1-1. This figure illustrates the feedback system between each component in the nursing process, depicting the typical flow of information by the dark lines and heavy arrows clockwise from assessment to diagnosis, plan, implementation, evaluation, and back to assessment. The small arrows in the opposite direction show that information from the succeeding components affects previous components by providing feedback. The lighter lines intersecting with the nurse-client relationship show that

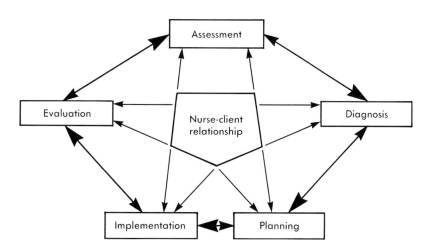

Figure 1-1 Nursing process: feedback system. (Developed by PJ Christensen.)

this relationship affects each component of the nursing process and that each component is dependent on all other components. The five components of the nursing process are described here and explained and illustrated more fully in Section II.

Assessment is a continuous process of collecting relevant data about the client's human responses, health status, strengths, and concerns. Critical thinking skills are used to distinguish essential, relevant information from irrelevant data, to validate important data, and to categorize and organize the information in a meaningful way. After initial information about the client's situation is obtained, a nursing model is chosen to guide the comprehensive data collection. The data are multifocal, reflecting historical and current data and representing a variety of sources. Interview, direct observation, and measurement are used to gather subjective and objective data. Data are systematically recorded and serve as the base for all other components in the nursing process. Data collection is ongoing throughout the nursing process. Because new data may alter other components, they should be communicated appropriately.

Diagnosis involves two phases: analysis/synthesis of the database into meaningful patterns, and writing diagnostic statements. The analysis begins by sorting the data into categories represented in the chosen model and identifying behavioral patterns. Critical thinking skills are required to recognize the client's patterns and establish meaningful relationships from the database. The client's behavioral patterns, including cues, signs, and symptoms, are compared with the model, health standards, and scientific or developmental norms to identify health concerns, strengths, and resources. Comparison of the client's patterns with health norms involves the use of critical thinking skills to recognize abnormal patterns or inconsistencies, make inferences, or assign meaning to the problem. Next the underlying cause of the client's problem is identified through critical thinking, forming the basis for the nursing diagnosis. Each diagnosis is validated with the client or health care professionals to verify the accuracy of the data interpretation.

The nursing diagnostic statements are written in clear, concise language. Each diagnosis is client-centered, specific, and accurate, and includes an etiological or descriptive statement. Nursing diagnoses reflect only those health concerns that can be treated by nurses. They provide direction for nursing interventions. The list of medical and nursing diagnoses represents the client's current health status and is updated as the client's condition changes.

The nursing diagnosis differentiates the practice of nursing from medicine. Medical care focuses on the disease pathology and a curative approach, whereas nursing focuses on human responses and caring. Nursing emphasizes the whole, unique person who is interacting with the environment and whose health state—not just the illness or disease—requires nursing intervention. Although the nursing and medical diagnoses are independent of one another, they are interrelated and should not be isolated from each other.

Planning occurs when the client and nurse identify the expected outcomes and actions to correct the nursing diagnoses. The phases in planning are: prioritize the nursing diagnoses, establish client health outcomes, identify appropriate nursing and client actions and scientific rationale, and establish the nursing care plan. The setting of the nurse-client interaction, whether it is the emergency room, clinic, hospital unit, home, or another site, directly influences planning.

The nursing diagnoses are *prioritized* according to their seriousness or life-threatening nature, which involves the use of critical thinking skills such as comparing and judging. After the health problems and concerns are prioritized, the client's *expected outcomes,* formerly known as long-term goals, are mutually established by the nurse and client. Each long-term expected outcome is based on a specific nursing diagnosis and reflects realistic resolution of the diagnosis. The expected outcomes must be achievable within the client's capabilities and limitations. These outcomes may include broad or specific criteria to measure the client's behavior during or after implementation of the plans. Identifying ways the chosen nursing model guides the desired outcomes and the strategies to achieve them are also part of critical thinking.

Short-term expected outcomes may be written as steps to achieve each long-term expected outcome. These outcomes are client-focused and reflect mutual planning with the client. They include specific criteria to measure the client's behavior and are written in the sequence in which they will be performed. Short-term expected outcomes must be realistic because they serve as the criteria against which nursing actions will be evaluated.

Next, the nurse focuses on achieving the client's expected outcomes by selecting appropriate *strategies and nursing interventions* to maintain and improve the client's health. Many critical thinking skills are used to choose effective nursing actions, such as generalizing from broad principles to specific actions, using knowledge from many sources, identifying criteria to measure achievement of the outcomes, and hypothesizing the effects of selected strategies.

Strategies are designed to prevent, reduce, or correct a client's health concern. The choice of a strategy is based on anticipated effectiveness in achieving the client's outcomes, the benefits and risks for the client, and the available resources, including people, equipment, time, finances, and facilities. To determine which potential strategy would be most effective, the nurse begins by identifying plausible actions, then analyzes the benefits, harms, and cost of each. Next, the nurse compares: (1) the benefits of each action with the potential harm (risks, side effects, inconvenience, and anxiety); (2) the expected outcomes, with possible costs in time, money, and involvement of others; and, (3) the availability of limited resources (equipment, health team members, and family, time, and money) with the benefits to be gained. Critical thinking involves the use of evaluating and judging the merits of each action, and requires the use of all forms of knowledge to make effective decisions and achieve the desired client-expected outcomes.

Nursing orders state who will do what within a given time period. They describe the client and nursing actions to achieve each outcome, as well as interdependent nursing actions. Nursing orders are stated in concise, specific terms in the appropriate sequence. They may include maintenance, promotion, and restorative aspects of care, along with coordination and collaboration with other health team members. The client's individuality and autonomy are incorporated in the nursing orders. The nursing orders support the medical regimen of care in addition to interdependent nursing actions. They are kept current and revised to describe alternate plans as necessary.

Scientific rationale describes the scientific basis for planning. The reason for each nursing order is clearly identified. The rationale may include principles, theory, research findings, and information from current literature. Critical thinking skills are used to identify the supporting rationale.

Implementation is performing the nursing orders designated in the plan by the client, nurse, or others. It may include collaboration with other health care providers in performing responsibilities. Application of knowledge from the sciences and humanities and hypotheses on the effect of nursing strategies are the essential critical thinking skills. The client's physical and psychological safety are considered and protected. Each action is performed with skill and efficiency and includes ongoing assessment. The nursing actions and the client's reactions or behaviors are recorded to verify that the plan was implemented and to evaluate the effectiveness of the plan.

Evaluation is comparing the client's current health status with the client's expected outcomes and determining the client's progress or lack of progress toward achievement of the outcomes. The nurse compares, judges, and evaluates as part of critical thinking. Criteria for measuring the client's level of achievement may be stated in short-term outcomes or evaluation. Evaluation is a continuous process that occurs during ongoing assessment and implementation of nursing care. While implementing orders the nurse makes ongoing evaluative judgments that describe the client's response or reaction to each nursing action and the respective outcome. The ongoing evaluation provides continuous data that may be used to change or modify the nursing diagnosis, plans, and implementation. Periodically a concluding evaluation is performed that compares the client's overall progress or lack of progress toward meeting the long-term expected outcomes.

Each component of the nursing process is explained in detail with examples in the chapters in Section II. Specific guidelines for each component and its phases are provided in Appendix B.

Purposes

The nursing process serves many purposes. The main purpose is to provide a systematic method for nursing practice: it unifies, standardizes, and directs nursing practice. The nurse's roles and functions are defined, and communication, collaboration, and synchronization of health team members are enhanced by the nursing process. Emphasis is placed either on health promotion, maintenance, and restoration or on enhancing a peaceful death, depending on the client's situation. Other purposes of the nursing process are to:

- Facilitate documentation of data, diagnoses, plans, client responses, and evaluation
- Evaluate the efficiency and effectiveness of care
- Give direction, guidance, and meaning to nursing care
- Provide for continuity of care and to reduce omissions
- Individualize client participation in care
- Promote creativity and flexibility in nursing practice

Accountability and responsibility to clients and the nursing profession can be demonstrated by use of the nursing process. As health care costs increase, both consumers and administrators of health care agencies are concerned about cost effectiveness and accountability. Service providers, including nurses, are watched by those paying for their services, namely consumers and third party payors, to determine the worth of their services. Nurses are expected to be accountable for their actions and to evaluate the effectiveness of their care. The nursing process enhances accountability to the client, service providers, and the agency/institution, and may be used to demonstrate cost effectiveness in these times of scarce resources.

Characteristics

Seven major characteristics of the nursing process enhance its usefulness in practice:

1. It is goal-directed toward client-centered health care.
2. It is systematic and provides an organized approach to nursing.
3. It is dynamic, focusing on the changing responses of the client during the ongoing process.
4. It is applicable to individuals, families, and community groups at any level of health.
5. It is adaptable to any practice setting or specialization, and the components may be used sequentially or concurrently.
6. It is interpersonal and based on the nurse-client relationship.
7. It is useful with any type of model, especially nursing.

History of Theory Development in Nursing

Until the 1960s nursing was principally derived from social, biological, and medical theories. With the exception of Florence Nightingale's work in the 1850s, nursing theory had its beginnings with the publication of Peplau's (1952) book, which described the interpersonal process between the nurse and the patient. The nature of the nurse's role came under scrutiny during this decade as nurse leaders debated the nature of nursing practice and theory development. Thereafter, several nurse leaders, namely Abdellah, Orlando, Wiedenbach, Hall, Henderson, Levine, and Rogers, developed and published their views of nursing, as shown in Table 1-2. Their descriptions of nursing and nursing models evolved from their personal, professional, and educational experiences and reflected their perception of "ideal" nursing practice. Several themes emerged as to the nature of nursing: it was described as an interpersonal process, as meeting the client's needs, or as providing nursing care.

During the 1970s a consensus developed among nursing leaders that the common elements of nursing include the nature of nursing (role/actions), the individual recipient of care (client), the context of nurse-client interactions (environment), and health (Fawcett, 1978). Nurses debated whether there should be one conceptual model for nursing or several models to describe the relationships among the nurse, client, environment, and health.

Several methods have been used to develop nursing models. Initially, as nurses acquired advanced education and became familiar with theories in other disciplines, they recognized that these theories would be useful in explaining nursing actions. Thus theories were borrowed from other disciplines. An example of this approach is the use of systems theory as the basis for Johnson's behavioral system model for nursing (1980). With recognition of the importance that theory plays in developing a scientific discipline, and awareness that theories in other disciplines were insufficient to describe nursing, nurses began to develop their own theories. Dickoff, James, and Weidenbach (1968) stimulated this trend by describing how theory is developed for a practice discipline. Although their approach has been debated, it sparked a growing commitment by nurses to develop their own models and theories. Some nurse theorists expanded or extended theories in other disciplines, such as Roy's (1984) work based on Helson's theory of adaptation. Other nurse theorists analyzed nursing practice situations to determine the theoretical underpinnings. King's (1981) work is representative of this approach, whereas Martha Rogers' (1970) work evolved from a philosophical and physics background.

Borrowing theories from other disciplines was criticized by some nurses as lacking originality and novelty. Also, some holistic nurses argued that current nursing models inadequately address the whole client and that a broader, phenomenological model was needed in nursing. Another criticism of nursing models is that they are relatively underdeveloped as theories in the strictest sense of the term. This problem may be related to the lack of clarity about what constitutes theory and theory testing in general and specifically the paucity of theory testing in nursing. Therefore, although some nursing models can describe and explain the nature of nursing, their ability to control and predict client outcomes is yet to be achieved. Developing a theory with such outcome control and predictability is the aim of some nurse theorists, but many nursing models reflect a synthesis of borrowed or expanded theories from other disciplines. Table 1-2 presents a chronology of events related to nursing theory development and nurse theorists' work.

Interrelationship of Nursing Theory, Practice, and Research

Nursing models are developed based on the theorist's assumptions, values, and beliefs about people, health, the environment, and nursing. Nursing theories derived from specific models describe and explain the relationships between clients, their health, the environment, and the role of the nurse. The theorist's definitions of each major concept, and the interrelationships of the concepts describe how nurses assist clients in attaining health within their environment. Both the theorist's concept definitions and the relationships serve to guide nursing practice and research.

Table 1-2	History of Nursing Theory Development	

Events	Year	Nurse theorists
	1860	Florence Nightingale Described nursing and environment

	1952	Hildegard E. Peplau
		  Nursing as an interpersonal process: patients with
		    felt needs

Scientific era: nurses questioned purpose of nursing	1960	Faye Abdellah (also 1965; 1973) Patient-centered approaches

	1961	Ida Jean Orlando
		  Nurse-patient relationship; deliberative nursing
		    approach

Process of theory development discussed among
  professional nurses
	1964	Ernestine Wiedenbach (also 1970; 1977)
		  Nursing: philosophy, purpose, practice, and art

	1966	Lydia E. Hall Core (patient), care (body), cure (disease)

	1966	Virginia Henderson (also 1972; 1978)
		  Nursing assists patients with 14 essential functions
		    toward independence

Symposium: theory development in nursing	1967	Myra Estrin Levine (also 1973) Four conservation principles of nursing
Symposium: nature of science and nursing Dickoff, James, and Weidenbach wrote "Theory in a Practice Discipline" in *Nursing Research*	1968	
Symposium: nature of science in nursing First nursing theory conference	1969	

Second nursing theory conference	1970	Martha E. Rogers (also 1980)
		  Science of unitary man: energy fields, openness,
		    pattern, and organization

Consensus on nursing concepts: nurse/nursing,
  health, client/patient/individual, society/environment
	1971	Dorothea E. Orem (also 1980; 1985)
		  Nursing facilitates patients' self-care

Discussion on what theory is: the elements, criteria,
  types, and levels, and the relation to research
	1971	Imogene King (also 1975; 1981)
		  Theory of goal attainment through nurse-client
		    transactions

NLN required conceptual frameworks in nursing education	1973	

Borrowed theories from other disciplines
Expanded theories from other disciplines
	1974	Sister Callista Roy (also 1976; 1980; 1984)
		  Roy's adaptation model: nurse adjusts patient's
		    stimuli (focal, contextual, or residual)

Recognized problems in practice and developed
  theories to test and use in practice
	1976	Josephine Paterson and L. Zderad
		  Humanistic nursing

Second nurse educator conference on nursing theory	1978	Madeleine Leininger (also 1980; 1981)
		  Transcultural nursing
		  Caring nursing

Articles on theory development in *ANS, Nursing Research,* and *Image*	1978	Jean Watson (also 1985)
	1979	Philosophy and science of caring; humanistic nursing

Books written for nurses on how to critique theory,
  how to develop theory, and describing application
  of nursing theories
	1980	Dorothy E. Johnson
		  Behavioral system model for nursing

Graduate schools of nursing develop courses in how
  to analyze and apply nursing theories
		Betty Neuman
		  Health-care systems model: a total person approach

Research studies in nursing identified nursing
  theories as framework for study
	1981	Rosemarie Rizzo Parse (also 1987)
		  Man-living-health: a theory of nursing

Numerous books published on analysis, application evaluation, and/or development of nursing theories	1982–present	

According to Fawcett (1988), nursing research begins with the creation of *basic* knowledge—the what, how, or why things occur. Next, basic knowledge may be studied to develop *applied* knowledge—the application of basic knowledge to practice. Lastly, further research studies may identify *clinical* knowledge—the application of applied knowledge to guide specific nursing practice situation. Thus theory, research, and practice are integrally related. Whereas the primary use of theory is to guide research, theory also interacts with and guides nursing practice; research studies serve to validate and modify nursing theory and to guide changes in nursing practice.

Current Trends in Nursing Science

The nursing discipline continually changes and evolves in response to major societal, political, and economic trends. Some of these trends include changes in consumers' needs, new developments in medical and human sciences and technology, shifts in professional nursing education and organizations, and health care reform with changes in the health care systems. Major trends which influence nursing science and practice are depicted in Fig. 1-2. Nursing science also evolves as more nurses become advanced practitioners, who develop, apply, and test nursing models and theories, and conduct nursing research.

Over the last two decades there has been a major paradigm shift in nursing from a reliance on the superiority of traditional empirical knowledge to a view of nursing science as examining *reality-based* changing life patterns and experiences of humans. Several nurse scholars claim that empirical science alone is not congruent with contemporary nursing science and that alternative research methods for developing nursing science are warranted (Schumacher and Gortner, 1992). Thus new views of nursing science are evolving that challenge the traditional methods of natural science and biomedical nursing, as shown in Table 1-3. Critical social theory and feminist perspectives have also contributed to a shift in the world views of nursing knowledge (Newman, 1992).

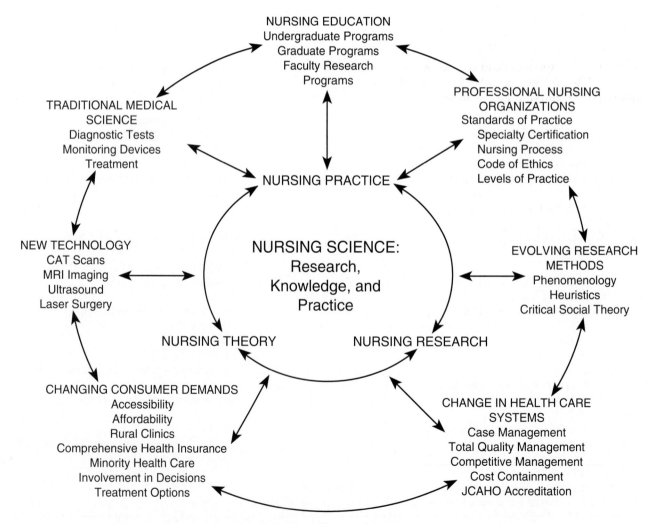

Figure 1-2   Major trends influencing the evolution of nursing science and nursing practice.

Table 1-3	Nursing Science's Shifting Perspectives (World Views)

Characteristics	Traditional natural science	Biopsychosocial integrative science	Humanistic / phenomenological
Types of knowledge	Reductionistic Mechanistic Objective	Multidimensional Organismic Subjective and objective	Holistic Contextual Relative Interactional
Research controls	Measurable Observable Verifiable	Desires objectivity, controllability, and predictability	Participant validation
Searches for	Laws and principles Linear causal relationships to predict and control	Probabilistic relationships and influential factors	Understanding of patterns and relationships
Change attributed to	Linear Causal and effect	Multifactorial Probabilistic	Unidirectional, unpredictable interactive processes
Views knowledge as	Verifiable facts, laws, and principles—a product	Contextual, relative, multifaceted, and interrelated	Personal interpretation of patterns, meanings Context of lived experience—a process of discovery

The Human Science Paradigm

In the last decade several alternative perspectives for nursing models, theories, and science were developed (Johnson, 1991; Newman, 1991). Based on the work of Dilthey (1988), nursing began to evolve as a human science paradigm (Mitchell and Cody, 1992). Dilthey believed that life must be understood as a process that is humanly lived—a living knowledge of "reflective" life that manifests itself in the dynamic unity of experience. This perspective views human beings as valued intentional, free-willed persons who are engaged in dynamic interaction with others and their environment. The person's lived experience is the focus of theory, practice and research. Four nurse theorists have developed new and different frameworks congruent with the human science paradigm. These frameworks are Paterson and Zderad's (1976) humanistic nursing, Newman's (1986) model of health as expanding consciousness, Parse's (1981) theory of human becoming (formerly man-living-health), and Watson's (1985) human science and human care.

As nurses embrace the human science paradigm, nursing practice, theory development, and research change to reflect this new perspective. Practitioners and researchers are regarded as coparticipants with clients in practice and in studies. A nurse practitioner who uses the human science approach examines clients' perceptions of reality and the meaning of their lives to develop insight into their living experiences of well-being and illness. This approach emphasizes understanding clients in terms of their lived experience and focuses on the meaning of the experience from the client's frame of reference. The nurse encourages clients to reveal their inner awareness and the contextual meaning of their daily lives, including past-present-future meanings and interpretations. The client's life-health-being is viewed in the living context without isolating any interacting variables. The nurse seeks to comprehend the essence and soul of clients and to understand their view of the total complex situation. In simplistic terms, the nurse is asking the client, "What does this health concern mean to you in relation to your life experiences (past and present) and how do you perceive it will affect your future?" According to Benner (1984), proficient and expert nurses recognize the effect of these interacting meanings on the client and develop a plan that takes these meanings into account.

Future Development of Nursing Models

Currently some nurse theorists, such as King, Roy, Parse, and Watson, continue to develop and refine their models in nursing, whereas others, like Orlando, Levine, and Orem, have developed their work as far as they had planned. In the future, nursing models must clearly differentiate activities that are unique to nursing and different from other health disciplines. Nursing must distinguish either a separate body of knowledge or a distinct manner of applying shared knowledge. Future nursing theories will strive to describe, explain, predict, and control client outcomes. Theories that facilitate the prevention of illness, and the maintenance, promotion, and restoration of the client's optimum health potential need further development.

Description of Theory

Structural Components

The terms *theory, theoretical framework,* and *conceptual model* are frequently used indiscriminately and interchangeably in nursing and other disciplines. These terms have been defined differently by various writers, which has led to much confusion. Different definitions of theory arise from a lack of consensus on what constitutes theory and what criteria must be met for something to be considered a theory. Although there is general consensus on the structural criteria required for a theory, there is less agreement on the functional criteria, which are based on values and beliefs of what constitutes a theory.

Several nurse scholars have described the process of theory development. As shown in Table 1-4, theory development is considered both a process with numerous activities and a product. According to Chinn and Kramer (1991), nursing theory development is a system or *process* that includes four interacting, sequential phases: analyzing concepts, constructing relationships, testing relationships, and validating relationships in practice. Each phase influences both the preceding and succeeding phases. Walker and Avant (1988) describe a similar process that begins with the development of concepts, statements, and then the-

ory, and is followed by theory testing with possible concept, statement, and/or theory revisions. This leads to further testing and contributions to nursing science. During theory development five *products* emerge: a philosophy of nursing, concept definitions, a conceptual model, a theoretical framework, and theories.

Initially theorists begin by defining their values, beliefs, and assumptions, which are expressed as their *philosophy of nursing.* Next, the major concepts in the philosophy are identified and defined. When the relationship among some concepts is explained by propositions or relational statements, the theorist's work is considered a *conceptual model.* As a network of concepts that are interrelated by relational statements is developed, the model may be called a *theoretical framework,* although further refinement is required for logical and empirical adequacy. Finally, when a theorist's work consists of a set of concepts logically interrelated and amenable to testing, it is considered a *theory.* However, the theory must be tested and validated in a variety of practice settings for support and acceptance. The terms commonly used to describe the system of theory development are explained in the following paragraphs and the process, activities, and products are shown in Table 1-4.

Table 1-4 Theory Development System: Process, Activities, and Product

Process	Activities	Product
Exploration	Identifies values, beliefs, and assumptions: What do nurses do (actions, skills) and for whom (individuals, families, community)? When (under what conditions)? Where (in what settings)? How (roles—practitioner, research)?	Philosophy of nursing
Concept analysis	Define and describe major concepts: Nursing—action, interactions, process Clients—individual, family, community Health—maintenance, prevention, restoration Environment—hospital, community, clinic	Concept identification
Construct relationships	Descriptive theory Describes some relationships between concepts, but the relationship is not clearly defined among *all* the concepts	Conceptual model
Test relationships	Explanatory theory Explains the interrelationship among the major concepts; however, the logical and empirical adequacy of the relationships requires further explication	Theoretical framework
Validate relationships in practice	Predictive and prescriptive theory Provides a set of interrelated concepts and relational statements that are logical and amenable to empirical testing and that explain or predict phenomena	Theory

Philosophy

Theory development begins with an examination and analysis of what a theorist believes about the nature of nursing: what is nursing, what does the nurse do, how, and to whom? A philosophy is the theorist's viewpoint: what the theorist assumes, believes, values, or holds to be true in relation to nursing.

Assumptions are beliefs that may have been tested or accepted as givens in other theories but are taken for granted by a theorist. They are the basis for the theorist's view and serve as a point of reference. Theorists may explicitly state their assumptions or they may imply their beliefs in their work. The more explicitly theorists state their assumptions, the less ambiguity there is in interpreting the theory. Assumptions are not tested; however, they lead to a set of propositions that can be tested. For example, Neuman (1982) assumes that a person is an open system interacting with the environment and responding to stressors.

A *concept* is an abstract word that conveys a mental image of a phenomenon. Concepts are names, labels, or categories for objects, persons, or events derived from one's perceptual experiences. Concepts are the basic building blocks of theory. A concept symbolically represents something but it is not the object or event itself. Concepts vary in degrees of abstractness: some concepts, such as anxiety or pain, are more abstract than others, such as medication or procedure. The more general a concept is, the more it transcends time and space, and the greater its abstractness. All concepts are intangible, descriptive terms that persons interpret according to their perceptions and experiences. Concepts must be specifically defined because people have different meanings for them. Alone, concepts are meaningless; they are judged according to their use in statements, such as propositions.

Conceptual Model

In the literature on theory, nursing continues to address the question of what the difference is between theory, theoretical frameworks, and conceptual models. What one person considers a theory another person may call a conceptual model. Without clear definitions and criteria for each, the argument is arbitrary and inconclusive. In this book the following definitions and descriptions are accepted.

In 1980 Johnson described a conceptual model for nursing practice as a systematically constructed, scientifically based, and locally related set of concepts. A conceptual model is a group of concepts or ideas that are related, but the relationship is not explicit. Models are an abstract perspective or framework representing reality. They use concepts to symbolize meanings, but they are not the real world. Conceptual models have a

"set of concepts"; however, the relational statements explaining the connection between the concepts are obscure and therefore are not amenable to testing. Models are more abstract with fewer specifically defined concepts than theories, and models do not explain how or why phenomena occur.

Some examples of conceptual models in nursing are: Orem's self-care model (1980), Roy's adaptation model (1984), and Johnson's behavioral system model for nursing (1980). The nursing process may also be considered a model because it is a group of related concepts.

Theoretical Framework

Theoretical frameworks consist of a set of defined concepts and relational statements; however, the relationship between some concepts is loosely described. A theoretical framework needs further explication of the specific relationships among *all* the major concepts to provide a systematic view of the phenomena. Although explicit relational statements in a theoretical framework may be tested, it is not considered a theory because the framework lacks a *set* of interrelated statements.

A *relational statement* is a proposition describing a specific relationship between two or more concepts. Relational statements are classified into two groups, associational and causal. *Associational propositions* show which concepts occur together and designate a positive, negative, or lack of relationship between two concepts. *Causal propositions* describe a cause and effect relationship; a change in one concept causes a change in another. Examples of these two types of statements are shown below:

> Associational: As anxiety increases, tension increases.
> As anxiety increases, perception decreases.
> Causal: High levels of anxiety cause decreased perception.

A theory contains two or more propositions—a *set*—that links the concepts and makes the interrelationship among the concepts explicit. The relationship between concepts in the proposition can be tested.

Some nurses believe that King's (1981) work in *A Theory for Nursing: Systems, Concepts, Process* is an example of a theoretical framework. Also, the work of Parse (1981) in *Man-Living-Health: A Theory of Nursing* is considered a theoretical framework because the interrelationships of the concepts are explicit and each concept is defined.

Theory

Theory is a highly complex term with arbitrary meanings. For some, theory may include ideas or hunches, whereas others believe that a theory must stand up to rigorous tests. In their book, Chinn and Jacobs (1983:70) define theory as

[a] set of concepts, definitions, and propositions that projects a systematic view of phenomena by designating specific interrelationships among concepts for purposes of describing, explaining, predicting, and/or controlling (prescribing) phenomena.

In a later edition, Chinn and Kramer (1991:73) define theory as "a creative and rigorous structuring of ideas that project a tentative, purposeful, and systematic view of phenomena."

Using the earlier definition, concepts, definitions, and propositions are required in a theory. Although there is a lack of consensus among the disciplines as to what a theory is, there is general agreement that theory consists of a set of defined concepts and a systematic, logical network of *relational statements or propositions. Set* means that a theory must contain two or more relationship statements that link the concepts, and the relationships among all the concepts must be explicit in the propositions. The statements linking the concepts can be tested. A theory symbolically represents reality but is not reality in itself. Theory is abstract and tentative; it varies in the degree of abstractness of the concepts and statements in the theory. Differences among models, frameworks, and theory are related to their levels of abstraction, degree of explication, and the level of theory development. All theories are models because they claim to represent some aspect of reality; however, all models are not necessarily theories. Conceptual models and theoretical frameworks usually precede and coexist with theory.

Some authors classify theories as descriptive, explanatory, or predictive (Stevens, 1983), as shown in Table 1-4. *Descriptive theory* identifies and describes the major concepts of phenomena but does not explain how or why the concepts are related. This is the first level of theory development. For example, descriptive nursing theory would provide definitions of concepts such as client, health, and nursing, as in Peplau's work (1952).

Explanatory theory, the next level of theory development, attempts to describe how or why concepts are related. It specifies the associations or relationships among some concepts, but further explication of the logical and empirical adequacy of these relationships is necessary. The theoretical frameworks or models by Johnson, King, Orem, and Roy are examples of explanatory theory.

Predictive theory is achieved when the conditions under which concepts are related are stated and the relational statements are able to describe future outcomes consistently. Selye's (1956) theory of stress and the general adaptation syndrome may be considered

predictive theory because it has been repeatedly tested and supported. In nursing and the social sciences it is generally accepted that predictive and prescriptive (controlling) theories are actively being pursued, but presently do not exist.

Within different disciplines, theories may be found at various stages of development. Some theories are developed as classifications or explanations of phenomena, whereas others serve the purpose of prediction, with or without control of phenomena. Depending on one's viewpoint, theory serves several different purposes. Some believe that the purpose of theory is to describe, explain, predict, and control outcomes, whereas others believe theory increases understanding and knowledge. In either case, theory is very useful in guiding nursing practice, research, and education.

Functional Components

The functional components of any theory are the major concepts and their definitions. These concepts are the focus of the theory or model. In the 1970s the nursing profession generally agreed that four major concepts are addressed in nursing models: the client, the nature of nursing (role/actions), the meaning of health, and the environment in which client-nurse interactions occur. However, each nurse theorist offers a unique perspective of these concepts in her model based on her assumptions and beliefs about humans, health, nursing, and the environment. Nurses who use these models must understand the unique ways in which each theorist defines these concepts and describes their interrelationships. Those who choose theory-based nursing practice must know the theorists' views on each of the following questions before applying their nursing models.

1. *Who is the client?* The client is the recipient of nursing care and may be defined as an individual, family, community, or an aggregate group. Theorists may define a client as a person with a need, an impaired health status, a self-care deficit, an adaptive person capable of change, or someone experiencing disharmony. Some theorists identify only individuals with health problems as the clients, whereas other theorists view any individual or family as care recipients within the scope of nursing.

2. *What is the nature of nursing—the nurse's role?* Nursing models generally describe nursing as a helping discipline that may involve cognitive acts, behavioral tasks, or interpersonal relationships between the client and the nurse. The nurse may act on the client's behalf, mutually with the client, or may teach the client how to carry out certain activities. One nursing model

defines the nurse's role as a self-care agent; other models view the nurse as reducing the client's stressors, promoting adaptation, or facilitating harmony between the client and their environment. The nurse's role in each model should be clearly understood by those who apply the model.

3. *What is the meaning of health?* Some theorists describe a health-illness continuum, whereas others refer only to ill health or the presence of health problems. Recently some theorists have described health as more than the absence of disease. They view health as a dynamic process that changes over time and varies with circumstances. Other theorists view health as interdependent with the changing environment or as a process that the person has some control over. Nurses must understand the theorist's view of health and determine whether that viewpoint is congruent with their own view of health.

4. *Where do client-nurse interactions occur?* What settings or environment are deemed appropriate for nursing? The *environment* may be defined as the central arena of nursing or the area of interchange with the client in the health setting. Some theorists limit the scope of nursing practice to hospital settings and/or outpatient clinics, whereas others include community concepts and some place no restrictions or limits on this concept.

General Perspectives of Nursing Models

The scope of nursing practice varies widely because of the multiple practice settings, the complexity of the client's health status and situation, and the role of the nurse. Nursing models each present a unique perspective on how to assist clients to attain optimal health. Models of nursing also vary in their levels of development, degree of abstractness, and clarity of concept definitions and relational statements. Most nursing models describe the four major concepts cited previously and some subconcepts. However, each model describes the major concepts and their interrelationships in a unique way. Also, some models are more applicable to a family or group, such as the models of Neuman and King, whereas other models, such as those of Roy, Johnson, Parse, and Watson, focus on individual clients.

Purposes

Knowledge and values about life, people, and events influence each person's perception, understanding, and behavior in the world. Viewing life events and people as separate facts or "bits of information" limit one's understanding of the world. Therefore disciplines construct theories, frameworks, and models to show relationships among events and people, to organize information, and to apply in practice. Nursing models represent several different views of nursing—perspectives about who is the client, what is health, what is the nurse's role or actions, and what is the environment in which nursing occurs.

The major purpose of nursing models is to guide theory-based nursing practice and direct theory development. Other purposes of nursing models are to:

- Provide a unique perspective to view the client situation
- Provide guidelines to organize thinking and observations, focus inquiry, interpret data, and communicate findings to others
- Guide the focus of nursing practice in each component of the nursing process
- Link nursing practice, theory, research, and education.

Conceptual models are used to guide theory-based nursing practice. Models are tools for systematically examining client situations. They assist nurses in organizing their thinking, observing, and interpreting. Therefore models are goal-directed and lead to more efficient and effective nursing practice. Models and theories also serve as the link between nursing practice, research, and education. Ideas for nursing theory may develop in practice, may be tested through research, and then serve to guide or explain practice. Models also serve as the basis for nursing research, both to test relationships in the models and to support various studies. In nursing education, nursing models may guide the curriculum and be applied throughout the nursing process.

Characteristics of Nursing Models

All nursing models have several general characteristics in common. Some of these characteristics are:

1. Nursing models represent the total nursing discipline—an image of the entire field of nursing.
2. Each model provides a unique and distinct perspective of the client, health, environment, and the nursing actions/roles. These essential concepts of nursing practice, together with their theoretical basis and values, are conveyed in each model.
3. Each model identifies and includes some relevant factors and excludes other irrelevant factors. However, no one model includes all factors that are relevant in all practice settings.
4. Models vary in their level of development, degree of abstractness, and level of specificity.

5. Nursing models provide direction for research development, generation of hypotheses, and guide data collection and theory development.
6. Collectively, nursing models provide a critical step in furthering theory-based nursing practice, research, education, and, ultimately, nursing science.

Categories

Nursing models not only reflect different world views but also may be categorized according to the discipline in which they were developed (Fawcett, 1989). Three ways to categorize models are developmental, systems, and interactional. *Developmental models* focus on the client's development through an orderly sequence to attain optimal health and greater degrees of self-responsibility. This approach is illustrated in Orem's and Rogers' models in which the nurse's role is to promote the client's restoration and growth. *Systems models* view clients as interrelated biological, psychological, and social systems. When an imbalance occurs in one system, it disrupts other systems. The nurse's role is to restore equilibrium or facilitate adaptation. Roy, Neuman, and Johnson use this approach in their nursing models. *Interactional models* emphasize the client-nurse interactions and the development of a relationship between the client and nurse to work toward the client's goal attainment. Examples of nursing models with this approach are the different models of Orlando, Peplau, and King. All nursing models contain some aspects of each of the three approaches; however, each model tends to emphasize one category over the others.

Application of Theory-Based Nursing Practice

Theory-based nursing practice is the application to clinical practice of knowledge of various theories, models, and principles from the scientific, behavioral, humanistic, and nursing disciplines. Nursing models provide a broad framework to interrelate various aspects of the client's complex health situation. With increasing clinical experience, nurses are able to use theoretical and clinical knowledge with their critical thinking skills to make better clinical decisions. Because individual, family, and community clients each present unique health concerns, nurses must select the model that is most congruent with the client's health situation. Each nursing model is based on different assumptions and has a unique perspective of the concepts—client, nursing, health, and environment—and their interrelationships.

Selection of an appropriate nursing model for a specific client situation requires both in-depth knowledge of nursing models and information about major variables affecting the client situation. First the nurse gathers preliminary information about the client's health concerns, age, lifestyle and activities of daily living to identify and understand the client's unique and common patterns. The client's health concerns are mutually identified and often redefined. Next the nurse considers relevant nursing models, their underlying assumptions, concept definitions, and the relationships among the concepts. The models are examined to determine how well each model "fits" with the client's health concerns, the nurse's own view of nursing, health, clients, and environment, and, the mission, goals, and philosophy of the employment agency. In other words, the nurse judges the *congruence* between the model's assumptions, beliefs, and definitions about people and their health concerns with the client's concerns and the views of the nurse, the clinical specialty, and the institution. Fawcett et al (1992) developed guidelines for selecting a conceptual model that would be the most appropriate for the client, rather than "forcing" the client to fit the model. To identify the best fit, nurses use their critical thinking skills, broad knowledge base, intuition, and experience to consider each of the following questions:

1. Does the nursing model address all the client's stated health concerns?
2. Is the goal of nursing proposed by the model congruent with the client's desired health outcomes?
3. Are the nursing interventions associated with the nursing model consistent with the client's expectations for nursing care? (Fawcett et al, 1992).

These questions serve to direct and prioritize further inquiry, organize the data into patterns, identify additional health concerns, and determine if the nursing model is most congruent with the nurse's beliefs and the client situation. Since each model is different, the nurse considers possible models that best fit the client's situation and the nurse's beliefs. The nurse must thoroughly understand differences among nursing models to answer the questions just listed and compare the client's health situation. Finally, the nurse chooses the most congruent model, one that addresses the client's health concerns, and includes relevant nursing actions. Some models apply better to individual clients with a chronic illness, whereas others apply more to a family crisis. Also, some models describe nursing as providing assistance, whereas others facilitate the client's self-care. Practice in applying models comes with clinical experience.

Table 1-5	Theory-Based Nursing Practice	
Component	**Nursing process** **Use**	**Nursing model** **Use**
Assessment	Describes *how to* collect data	Guides *what* data to collect
Diagnosis	Describes *how to* process data	Guides organizing, categorizing, and interpreting data
	Provides format for nursing diagnosis	Provides concepts for nursing diagnosis
Plan	Describes *how to* plan	Guides *what* to plan
	Facilitates development of care plan unique to client	Designates appropriate types of nursing interventions
Implementation	Describes phases of implementation	Directs model-specific nursing actions
Evaluation	Identifes *how to* evaluate	Guides *what to* evaluate
General	Requires accountability through use of systematic approach to nursing practice	Enhances accountability of theory-based practice
	Process enhances continuity of care	Provides a comprehensive, coherent approach to care of client

Adapted with permission from Wealtha Y. Helland

The chosen model has a major influence on nursing practice and each component of the nursing process, as shown in Table 1-5. The major concepts and subconcepts in the model guide the collection of data. For example, using Roy's model, the nurse would collect data about the client's physiological needs, self-concept, role mastery, and interdependence, along with related stimuli. Next the model is used to organize and categorize the client data and to identify behavioral patterns. The nurse using Johnson's model would organize the data into the seven subsystem categories and identify behavioral responses. The model also provides the structure for analyzing and interpreting the data. The nurse using Orem's model would identify universal and developmental self-care requisites and deficits. Health concerns are stated as nursing diagnoses, based on concepts from the model. The plans, which consist of expected outcomes, strategies, and orders, evolve from the chosen model. The model identifies what to plan, guides selection of strategies, and may serve as the rationale. The nurse using Johnson's model would consider nurturance, protection, or stimulation strategies, whereas Neuman's model would suggest reducing stressors within the three levels of prevention. The model also serves as the basis for nursing implementation by directing specific actions. Evaluation of the client's progress is based on the client's expected outcomes, which were derived from the chosen model. The model directs the outcomes, thus enhances achievement of positive outcomes. Use of nursing models enables nurses to demonstrate accountability for their actions through scientific explanation and provides a coherent approach to theory-based nursing practice.

Summary

Professional nursing has evolved into a scientific discipline that supports the integration of theory, research, and practice. The nursing process, the core of practice, was legitimized in the *Standards of Clinical Nursing Practice* (ANA, 1991) and is tested by state board exams. The five components of the nursing process are assessment, diagnosis, planning, implementation, and evaluation. With the development of nursing models, nurses are learning to apply these models in the nursing process.

The future of nursing is theory-based nursing practice, applying critical thinking skills and nursing models to guide practice. Presently there are many nursing models, some of which continue to be tested and refined by theorists and others. These models are used in theory-based nursing practice and are applied in each component of the nursing process. Models provide a broader understanding of a client's complex situation and guide the collection, organization, and interpretation of data about the client. Models also guide the nursing diagnoses, plans, implementation, and evaluation. They provide a logical basis for explaining how nurses assist clients toward optimum health. Today professional nurses use critical thinking skills and theory-based practice to justify each component in the nursing process and to demonstrate the nurse's accountability to the client, the health team, and the agency.

This book describes how different models are applied in each component of the nursing process. Chapter 2 provides an overview of various nursing models, developmental models, family models, and broad general models. Readers will find it helpful to review these models before reading succeeding chapters. Section II describes the components of the nursing process. These chapters should be read in sequence, as each provides the basis for subsequent chapters. Each component of the nursing process is fully described and illustrated with the application of different models. The chapters in Sections I and II provide the foundation for understanding the case studies in Section III. These case studies illustrate the complete nursing process applied to a specific client situation using a selected nursing model.

Critical Thinking Exercises BY ELIZABETH S. FAYRAM

1. Describe the benefits of *theory-based* nursing practice.
2. Explain how you use the four patterns of knowing (empirical, ethical, esthetic, and personal knowledge) in your nursing practice. Describe specific client situations in your explanation.
3. Compare and contrast a *novice* nurse with a *proficient* nurse in terms of knowledge, experience, and expertise. Discuss how nurses develop to the level of proficient nurse or beyond.
4. Discuss ways nurses can be advocates for clients. Describe specific client situations when possible.
5. Identify consequences that may occur when a nurse does not use the nursing process in practice.
6. Identify current trends that are influencing your nursing practice.

REFERENCES AND READINGS

Adam E: Toward more clarity in terminology: frameworks, theories, and models, *J Nurs Ed* 24:151, 1985.

Aggleton P and Chalmers H: Models of nursing, nursing practice, and nursing education, *J Adv Nurs* 12:573, 1987.

Aguilera DC and Messick JM: *Crisis intervention: theory and methodology,* ed 6, St Louis, 1990, Mosby.

Alfaro R: *Application of nursing process: a step-by-step guide,* ed 2, Philadelphia, 1990, Lippincott.

American Nurses Association: *Standards of nursing practice,* Kansas City, Mo., 1973, The Association.

American Nurses Association: *Standards of clinical nursing practice,* Kansas City, Mo., 1991, The Association.

Barnum BJ: Holistic nursing and nursing process, *Holistic Nurs Pract* 1:27, 1987.

Barnum BJ: *Nursing theory: analysis, application, evaluation,* ed 3, Glenview, Il., 1990, Little, Brown.

Becker PH: Advocacy in nursing: perils and possibilities, *Holistic Nurs Pract* 1:54, 1986.

Benner P, Tanner C, and Chesla C: From beginner to expert: gaining a differentiated clinical world in critical care nursing, *ANS* 14:13, 1992.

Benner P and Tanner C: Clinical judgment: how nurses use intuition, *AJN* 87:23, 1987.

Benner P: From novice to expert, *AJN* 82:402, 1982.

Benner P: *From novice to expert,* Menlo Park, Calif., 1984, Addison-Wesley.

Benner P and Tanner C: How expert nurses use intuition, *Am J Nurs* 87:23, 1987.

Bottorff J: Nursing: a practical science of caring, *ANS* 14:26, 1991

Botha ME: Theory development in perspective: the role of conceptual frameworks and models in theory development, *J Adv Nurs* 14:49, 1989.

Buchanan BF: Conceptual models: an assessment framework, *J Nurs Adm* 17:22, 1987.

Capers CF: Some basic facts about models, nursing conceptualizations, and nursing theories, *J Cont Ed Nurs* 16:149, 1986.

Carper BA: Fundamental patterns of knowing in nursing, *Adv Nurs Sci* 1:13, 1978.

Chance KS: Nursing models: a requisite for professional accountability, *Adv Nurs Sci* 4:57, 1982.

Chinn PL: *Advances in nursing theory development,* Rockville, Md., 1983, Aspen.

Chinn PL: Debunking myths in nursing theory and research, *Image* 17:45, 1985.

Chinn PL and Kramer MK: *Theory and nursing: a systematic approach,* ed 3, St Louis, 1991, Mosby.

Clark J: Development of models and theories on the concept of nursing, *J Adv Nurs* 7:129, 1982.

Correnti D: Intuition and nursing practice implications for nurse educators: a review of the literature, *J Con Ed Nurs* 23:91, 1992.

Craig SL: Theory development and its relevance for nursing, *J Adv Nurs* 5:349, 1980.

Dickoff J, James, P, and Weidenbach E: Theory in a practice discipline. I. Practice oriented theory, *Nurs Res* 17:415, 1968.

Donaldson SK and Crowley DN: The discipline of nursing, *Nurs Outlook* 26:113, 1978.

Donnelly GF: The promise of nursing process: an evaluation, *Holistic Nurs Pract* 1:1, 1987.

Duvall EM: *Marriage and family development,* ed 5, Philadelphia, 1977, Lippincott.

Erikson E: *Childhood and society,* ed 2, New York, 1963, Norton.

Fawcett J: The relationship between theory and research: a double helix, *Adv Nurs Sci* 1:49, 1978.

Fawcett J: *Analysis and evaluation of conceptual models,* ed 2, Philadelphia, 1989, FA Davis.

Fawcett J: Conceptual models and theory development, *JOGNN* 17:400, 1988.

Fawcett J, Archer CL, Becker D, et al: Guidelines for selecting a conceptual model of nursing: focus on the individual patient, *Dimen Crit Care Nurs* 5:268, 1992.

Field PA: The impact of nursing theory on the clinical decision making process, *J Adv Nurs* 12:563, 1987.

Fitch M, Rogers M, Ross E, et al: Developing a plan to evaluate the use of nursing conceptual frameworks, *CJNA* 4:22, 1991.

Fitzpatrick JJ: Use of existing nursing models, *J Gerontol Nurs* 13:8, 1987.

Fitzpatrick JJ and Whall A: *Conceptual models of nursing: analysis and application,* ed 2, Norwalk, Conn., 1989, Appleton & Lange.

Gerrity PL: Perception in nursing: the value of intuition, *Holistic Nurs Pract* 1:63, 1987.

Henderson V: Nursing process—a critique, *Holistic Nurs Pract* 1:7, 1987.

Huch MH: Theory-based practice: structuring nursing care, *Nurs Sci Q* 1:6, 1988.

Huckabey LM: The role of conceptual frameworks in nursing practice, administration, education, and research, *Nurs Admin Q* 15:17, 1991.

Iyer PW, Taptich BJ, and Bernocchi-Losey D: Nursing process and nursing diagnosis, ed 2, Philadelphia, 1991, Saunders.

Johnson DE: Professional practice in nursing. In *The shifting scene: directions for practice*, NLN Pub. No. 15-1252, New York, 1967, National League for Nursing.

Johnson DE: The behavioral system model for nursing. In Reihl JP and Roy C Sr., ed: *Conceptual models for nursing practice*, ed 2, New York, 1980, Appleton-Century-Crofts.

Johnson JL: Nursing science: basic, applied, or practical? Implications for the art of nursing, *ANS* 14:7, 1991.

Kelly K: Clinical inference in nursing, *Nurs Res* 15:23, 1966.

Kenney JW: The evolution of nursing science and practice. In Deloughery G, ed.: *Issues and trends in nursing*, ed 2, St. Louis, 1994, Mosby.

King IM: *A theory for nursing: systems, concepts, process*, New York, 1981, Wiley & Sons.

Knowles LN: Decision making in nursing: a necessity for doing, ANA Clinical Sessions 1966, New York, 1967, Appleton-Century-Crofts.

Krieger D: Foundations of holistic health nursing practice, Philadelphia, 1981, Lippincott.

Kristjanson LJ, Tamblyn R, and Kuypers JA: A model to guide development and application of multiple nursing theories, *J Adv Nurs* 12:523, 1987.

Leddy S and Pepper JM: *Conceptual bases of professional nursing*, Philadelphia, 1984, Lippincott.

Maslow A: *Motivation and personality*, ed 2, New York, 1970, Harper & Row.

Mayberry A: Merging nursing theories, models, and nursing practice: more than an administrative challenge, *ANS* 15:44, 1991.

McHugh M: Nursing process: musings on the method, *Holistic Nurs Pract* 1:21, 1986.

Meleis AI: *Theoretical nursing: development and process*, ed 2, Philadelphia, 1991, Lippincott.

National League for Nursing: *Theory development: what, why and how*, New York, 1978, Pub. # 15-1708, The League.

Neuman B: *The Neuman systems model*, ed 2, New York, 1989, Appleton & Lange.

Newman MA, Sime AM, and Corcoran-Perry SA: The focus of the discipline of nursing, *ANS* 14:1-6, 1991

Newman MA: Prevailing paradigms in nursing, *Nurs Outlook* 40:10, 1992.

Orem DE: *Nursing: concepts of practice*, ed 3, New York, 1985, McGraw-Hill.

Orlando IJ: *The dynamic nurse-patient relationship: function, process and principles*, New York, 1961, Putnam.

Parse RR: *Man-living-health: a theory of nursing*, Philadelphia, 1981, Wiley.

Parse RR: *Nursing science: major paradigms, theories, and critiques*, Philadelphia, 1987, Saunders.

Paterson JG and Zderad LT: *Humanistic nursing*, New York, 1976, Wiley.

Peplau H: *Interpersonal relations in nursing*, New York, 1952, Putnam.

Pinnell NN and deMeneses M: *The nursing process: theory, application, and related processes*, Norwalk, Conn., 1986, Appleton-Century-Crofts.

Rew L and Barrow EM: Intuition: a neglected hallmark of nursing knowledge, *Adv Nurs Sci* 10:49, 1987.

Rogers ME: *The theoretical basis of nursing*, Philadelphia, 1970, FA Davis.

Rogers ME: Creating a climate for the implementation of a nursing conceptual framework, *J Cont Ed Nurs* 20:112, 1989.

Roy Sr C: *Introduction to nursing: an adaptation model*, ed 2, Englewood Cliffs, N.J., 1984, Prentice-Hall.

Ruffing-Rahal MA: Personal documents and nursing theory development, *Adv Nurs Sci* 8:50, 1986.

Schlotfeldt R: Structuring nursing knowledge: a priority for creating nursing's future, *Nurs Sci Q* 1:35, 1988.

Schultz PR and Meleis A: Nursing epistemology: traditions, insights, questions, *Image: J Nurs Scholarship* 20:217, 1989.

Selye H: *The stress of life*, New York, 1956, McGraw-Hill.

Shea H, Rogers M, Ross E, et al.: Implementation of nursing conceptual models: observations of a multi-site research team, *CJNA* 2:15, 1989.

Silva MC: Research testing nursing theory: state of the art, *Adv Nurs Sci* 9:1, 1986.

Smith MJ: Perspectives on nursing science, *Nurs Sci Q* 1:80, 1988.

Stevens BJ: *Nursing theory: analysis, application, evaluation*, ed 2, Boston, 1983, Little, Brown.

Swanson K: Empirical development of a middle range theory of caring, *Nurs Research* 40:161, 1991.

Walker KO and Avant K: *Strategies for theory construction in nursing*, ed 2, New York, 1988, Appleton & Lange.

Walker L: The future of theory development: commentary and response, *Nurs Sci Q* 2:118, 1989.

Watson J: Nursing—human science and human care: a theory of nursing, Norwalk, Conn., 1985, Appleton-Century-Crofts.

Wilkinson JM: *Nursing process in action: a critical thinking approach*, Menlo Park, Calif., 1992, Addison-Wesley.

Visintainer MA: The nature of knowledge and theory in nursing, *Image: J Nurs Scholarship* 18:32, 1986.

Young CE: Intuition and nursing process, *Holistic Nurs Pract* 1:52, 1987.

Yura H and Walsh MB: *The nursing process: assessing, planning, implementing, evaluating*, New York, 1967, Appleton-Century-Crofts.

Yura H and Walsh MB: *The nursing process: assessing, planning, implementing, evaluating*, ed 5, Norwalk, Conn., 1988, Appleton & Lange.

CHAPTER 2

OVERVIEW OF SELECTED MODELS

Janet W. Kenney

T his chapter presents an overview of selected models commonly used in the nursing process. Generally these models are well known and the major concepts are defined. Some models have been tested in research studies. The chapter is organized into three categories of models: general, nursing, and family models. The major concepts of each model are defined, and the basic structure and essence are described and illustrated. This chapter will familiarize readers with various models that will be applied in the nursing process components in the following chapters. However, readers are strongly encouraged to review primary sources in the literature to fully understand any model before applying it in the nursing process. This chapter presents the following models in the order listed below:

General Models

Maslow's hierarchy of needs

Erikson's eight stages of development

General systems

Aguilera and Messick's crisis intervention

Nursing Models

Johnson's behavioral systems model

King's theory of goal attainment

Leininger's transcultural nursing model

Neuman's health-care systems model

Orem's self-care nursing model

Parse's man-living-health model

Peplau's interpersonal model

Rogers' science of unitary human beings

Roy's adaptation model

Watson's human caring model

Family Models

Duvall

Stevenson

Satir

Friedman

Calgary

First, four general models are described; these may be familiar to the reader. Next, nine nursing models are presented, beginning with each theorist's definition of the four major concepts. The unique concepts and subconcepts of each theorist are defined and the relationships between concepts are illustrated. Some nursing models are developed for individual clients; others can be applied to a family or community. The strengths, limitations, and applications in the nursing process are discussed. Three of the five family models presented here were developed by nurses. Models that can be applied to a community are the general systems model and Neuman's Health Care Systems Model. (A third community model, developed by Goeppinger and Schuster, is presented in Chapter 6.) Application of these models in each component of the nursing process is shown in Sections II and III.

General Models
Maslow's Hierarchy of Needs

Advocates of human needs theory view individuals as integrated, whole beings who are motivated by internal and external needs that create tension. To reduce this tension, an individual seeks to meet specific needs through goal-directed behavior. Abraham Maslow (1970) classified human needs into five categories of predominance and placed them in a hierarchy. This hierarchy of human needs begins with basic fundamental needs of the individual that must be satisfied before proceeding to the next higher level. Throughout life the individual strives to satisfy needs at each level, but at different periods needs within one or more categories may predominate. The desire to gratify human needs at each level motivates the individual and strengthens goal-directed behaviors. Generally, basic physiological needs and safety needs must be relatively satisfied in the individual before he or she can strive for higher level needs (Fig. 2-1).

Physiological Needs

A variety of fundamental physical needs have been identified, including air, food, sleep, sex, fluids, exercise, elimination, and stimulation. For survival and satisfactory functioning, every individual must have these basic physiological needs met. The extent or degree to which each of these needs is met varies with the individual. Some people require more sleep or food than others, but individuals must satisfy these needs at their own specific levels.

Safety

When basic physical needs are relatively satisfied, safety needs emerge; these include security, stability, order, physical safety, freedom from fear, protection, and sometimes dependency. These needs reflect self-protection through the establishment of structure, law, order, and limits.

Needs for safety and protection from harm may become more prominent when the individual is threatened by bodily harm, as in physical illness or potential injury. Safety needs involve both imminent danger or concerns and potential loss, such as loss of the security of a spouse or an occupational position.

Love and Belonging

As physical and safety needs are reasonably satisfied, the need for love and belonging emerges. Within this category are needs for affectionate relationships, identification within various groups (family, church, and work), and companionship. These needs may be expressed through contact with significant others, tenderness, affection, and intimacy in sharing time spent together. Love and belonging needs may include contact with and affection for family members, friends, and associates of all age groups and both sexes. When love and belonging needs remain unsatisfied, the individual may feel alone, alienated, estranged, and distant from friends and relatives. The need for love encompasses mutual giving and receiving.

Esteem and Recognition

When the needs just mentioned have been gratified, the individual's need for esteem and recognition arise. These needs include self-respect, self-esteem, prestige, respect, and esteem from others. An individual may be motivated by the desire to achieve fame, recognition, strength, competency, independence, or an outstanding reputation. This desire for esteem and recognition motivates individuals toward goal-directed behaviors to achieve or gratify these needs in their own unique ways. As this need is relatively satisfied, the individual experiences a sense of adequacy, self-worth, self-fulfillment, and contentment.

Self-Actualization

When the lower needs in the hierarchy have been relatively satisfied, an individual strives toward self-actualization. Young people may grow toward self-actualization but usually must reach maturity before they have a sense of self-actualization. Self-actualization means that the individual is relatively satisfied with most aspects of life. This includes what the person thinks of self and the level of achievement reached or the ability to fulfill that designated purpose in life. Some adults continue working toward self-actualization all their lives; others arrive at a sense of fulfillment or accomplishment in midlife. The individual feels a sense of having achieved a purpose in life and having developed capabilities to the fullest.

Maslow's hierarchy of needs is a broad model that can be applied to all components of the nursing process, especially to assessment and prioritization of nursing diagnoses. It is applicable to individual and family clients. Although the nurse can assist clients to meet the first four needs, the fifth need, self-actualization, is generally left to the client to meet after other needs are met.

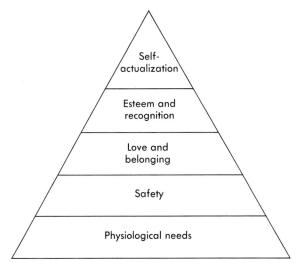

Figure 2-1 Maslow's hierarchy of needs.

Erikson's Developmental Model

Erik Erikson (1963) is a lay psychoanalyst who extended Freud's theories on man. He emphasized the influence of sociocultural and biophysical dimensions on the individual's development. In Erikson's model, human development is interrelated with cultural and physical growth over eight distinctive stages. Each stage represents a developmental task: a foundation for the next stage as shown in Table 2-1. Each task is never fully resolved and may resurface in later years. The critical task at each stage holds a zenith position at that period of development; it becomes less dominant later but may arise again. If the specific task is not accomplished during the critical period, Erikson notes the consequences in the development of undesirable behaviors.

Erikson's Eight Stages of Development
Trust versus Mistrust

In infancy the central task is to develop a sense of trust that basic needs will be adequately met. As these needs are met, the infant learns that the world is a safe place to live in. Others' behaviors result in a predictable pattern that can be trusted. Mistrust in the safety and predictability of life occurs when the infant's needs are not satisfactorily met.

Autonomy versus Shame and Doubt

The toddler who has learned to trust begins to test the environment, determining the extent to which the environment can be manipulated. Autonomy develops as the toddler explores and learns control of self and the environment. If independent actions are thwarted or are unacceptable to others, the toddler experiences shame. When attempts to manipulate the environment are ineffectual, the toddler may develop doubt.

Initiative versus Guilt

As the preschooler tries to be assertive during interactions with others and the environment, approval from others foster initiative. When the preschooler's

actions are not permitted or are disapproved of by others, the child develops a sense of guilt.

Industry versus Inferiority

The school-age child directs energy toward learning knowledge and skills applicable in the real world. The child who receives satisfaction from those efforts continues to be industrious. The child who has difficulty and whose efforts go unrewarded may feel inferior and inadequate.

Identity versus Role Diffusion

During adolescence the individual searches for current and future identities in an attempt to integrate life experiences into a sense of self. To master identity the adolescent must feel an internally consistent self-image, which must agree with others' views. The adolescent who is unable to integrate life experiences and self-image into a consistent identity experiences role diffusion. Feelings of being lost or confused may occur.

Intimacy versus Isolation

The young adult seeks relationships with others to acquire a sense of sharing, caring, and intimacy. An individual who is unable to share close relationships and feel comfortable in intimate relationships may have a sense of isolation from friends or family members.

Generativity versus Stagnation

In adulthood the primary task is satisfaction with productivity, including work, family, home, and citizenship. These activities and a sense of accomplishment provide the individual with intrinsic rewards, but the adult who is dissatisfied in these areas may feel stagnation. With lack of productivity, the adult may indulge in self-absorption and develop derogatory attitudes toward others.

Integrity versus Despair

The older adult, satisfied with life and its meaning and believing that life is fulfilling and successful, has integrity. A sense of despair develops when the adult fears death and finds failure with self and others.

Erikson's developmental model depicts eight psychosocial stages in the life cycle. It identifies critical developmental tasks at each stage and the consequences when a critical task remains unaccomplished. Although each task is age-appropriate, the tasks are never completely resolved and may arise at any time in the life cycle. This developmental model has limited use in the nursing process. Each client should be assessed and analyzed according to the age-appropriate developmental level. The model is used in conjunction with other, broader models that include biopsychosocial concepts.

◤ *Table 2-1*	**Erikson's Stages of Development**
Stages of development	**Age level**
Trust versus mistrust	Infancy
Autonomy versus shame and doubt	Toddler
Initiative versus guilt	Preschool
Industry versus inferiority	School age
Identity versus role diffusion	Adolescence
Intimacy versus isolation	Young adult
Generativity versus stagnation	Adulthood
Integrity versus despair	Older adult

General Systems Theory

General systems theory serves as a model for viewing people as interacting with the environment. One of the first theorists to develop systems theory was Ludwig von Bertalanffy (1968), who synthesized the following abstract laws in systems theory development:

1. Systems are organized complexities in which behavior is determined by interaction among various components.
2. No system repeats its interaction, but continuous interaction among variables infinitely produces unique, dynamic situations.
3. Evolution proceeds from a less to a more differentiated state; dynamic interaction between individuals and the environment results in increasing complexity for both.
4. Regular changes are found in the evolution of all systems as they move toward higher states of order, differentiation, and probability.
5. People are living, open (metabolizing) systems exhibiting self-differentiation, providing energy, and having a stored information system (genetic code) to steer the process.

A *system* consists of a set of interacting components within a boundary that filters the type and rate of exchange with the environment. Systems are composed of both structural and functional components. *Structure* refers to the arrangements of the parts at a given time; *function* is the process of continuous change in the system as matter, energy, and information are exchanged with the environment.

All living systems are *open* in that there is continual exchange of matter, energy, and information (Fig. 2-2). Open systems have varying degrees of interaction with the environment from which the system receives input and gives back output in the form of matter, energy, and information. Theoretically no closed systems exist, as they would be totally isolated from interacting with the environment.

The universe consists of a *hierarchy of systems* (numerous suprasystems, systems, and subsystems), and each system may be viewed as having one or more suprasystems and subsystems. For example, the individual as a system belongs to suprasystems in a family, community, and region. An individual's subsystems are composed of organ systems or biopsychosocial components.

Each system has discrete, definable *boundaries* that filter and regulate the flow of input and output exchange with the environment. Boundaries may consist of physical or abstract lines of demarcation that separate the system from the surrounding environment. The boundary filter may be very permeable or fairly impermeable, depending on the component it is screening in or out of the system. For survival all systems must receive varying types and amounts of matter, energy, and information from the environment. Through the process of selection, the system regulates the type and amount of *input* received.

The system uses the input through self-regulation to maintain the system's equilibrium or homeostasis. Some types of inputs are used immediately in their original state, whereas others require complex transformation *(throughput)* for use. Matter, energy, and information are continuously processed through the system and released as outputs. After processing input, the system returns *output* (matter, energy, and information) to the environment in an altered state, affecting the environment.

The system continuously monitors itself and the environment for information to guide its operation. This *feedback* information of environmental responses to the system's output is used by the system in adjustment, correction, and accommodation to the interaction with the environment. Feedback may be positive, negative, or neutral.

Substances that occupy space and can be exchanged between the system and environment are considered *matter*.

The ability to perform, carry out tasks, and overcome resistance in a physical and emotional sense may be considered *energy*.

Through dynamic interaction with the environment, the system exchanges *information* in different forms, such as verbal and behavioral communication, visual media, taste, smell, and touch. Information is used by the system in the process of selection and decision making.

For survival a system must achieve a balance internally and externally. *Equilibrium* depends on the ability of the system to regulate input and output with the environment to achieve a balanced relationship of the interacting parts. Because balance is continually changing, a self-regulating mechanism within the system monitors the interaction of inputs and outputs with the environment by using information from feedback. Through interactions with the environment the system uses various *adaptation* mechanisms to maintain equilibrium. Adaptation may occur through accepting or rejecting the matter, energy, or information and by accommodating the input and modifying the system's responses to maintain or regain equilibrium.

Systems theory is applicable in the nursing process of the individual, family, and community client. It is frequently used to assess and analyze a community. However, because it is so broad, supplemental models are often required to delineate input, throughput, and output.

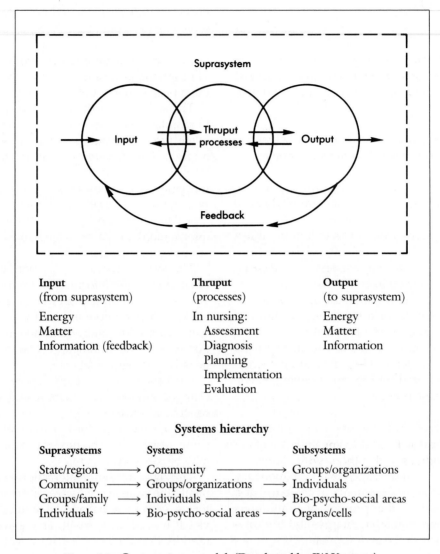

Figure 2-2 Open systems model. (Developed by JW Kenney.)

Aguilera and Messick's Crisis Intervention Model

Donna Aguilera and Janice Messick (1990) synthesized the views of several behaviorists in their crisis intervention model. They consider *crisis* a stressful event or change in the individual's life involving loss or threat of loss, which disrupts the individual's equilibrium. Crises are categorized as maturational or situational. Maturational crises are those events that occur routinely. They include marriage, pregnancy, going away to school, and the death of a friend or spouse. Situational crises are unexpected events, such as failing an examination, losing a job, receiving a promotion, and sustaining an injury.

These authors describe three balancing factors, each of which must be present in a threatening situation to avert a crisis. These factors reduce the risk of a crisis and help the individual maintain equilibrium. The three factors are realistic perception of the event,

adequate situational supports, and adequate coping mechanisms, as shown in Fig. 2-3.

Realistic Perception of the Event

The meaning an individual attaches to an event influences the perception of it. Sometimes past experiences evoke feelings unrelated to the event; these feelings may distort the individual's perception and magnify the consequences of the event. When an individual attaches great significance to an event, a distorted perception is likely. The individual's feelings and emotions may create an unrealistic picture of the present and future, which hinders effective decision-making and may lead to crisis. Those with a realistic perception of the event are able to view the situation in perspective, which reduces the chance that their emotions will cloud decision-making. A realistic perception of the event may avert a crisis.

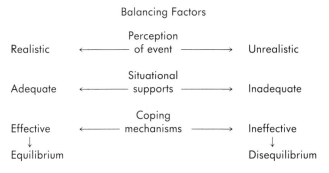

Situational or maturational events

Balancing Factors

	Perception	
Realistic	←——— of event ———→	Unrealistic
	Situational	
Adequate	←——— supports ———→	Inadequate
	Coping	
Effective	←——— mechanisms ———→	Ineffective
↓		↓
Equilibrium		Disequilibrium

Figure 2-3 Aguilera and Messick's crises intervention model.

Adequate Situational Supports

Individuals rely on others to assist them in times of need. Significant others reflect an appraisal of the individual's self-worth and the meaning of the event. When faced with a loss or threat of loss, individuals share the meaning of the event with significant others. This sharing helps the individual place the event in perspective. Situational supports are considered adequate when individuals feel they can share the concern with and receive support from significant others. Sometimes an individual cannot share the concern with others for fear of losing respect or esteem. When individuals lack others with whom to share events or concerns, their situational supports are inadequate. This may cause disequilibrium and lead to a crisis.

Adequate Coping Mechanisms

From life experiences, individuals learn a repertoire of coping responses or patterns. These patterns assist individuals in reducing tension, in adapting to daily stressful events, and in maintaining equilibrium. Occasionally a stressful event occurs that overwhelms the individual. It may be an unfamiliar situation, the magnitude of the concern, or several concerns occurring simultaneously. When usual coping responses are ineffective, disequilibrium and crisis may occur.

Aguilera and Messick's crisis intervention model describes three balancing factors: realistic perception of the event, situational supports, and coping mechanisms. Each factor must be adequately present to maintain equilibrium and avoid a crisis. In crisis intervention each factor is assessed and, if one factor is missing or inadequate, means are sought to enhance or develop that factor. This crisis model is excellent for individuals or families experiencing situational or maturational crises, such as unwanted pregnancy, loss of a family member, rape or abuse, or a chronic health problem.

◆

Johnson's Beliefs

Nursing: regulation of external forces to stabilize client's behavioral system and restore, maintain, or attain balance

Client: a behavioral system (person) threatened or potentially threatened by illness (imbalance) and/or hospitalization

Health: an efficient and effectively functioning behavioral system (person) who maintains balance/stability by adapting/adjusting to outside forces

Environment: no specific setting is identified

Nursing Models

Ten nursing models were selected for presentation in alphabetical order. For purposes of comparison, a brief description of each theorist's four major concepts is shown in Table 2-2. In the table the term *nursing* refers to the nurse's role or actions; *client* is the recipient of nursing care or one who qualifies for nursing care; *health* refers to the theorist's view of what constitutes health; and *environment* is the setting in which nursing occurs.

Johnson's Behavioral System Model

Dorothy Johnson's (1980, 1990) model is a synthesis of theories and concepts from the behavioral and biological sciences, integrated into a systems framework. Stress and adaptation theories are emphasized in this model.

Each person is viewed as a behavioral system composed of seven subsystems. The subsystems interact and are interdependent. Each person strives to achieve balance and stability both internally and externally and to function effectively by adjusting and adapting to environmental forces through learned patterns of response. When these forces are too great and the person is unable to adapt or achieve optimum functioning, behavioral instability develops in one or more of the subsystems, reducing functional capacity and efficiency and depleting energy.

Nurses assist any person threatened or potentially threatened by behavioral system imbalance to maintain efficient and effective functioning. They regulate external forces to preserve the client's behavioral (biopsychosocial) system at an optimum level by imposing external regulations or controls, changing structural elements in desirable directions, or fulfilling functional requirements of the subsystems.

Johnson's model is based on the interaction of the person's behavioral system and subsystems with the environment, as shown in Figs. 2-4 and 2-5.

Table 2-2	Major Concepts of Ten Nursing Theorists

Theorist	Nursing	Client	Health	Environment
Johnson's behavioral system model	Regulation of external forces to stabilize client's behavioral system and restore, maintain, or attain balance	A behavioral system (person) threatened or potentially threatened by illness (imbalance) and/or hospitalization	An efficient and effectively functioning behavioral system (person) who maintains balance/stability by adapting/adjusting to outside forces	No specific setting is identified
King's theory of goal attainment	An interaction process between client and nurse whereby during perceiving, setting goals, and acting on them, transactions occur and goals are achieved	An individual (personal system) or group (interpersonal system) unable to cope with an event or a health problem while interacting with the environment	An ability to perform the activities of daily living in one's usual social roles; a dynamic life experience of continuous adjustment to environmental stressors through optimum use of resources	Any social system in society; social systems are dynamic forces that influence social behavior integration, perception, and health, such as hospitals, clinics, community agencies, schools, and industry
Leininger's transcultural nursing model	A humanistic and scientific mode of helping a client through specific cultural caring processes (cultural values, belief, and practices) to improve or maintain a health condition	An individual family, group, society, or community with possible physical, psychological, or social needs, within the context of their culture, who is a recipient of nursing care	Defined by specific culture and the local people's viewpoint; technology-dependent cultures view health and health care differently from non–technology-dependent societies	Any culture or society worldwide where ethnocaring is practiced by nurses assisting clients
Neuman's health care systems model	Assists clients toward stability by reducing stress factors and adverse conditions that reduce optimum functioning	Individual, family, or group with an identified or suspected stressor that may disrupt normal wellness or system stability	A dynamic stability state of the normal lines of defense. This varies with the amount of available energy stored and/or used to maintain system stability	Internal and external stressors and resistance factors surrounding the client at the time; nurse-client settings are not described
Orem's self-care model	A service of deliberately selected and performed actions to assist individuals or groups to maintain self-care, including structural integrity, functioning, and development	Individual or group unable to continuously maintain self-care in sustaining life and health, in recovering from disease or injury, or in coping with their effects	Individual or group's ability to meet self-care demands that contribute to maintenance and promotion of structural integrity, functioning, and development	Any setting in which a client has unmet self-care needs/requisites and in which a nurse is present is implied but not specified
Parse's man-living-health model	Guiding individuals and families to share and uncover the personal meaning of their living-health situation	Any person or family concerned with their quality of life situation; man is viewed as an open whole being, influenced by past and present lived experiences, who interacts with the environment through choices and responsibility for those choices	Process of lived experiences, unfolding, continually changing, including a synthesis of values and way of living	Undefined setting, but any health-related setting is implied
Peplau's interpersonal model	Goal-directed interpersonal process to promote clients' forward movement of their personality and personal living	Any individual who feels or recognizes unmet needs	Ability to accomplish interpersonal activities and developmental tasks within a productive level of anxiety	Any health-related setting is implied but not defined

Table 2-2	Major Concepts of Ten Nursing Theorists—cont'd			
Theorist	**Nursing**	**Client**	**Health**	**Environment**
Rogers' science of unitary human beings	Science and art to facilitate and promote symphonic interaction between human beings and their environment	Any human being or individual and his or her environment	Expression of the life process characterized by behaviors emerging from mutual, simultaneous interaction between human beings and their environment; a continuum based on value judgments	Four-dimensional negentropic energy field identified by pattern and organization and encompassing all that is outside any given human field; any setting worldwide where nurse and client meet
Roy's adaptation model	Promotion of the client's adaptation in the four modes to enhance health using the nursing process	Person, family, group, or community with unusual stresses or ineffective coping mechanisms	State and process of being and becoming an integrated and whole person	All conditions, circumstances, and influences surrounding and affecting the development and behavior of persons or groups; any health-related situation is implied as the setting
Watson's human caring model	Application of the art and human science through transpersonal caring transactions to help persons achieve mind-body-soul harmony, which generates self-knowledge, self-control, self-care, and self-healing	A person or group experiencing mind-body-soul disharmony who needs assistance with health-illness decisions to promote harmony, self-control, choice, and self-determination	Unity and harmony within the mind-body-soul between self and others and self and nature	Wherever transpersonal caring interactions transpire between a client and nurse

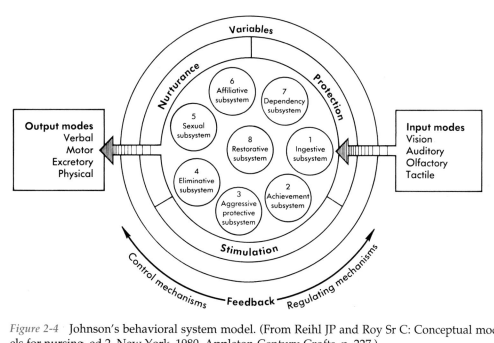

Figure 2-4 Johnson's behavioral system model. (From Reihl JP and Roy Sr C: Conceptual models for nursing, ed 2, New York, 1980, Appleton-Century-Crofts, p. 227.)

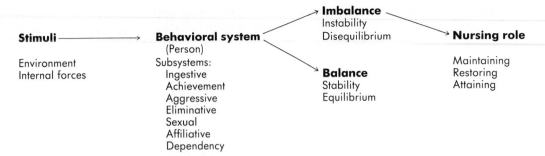

Figure 2-5 Responses of behavioral system to stimuli. (Modified from Fitzpatrick JJ and Whall AI: Conceptual models in nursing: analysis and application, Bowie, Md., 1983, Robert Brady, p. 121.)

Behavioral System

In systems theory a *system* is a whole with interdependent parts. The parts have a structure and a process or pattern of behavior. Systems are characterized by organization, interaction, interdependence, and integration of the parts. Through interaction both within the subsystems and with the external forces acting on it, the system strives to maintain balance and stability by adjusting and adapting.

Subsystems

Johnson's model has seven interdependent subsystems. A disturbance in one may affect the others. Each subsystem has a unique function or special task necessary for an integrated performance of all the subsystems, and each has both structure and function. Four structural elements influence each subsystem. First is the *goal* or *drive,* defined as the purpose of the behavior and the consequences achieved. In general the goal of each subsystem is universal, but individual variations exist. Second, an individual's subsystem *set* reflects the "person's predisposition to act with reference to the goal" (Johnson, 1990). Set distinguishes the range of behaviors available to the individual to achieve a particular goal. Preferred behaviors are developed through learning, maturation, and experience. Third, each subsystem has a *choice* of alternative behaviors to achieve specific goals. The goal is achieved by the individual's subsystem *behavior,* which is the only observable aspect of each subsystem. This behavior is examined for its efficiency in achieving the goal.

Each subsystem has an established set of behavioral responses or tendencies toward a common goal or drive. These responses are developed through maturation, experience, and learning. They are influenced by biopsychosocial factors. Over time, responses may be modified, but an observable recurrent pattern of responses continues.

Each of the seven subsystems has a unique goal:

1. Ingestive—to take in from the environment needed resources to maintain integrity, achieve pleasure, and internalize the external environment (Grubbs, 1980)
2. Achievement—to master or control self or environment through seeking some standard of excellence, such as physical, social, or creative skills
3. Aggressive—to protect self and others from potentially threatening objects, persons, or ideas; serves as a self-preservation mechanism
4. Eliminative—to expel biological waste from the system
5. Sexual—to procreate and gratify feeling attractive to and cared about by others
6. Affiliative or attachment—to relate to or belong to something or someone. Its purpose is to achieve social inclusion, intimacy, and strong social bonds for security and ultimately for survival
7. Dependency—to obtain resources needed for assistance, attention, reassurance, and security; aids in gaining approval, attention, trust, and reliance

System Requirements

Each subsystem requires that functional needs be met and regulating mechanisms be intact to maintain stability and balance. Functional requirements are met through the individual's own efforts or through assistance from the environment. These requirements include protection, nurturance, and stimulation. *Protection* refers to safeguarding the individual from noxious influences with which the system cannot cope, defending the individual from unnecessary threats, and coping with a threat on the individual's behalf (Grubbs, 1980). *Nurturance* means supporting the individual's adequate adaptive behaviors through

Table 2-3	**Characteristics of King's Concepts**

Personal system

Perception	Growth and development
Self	Time
Body image	Space

Interpersonal system

Role	Communication
Human interaction	Transactions
	Stress

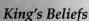

King's Beliefs

Nursing: an interaction process between client and nurse whereby during perceiving, setting goals, and acting on them, transactions occur and goals are achieved

Client: an individual (personal system) or group (interpersonal system) unable to cope with an event or a health problem while interacting with the environment

Health: an ability to perform the activities of daily living in one's usual social roles; a dynamic life experience of continuous adjustment to environmental stressors through optimum use of resources

Environment: any social system in society; social systems are dynamic forces that influence social behavior, interaction, perception, and health, such as hospitals, clinics, community agencies, schools, and industry

nourishment, training, and conditions that support appropriate behaviors. *Stimulation* promotes continued growth and development. Different forms of stimulation are used for different purposes to maintain or enhance behavioral stability.

Individuals use a variety of *regulating and controlling mechanisms* to evaluate and choose desirable behavior. These mechanisms are learned through experience in childhood and are usually internalized by adulthood. The three major types of regulating and controlling mechanisms that individuals use are biophysiological, psychological, and sociocultural. These mechanisms provide a monitor and feedback to the system. They guide behavioral alterations and coordination among the subsystems.

Behavioral Patterns

Each system and subsystem develops patterned, repetitive, and purposeful responses to form an organized and integrated functional unit. These patterned responses determine the interaction of the subsystems, the system, and the environment. The behavioral patterns establish the relationship of the system or person to objects, events, and situations in the environment. These patterns are orderly, purposeful, and predictable, maintaining efficient functioning of the system.

In Johnson's view the goal of nursing is to maintain, restore, or attain a balance of stability in the client's behavioral system. When the person's system cannot adapt or adjust to external environmental forces, the nurse acts as an external regulatory force to modify or change the structure or guide functional requirements to restore stability.

This model applies only to an individual whose behavioral system is threatened or potentially threatened with instability. The model is useful in the nursing process for ill individuals. It includes biopsychosocial aspects of health; however, a developmental model may also be required for a complete nursing assessment and analysis. Johnson's model does not specify the environmental setting in which nursing occurs, nor does it address a person's health maintenance and promotion requirements.

King's Theory of Goal Attainment

In 1971 Imogene King introduced a conceptual model consisting of three interacting systems. Over the years she further refined and developed her model (King, 1981, 1990). King's latest model of nursing incorporates three dynamic interaction systems—personal, interpersonal, and social—that lead to development of a theory of goal attainment.

According to this theory, individuals (personal systems) form groups (interpersonal systems) and groups compose a society (social systems). The major characteristics of these three concepts and King's theory are shown in Table 2-3; the subconcepts are described later.

In King's view, nurses and individuals are personal systems who interact when the individual (or group/interpersonal system) is unable to cope with an event or a health problem. These personal systems enter the health care system (social system) or request services from a health professional and interactions occur, leading to transactions and goal attainment for the individual or group. Interactions between the nurse and the client include assessment, analysis, and interpretation for planning, which may or may not be purposeful and systematic and lead to goal attainment. However, when transactions occur, such as nurse or client goal-directed behaviors, then goals are achieved.

The major concepts in King's model and theory of goal attainment are described here:

- *Personal systems* are individuals/clients viewed as open, interacting, and exchanging matter, energy, and information with the environment. Individuals are social, sentient, rational, reacting, perceiving, controlling, purposeful, action oriented, and time oriented, with rights and responsibilities. The personal system is understood by examining the interaction of six concepts: perception, self, body image, growth and development, time, and space.

- *Interpersonal systems* are two or more individuals or groups interacting. These interactions are understood by exploring such concepts as role, interaction, communication, transaction, and stress.
- *Social systems* are dynamic forces composing society and the environment. They influence social behavior, interaction, perception, and health. Health delivery organizations are a form of social system and can be understood by examining concepts such as: organization; power, authority, and status; and decision-making.

King's theory of goal attainment was primarily derived from the interpersonal system, which interacts with the personal and social systems. In this theory King (1981:145-148) defines her subconcepts as:

- *Interaction*—process of perception and communication between person and environment and between person and person, represented by verbal and nonverbal behaviors that are goal-directed
- *Perception*—each person's representation of reality; it involves (1) taking energy from the environment organized by information, (2) changing energy, (3) processing information, (4) storing information, and (5) giving information in overt behaviors
- *Communication*—process whereby information is given from one person to another, either directly in face-to-face meetings or indirectly through telephone, television, or the written word
- *Transaction*—observable behavior of human beings interacting with their environment
- *Role*—set of behaviors expected of persons occupying a position in a social system; rules that define rights and obligations in a position; relationship with one or more individuals interacting in a specific situation for a purpose
- *Stress*—dynamic state whereby a human being interacts with the environment to maintain balance for growth, development, and performance
- *Growth and development*—continuous changes in individuals at the cellular, molecular, and behavioral levels of activities
- *Time*—continuous flow of events in successive order that implies change, a past, and a future
- *Self*—personal system that is a complex, unified whole who perceives, thinks, desires, imagines, decides, identifies goals, and selects means to achieve them
- *Space*—physical area called *territory*, existing in all directions, defined by the behavior of individuals with boundaries that identify personal space

In her theory of goal attainment, King (1981:149) provides the following propositions, which show the relationships between her major concepts:

1. If perceptual accuracy is present in nurse-client interactions, transactions will occur.
2. If nurse and client make transactions, goals will be attained.
3. If goals are attained, satisfactions will occur.
4. If goals are attained, effective nursing care will occur.
5. If transactions are made in nurse-client interactions, growth and development will be enhanced.
6. If role expectations and role performance as perceived by nurse and client are congruent, transactions will occur.
7. If role conflict is experienced by nurse or client or both, stress in nurse-client interactions will occur.
8. If nurses with special knowledge and skills communicate appropriate information to clients, mutual goal-setting and goal attainment will occur.

King's model views nurses as interacting with clients who are unable to cope with environmental stressors through perception and communication to achieve transactions. The nurse and client establish mutual goals and explore and agree on means to achieve the goals. When transactions occur, goals are achieved, as shown in Fig. 2-6.

The focus of King's model is the nurse-client interaction within a systems approach. Strengths of this model include active client participation in mutual goal-setting, decision-making, and interactions to achieve the client's goals. Also, the model can be applied in numerous health care settings and includes the importance of collaboration among health professionals. This model can be applied to individuals, families, or groups; major psychological, sociocultural, and interpersonal concepts are addressed. However, an individual's physiological status also needs to be considered for a holistic approach. This model may not be useful for clients who cannot communicate appropriately, such as small children and comatose or psychotic clients, other than for use with their families.

Leininger's Transcultural Nursing

Madeleine Leininger initially described transcultural nursing in the 1970s; in 1978 she presented a theory-generating model for the study of transcultural nursing theory and practice. She defines transcultural nursing as

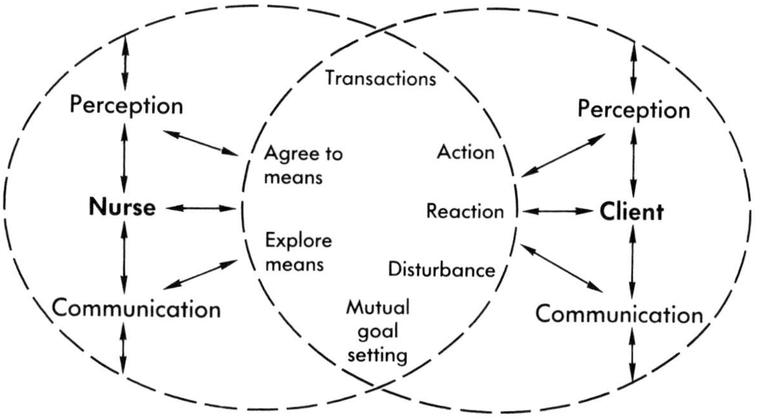

Figure 2-6 Schema of King's theory of goal attainment. (From King IM: A theory for nursing: systems, concepts, process, New York, 1981, Wiley, p. 157.)

Leininger's Beliefs

Nursing: a humanistic and scientific mode of helping a client through specific cultural caring processes (cultural values, beliefs, and practices) to improve or maintain a health condition

Client: an individual, family, group, society, or community with possible physical, psychological, or social needs within the context of their culture, who is a recipient of nursing care

Health: defined by the specific culture and the local people's viewpoint; technology-dependent cultures view health and health care differently from non-technology—dependent societies

Environment: any culture or society worldwide in which ethnocaring is practiced by nurses assisting clients

---

a subfield of nursing which focuses upon a comparative study and analysis of different cultures and subcultures . . . with respect to their caring behavior; nursing care; and health-illness values, beliefs and patterns of behavior with the goal of developing a scientific and humanistic body of knowledge . . . to provide culture-specific and culture-universal nursing care practices (1978:8).

More recently, Leininger (1981, 1984, 1991) has shifted her emphasis to describing care, both transcultural and ethnocaring. The major focus of her work is the "humanistic and scientific study of all people from different cultures . . . [in] ways the nurse can assist people with their daily health and living needs" (1981:8).

In Leininger's view, nursing is synonymous with "caring," which she believes is the central focus. She has classified 28 ethnocaring and nursing care constructs, as shown in Fig. 2-7, that are related to caring behaviors, processes, needs, consequences, conflicts, and gaps.

Ethnocaring is defined as "the systematic study and classification of nursing care beliefs, values, and practices as cognitively perceived by a designated culture through their local language, experiences, beliefs, and value system" (Leininger, 1978:15). *Ethnonursing* is the use of knowledge about the local cultural or subcultural group's values, beliefs, and practices related to health and nursing.

Nursing is the humanistic and scientific application of knowledge in "caring" for individuals, families, and communities, with emphasis on their unique cultural values, beliefs, and health practices. Leininger (1981:13) lists 28 caring constructs that are applicable to all health professionals, including comfort, compassion, coping behaviors, empathy, involvement, love, protective and restorative behaviors, support, and trust. Nurses assist individuals and groups to improve or maintain human conditions by applying knowledge of culturally sanctioned caring modes of intervention. *Transcultural nursing* involves integrating cultural views, knowledge, and experiences in planning and implementing care specific for individuals of a culture.

Leininger's work is unique for nursing because it is considered a theory-generating model rather than a model to guide nursing practice. The 28 care constructs are applicable in nursing but also can be used by any health professional. The model emphasizes a world view, with consideration for cultural differences. It is useful for nurses working with individuals, groups, families, or communities with unique cultural beliefs, values, and practices. Transcultural nursing involves integrating cultural views, knowledge, and experiences in all areas of the nursing process; however, this model does not provide a specific guide to assess clients—individuals, groups, or communities—nor does it guide nursing diagnoses, planning, or intervention. The model provides a guide to generate theories for nursing practice in specific cultures.

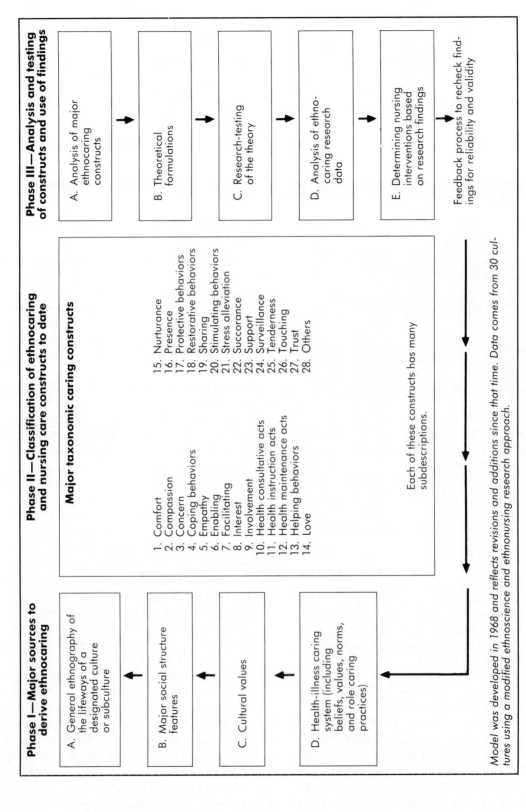

Phase I—Major sources to derive ethnocaring

A. General ethnography of the lifeways of a designated culture or subculture

B. Major social structure features

C. Cultural values

D. Health-illness caring system (including beliefs, values, norms, and role caring practices)

Phase II—Classification of ethnocaring and nursing care constructs to date

Major taxonomic caring constructs

1. Comfort
2. Compassion
3. Concern
4. Coping behaviors
5. Empathy
6. Enabling
7. Facilitating
8. Interest
9. Involvement
10. Health consultative acts
11. Health instruction acts
12. Health maintenance acts
13. Helping behaviors
14. Love

15. Nurturance
16. Presence
17. Protective behaviors
18. Restorative behaviors
19. Sharing
20. Stimulating behaviors
21. Stress alleviation
22. Succorance
23. Support
24. Surveillance
25. Tenderness
26. Touching
27. Trust
28. Others

Each of these constructs has many subdescriptions.

Phase III—Analysis and testing of constructs and use of findings

A. Analysis of major ethnocaring constructs

B. Theoretical formulations

C. Research-testing of the theory

D. Analysis of ethnocaring research data

E. Determining nursing interventions based on research findings

Feedback process to recheck findings for reliability and validity

Model was developed in 1968 and reflects revisions and additions since that time. Data comes from 30 cultures using a modified ethnoscience and ethnonursing research approach.

Figure 2-7 Leininger's conceptual and theory-generating model to study transcultural and ethnocaring constructs. (From Leininger M: Caring: an essential human need, Thorofare, N.J., 1981, Charles B. Slack.)

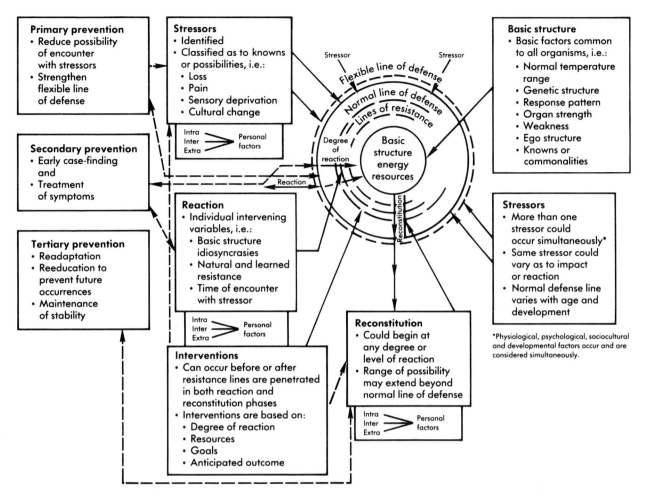

Figure 2-8   The Neuman model of health care systems. (From Neuman B, ed: The Neuman systems model: application to nursing education and practice, Norwalk, Conn., 1982, Appleton-Century-Crofts.)

Neuman's Health-Care Systems Model

Betty Neuman first described her model in 1974 and refined it in later publications (Neuman, 1982, 1989). This complex model views clients holistically and multidimensionally, with a focus on stress reactions and stress reduction. The model was developed for use by any health profession, not just nursing.

This comprehensive model, as shown in Fig. 2-8, depicts the client as a core circle with several protective layers. The client is continuously exposed to internal and external *stressors* that require *lines of defense* and *reactions*. Nursing *interventions* can occur before or after stressors and at three levels of *prevention*.

The *person* is viewed as an open system interacting with the environment through interpersonal and extrapersonal factors. Each individual is a dynamic composite of physiological, psychological, sociocultural, developmental, and spiritual variables that influence the state of wellness or illness. Individuals are continuously exposed to various stressors in the environment, both beneficial and noxious, and respond by adjusting to the environment or adjusting

Neuman's Beliefs

Nursing: assists clients toward stability by reducing stress factors and adverse conditions that reduce optimum functioning

Client: individual, family, or group with an identified or suspected stressor that may disrupt normal wellness or system functioning

Health: a dynamic stability state of the normal lines of defense that varies with the amount of available energy stored and/or used to maintain system stability

Environment: internal and external stressors and resistance factors surrounding the client at the time; nurse-client settings are not described

the environment. Through interactions and adjustments the individual maintains system harmony and balance, both internally and externally.

The individual is composed of a central core or basic structure with three protective layers. The central core consists of normal temperature range, organ strength, weakness, ego structure, and knowns or commonalities. The three surrounding layers protect the individual from stressors. First, a *flexible line of defense,* the outer layer, acts as a dynamic, rapidly changing buffer of stressors, but is highly vulnerable to internal factors such as loss of sleep or hunger. The second layer, or *normal line of defense,* evolves over time to maintain a steady state. It consists of coping patterns, lifestyle, and the individual's usual ways of handling stress. The innermost layer, *lines of resistance,* consists of internal factors that attempt to stabilize the individual and restore the normal line of defense when a stressor breaks through.

Health is viewed as a continuum of well-being and illness and is reflected in the harmony or balance of the individual's interaction and adjustment to the environment. Health is a level of wellness in which all needs are met and more energy is built and stored than is expended. Health is evident in clients with optimal system stability. Illness occurs in varying degrees when needs are not sufficiently satisfied and more energy is needed and expended than is available.

Stressors are noxious or beneficial stimuli that produce tension and have the potential to disrupt system stability and harmony. Stressors are categorized as intrapersonal—forces operating within the individual; interpersonal—forces operating between the individual and others; and extrapersonal—forces outside the individual. Stressors vary in nature, timing, degree, and potential for change, and require energy to cope and to return to stability. They are considered to be any situation, condition, force, or potential source that is capable of creating instability within the individual or reducing the individual's lines of defense or resistance.

Nursing is concerned with maintaining the client's stability by reducing reactions or possible reactions to stressors. The goals of nursing actions are to attain or maintain the client's system balance and conserve energy by vigorously controlling variables affecting the client. Nursing intervention is initiated when a stressor is suspected or identified. Interventions are based on four factors: the client's degree of reaction, resources, goals, and anticipated outcomes. Neuman describes nursing interventions as three levels of prevention: primary, secondary, and tertiary. *Primary prevention* consists of interventions initiated before or after an encounter with a stressor; it includes decreasing the possibility of encounter with stressors and strengthening the flexible lines of defense in the presence of stressors. *Secondary prevention* consists of interventions initiated after encounter with a stressor; it including early casefinding and treatment of symptoms following a reaction to a stressor. *Tertiary prevention* consists of interventions generally initiated after treatment, it focusing on readaptation, reeducation to prevent future occurrences, and maintenance of stability.

Neuman's model is applicable in all components of the nursing process. It is especially useful for individuals and families because it views the client as a composite of physiological, psychological, sociocultural, and developmental variables. This model may also be applied to a community, as shown in Chapter 6. It is a holistic approach because each system or subsystem cannot be isolated; rather the influence of each system on the whole must be considered. The three levels of prevention are useful guides for planning nursing interventions. This model can also be applied across all clinical areas. An example of how Neuman's model can be applied to a family case study is provided in Chapter 15.

Orem's Self-Care Nursing Model

Dorothea Orem first published her concepts of nursing in 1959, then further developed and later refined the model (Orem, 1980, 1985, 1990, 1991). Originally she designed her model for nursing curricula to differentiate nursing actions. This model focuses on identifying client's self-care requisites or needs and nursing actions to meet the client's requisites. Several nurses have described application of her model in practice settings (Feathers, 1989; Gast et al, 1989; Riehl-Sisca, 1989; Taylor, 1990; Morales-Mann and Jiang, 1993).

Orem's model is based on three major constructs: self-care requisites, self-care and nursing systems (see Table 2-4). Central to Orem's model is the belief that individuals function and maintain life, health, and

◆

Orem's Beliefs

Nursing: a service of deliberately selected and performed actions to assist individuals or groups to maintain self-care, including structural integrity, functioning, and development

Client: individual or group unable to continuously maintain self-care in sustaining life and health, in recovering from disease or injury, or in coping with their effects

Health: individual or group's ability to meet self-care demands that contribute to the maintenance and promotion of structural integrity, functioning, and development

Environment: any setting in which a client has unmet self-care needs/requisites and in which a nurse is present is implied but not specified

well-being by caring for themselves. When an individual or group is unable to meet their needs (self-care requisites), self-care deficits occur and therapeutic self-care demands arise, which lead to nursing assistance. The three *self-care requisites* are universal, developmental, and health-deviation. Orem defined three *nursing systems* according to the degree of nursing assistance required by the client: wholly compensatory, partly compensatory, and supportive-educative.

Self-Care Requisites

Self-care activities are behaviors that the individual or guardian personally initiates and performs to maintain life, health, and well-being. These requisites describe the individual's purpose for self-care.

Universal self-care requisites are those activities necessary to meet the basic needs of daily living. They are common to everyone throughout life and are adjusted for age, developmental stage, environment, and other factors. They are associated with maintaining life processes, structural integrity, and functioning. Individuals who are able to meet their universal self-care needs are at one end of the continuum, and those who require total assistance are at the other end. Orem's universal self-care requisites are:

1. Maintenance of sufficient air, water, and food
2. Balance between activity and rest
3. Balance between solitude and social interaction
4. Provision of care associated with elimination processes and excrements
5. Prevention of hazards to human life, functioning, and well-being
6. Promotion of human functioning and development within social groups

Developmental self-care requisites are associated with developmental processes and conditions occurring during the life cycle. The two categories of developmental self-care are, (1) maintaining conditions that support life processes and promote development, and (2) preventing harmful effects on human development and providing care to overcome these effects.

Health-deviation self-care requisites are associated with individuals who are ill or injured or have a pathological condition and are receiving medical care.

Orem identified six requisites for individuals with health deviations:

1. Seeking and securing appropriate medical assistance
2. Recognizing and taking care of these conditions
3. Implementing prescribed diagnostic, therapeutic, and rehabilitative measures
4. Recognizing and regulating the effects of treatment
5. Modifying self-concept and acceptance of the condition
6. Learning to live with the condition in a lifestyle that promotes continued development

Self-Care

When the self-care *demands* exceed an individual's self-care *capabilities*, self-care *deficits* occur, which may require nursing intervention. Therapeutic self-care demands are those universal and developmental requisites, and possibly health-deviation self-care requisites necessary for life, health, and well-being. Capabilities refers to the individual's ability to acquire knowledge for action and to act on that knowledge to meet one's self-care requisites. Self-care deficits occur when an individual is unable to perform the necessary actions to meet one's self-care requisites.

Nursing Systems

Nursing is a human service consisting of "actions deliberately selected and performed . . . to help individuals or groups under their care to maintain or change conditions in themselves or their environments" (Orem, 1980:5). Nurses assist individuals with self-care activities that they are unable to perform for themselves; the goal is guiding clients to perform their own self-care.

To determine which nursing system would be appropriate, the nurse first calculates the therapeutic self-care demands of the individual or group by examining each universal, developmental, and health-deviation self-care requisite. The nurse also considers factors affecting these requisites and the interrelationships among the requisites. Based on the type of self-care deficits the client cannot meet, the nurse determines which nursing system would be most effective. Orem described three nursing systems.

The *wholly compensatory* nursing system is used with clients who are unable to engage in any form of deliberate action, who cannot or should not perform actions, or who are unable to attend to themselves and make rational decisions about self-care. The nursing actions consist of performing the clients' therapeutic self-care, compensating for their inability, and supporting and protecting the clients.

The *partly compensatory* nursing system is for clients

Table 2-4	Orem's Major Concepts		
Self-care requisites	**Self-care**	**Nursing systems**
Universal self-care	Demands	Wholly compensatory
Developmental self-care	Capabilities	Partly compensatory
Health deviation self-care	Deficits	Supportive-educative

who are unable to perform some self-care activities, such as those with actual or medically prescribed limitations, inadequate scientific or technical knowledge or skills, or impaired readiness to learn or perform special activities. The nurse may perform some self-care activities to compensate for client limitations or may assist the patient as required.

The *supportive-educative* nursing system assists clients who are able or can learn to perform therapeutic self-care, yet require assistance in decision-making, behavior control, or acquiring knowledge or skills. The nurse may assist the client through guidance, support, teaching, or environmental change.

Orem's model is widely used in nursing education and practice. It is a comprehensive model for assessment and analysis of an individual, especially in the physiological, social, and developmental areas. The nursing systems are also excellent guides to plan and implement nursing care. This model is very useful for chronically ill clients in the hospital or in other settings. It can easily be adapted to groups with similar self-care deficits, but the model is not appropriate for families. Also, this model limits the nurse's role to working only with clients who are unable to provide their own self-care requisites, which does not include health maintenance and prevention of illness.

Parse's Man-Living-Health Model

Rosemary Parse first described her existential-phenomenological view of man (humans) and health in 1981. Since then she has tested and further explicated her model in more recent publications (Parse, 1987, 1989). Her work is based on Martha Rogers' (1970) view of unitary man (person) as more than the sum of parts, and on Rogers' principles of nursing science: helicy, complementarity, and resonancy. Parse also incorporates Rogers' concepts of energy field, openness, pattern and organization, and four-dimensionality in her work. These principles and concepts are

◆

Parse's Beliefs

Nursing: guiding individuals and families to share and uncover the personal meaning of their living-health situation

Client: any person or family concerned with their quality of life situation; man is viewed as an open whole being, influenced by past and present lived experiences, who interacts with the environment through choices and responsibility for those choices

Health: process of lived experiences, unfolding, continually changing, including a synthesis of values and way of living

Environment: undefined setting, but any health-related setting is implied

synthesized with the existential and phenomenological views of Kierkegaard, Sartre, Dilthey, and others in Parse's concepts, principles, and theoretical structures (Figs. 2-9 and 2-10).

Man (person) is viewed as an open, whole being, coexisting and participating with the environment while continuously coconstituting patterns of relating. As an open being, man freely chooses situations, attaches meaning to those situations, and bears the responsibility for decisions. Man is involved in becoming and reaching beyond self to achieve potentials and possibilities. Through coparticipating with the environment and freely choosing to live certain values, man coconstitutes by creating meaning with others and the world and cocreates self in becoming. Man lives with predecessors, contemporaries, and successors all at once in coexistence, which gives meaning to becoming.

Health is viewed as an open process of becoming through rhythmically unfolding in the man-environment relationship. It is an incarnation of man's choosing and man's patterns of relating value priorities. Health is a continuously changing process of interacting with the environment, transcending with the possibilities, and reaching beyond in a negentropic unfolding. Man is viewed as a composite of more than the sum of parts, a wholeness of biological, social, psychological and spiritual aspects within the context of the environment and lived experiences. Health is *not* good, bad, more, or less, nor is health adapting, coping, or a steady state.

The theory of man-living-health is derived from these views and is reflected in three principles:

- *Principle 1.* Structuring meaning multidimensionally is cocreating reality through the language of valuing and imaging. This principle asserts that reality is continuously cocreated by assigning meaning based on past, present, and future and is expressed through language by means of values and images or symbols.
- *Principle 2.* Cocreating rhythmic patterns of relating is living the paradoxical unity of revealing-concealing and enabling-limiting while connecting-separating. This principle means that man continually has an unfolding cadence of coconstituting patterns of interacting with the world, including revealing-concealing (simultaneously disclosing some aspects of self while hiding others), enabling-limiting (as man moves in one direction, man is limited in movement in another), and connecting-separating (as man links with one phenomenon, man unlinks with another, leading to greater complexity).
- *Principle 3.* Cotranscending with the possibles is powering unique ways of originating in the process of transforming. This principle asserts

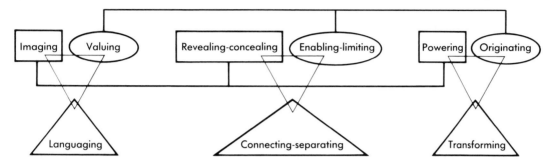

Principle 1: Structuring meaning multidimensionally is cocreating reality through the languaging of valuing and imaging.

Principle 2: Cocreating rhythmical patterns of relating is living the paradoxical unity of revealing-concealing and enabling-limiting while connecting-separating.

Principle 3: Cotranscending with the possibles is powering unique ways of originating in the process of transforming.

Relationship of the concepts in the **squares:** **Powering** is a way of **revealing and concealing imaging.**

Relationship of the concepts in the **ovals:** **Originating** is a manifestation of **enabling and limiting valuing.**

Relationship of the concepts in the **triangles:** **Transforming** unfolds in the **languaging of connecting and separating.**

Figure 2-9 Relationship of principles, concepts, and theoretical structures of man-living-health. (From Parse RR: Man-living-health: a theory of nursing, New York, 1981, Wiley, p. 69.)

Assumptions

1. Man is coexisting while coconstituting rhythmical patterns with the environment.
2. Man is an open being, freely choosing meaning in situation, bearing responsibility for decisions.
3. Man is a living unity continuously coconstituting patterns of relating.
4. Man is transcending multidimensionally with the possibles.
5. Health is an open process of becoming, experienced by man.
6. Health is a rhythmically coconstituting process of the man-environment interrelationship.
7. Health is man's patterns of relating value priorities.
8. Health is an intersubjective process of transcending with the possibles.
9. Health is unitary man's negentropic unfolding.

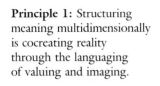

Man-Living-Health

Principles	Structuring meaning multidimensionally	Cocreating rhythmical patterns of relating	Cotranscending with the possibles
Concepts	Imaging Valuing Languaging	Revealing-concealing Enabling-limiting Connecting-separating	Powering Originating Transforming
Theoretical structures	**Powering** is a way of **revealing and concealing imaging.** **Originating** is a manifestation of **enabling and limiting valuing.** **Transforming** unfolds in the **languaging of connecting and separating.**		

Figure 2-10 Parse's theory of man-living-health. (From Parse RR: Man-living-health: a theory of nursing, New York, 1981, Wiley, p. 73.)

that man goes beyond the actual in interrelationships with others and propels into the future by incarnating intentions and actions in moving toward possibilities. Transforming occurs through originating and powering, a process of man-environment-energy interchange with recognition of continuous affirmation of self.

Nursing focuses on guiding individuals and families in sharing the meaning of the changing health process and in making choices. The goal of nursing is to enhance the quality of life as perceived by the individual and the family. Parse describes three dimensions of health: illuminating meaning, synchronizing rhythms, and mobilizing transcendence.

Illuminating meaning occurs as the nurse guides the client and the family to relate the personal meaning of the health situation from their viewpoint through explicating. *Synchronizing rhythms* of the client and the family occurs as the nurse "dwells with" them, moves with their rhythm, and leads them to recognize the harmony of the lived experience in context. *Mobilizing transcendence* occurs as the nurse guides the client to visualize the future possibilities and to move beyond and plan for changing the lived health patterns.

In Parse's view, nursing is not offering professional advice nor assisting the client to adapt to or change the health situation. It is the interpersonal interrelationship of the client and nurse to promote health and quality of life by moving beyond present health patterns.

Parse's model is complex and existential, making it difficult for a novice to understand and apply. Parse states that her model is not congruent with the commonly accepted form of the nursing process, which assumes that the nurse is an authority on health (Parse, 1987). Although the model is difficult to apply in the nursing process and probably more appropriate for the "expert" clinician because it does not provide specific guidelines or rules, it is a model that can guide the nurse. The model emphasizes understanding the client and family's perception of the personal meaning of their health situation and guiding them to recognize and act on future possibilities for changing their lived health situation. The model could be applied to any family and to any individual who is coherent and able to communicate.

Peplau's Interpersonal Model

In 1952 Dr. Hildegard Peplau described her major concepts of nursing. In later publications some of these concepts were modified (Blake, 1980; Nordal and Sato, 1980; Forchuk, 1992). Peplau views the *individual* as a developing self-system with unique biochemical, physiological, and sociopsychological characteristics and needs. Throughout life individuals encounter anxiety-producing experiences that create

◆

Peplau's Beliefs

Nursing: goal-directed interpersonal process to promote clients' forward movement of their personality and personal living

Client: any individual who feels or recognizes unmet needs

Health: ability to accomplish interpersonal activities and developmental tasks within a productive level of anxiety

Environment: any health-related setting is implied but not defined.

tension and can be transformed into either health-promoting or health-debilitating behaviors. Peplau believes that an individual's behaviors are purposeful and directed toward self-maintenance, reduction of anxiety arising from unmet needs, and achievement of higher needs. When unmet needs are felt or recognized, individuals may seek professional assistance.

Health is viewed as a continuum with varying degrees of anxiety. Peplau defines health as "forward movement of personality and other ongoing human processes in the direction of creative, constructive, productive, personal, and community living" (1952:12). Health is the relief of anxiety and tension and the redirecting of energy to facilitate need satisfaction, self-awareness, and the integration of meaningful life experiences.

Nursing is "a significant, therapeutic, interpersonal process . . . an educative instrument, a maturing force, that aims to promote forward movement of [the] personality" (Peplau, 1952:16). This process is initiated when a person expresses a felt need. The nurse-client relationship facilitates the patient's identification and resolution of unmet needs while simultaneously promoting growth and development of both, within the therapeutic relationship. Peplau identifies six roles that nurses may assume while working with clients: teacher, resource, counselor, leader, technical expert, and surrogate. These roles are used in the four phases of the goal-directed interpersonal relationship to assist clients to (1) examine their interpersonal relationships, felt needs, and problems and (2) define, understand, and productively resolve those problems. During the relationship, the attitudes toward the client and the relationship are also examined by the nurse to understand their interpersonal dynamics and develop therapeutic use of self. Nurses use communication techniques, unconditional acceptance, and empathy. These skills promote a trusting relationship, the client's self-reliance, and independent decision-making. The four phases in the nurse-client relationship are described here.

Orientation refers to the initiation of the relationship when the client recognizes a felt need or difficulty and seeks professional assistance. Upon mutual agreement, the nurse defines the nature of the reciprocal relationship and its purposes. The nurse explains that the collaborative role is to identify, examine, and find ways to resolve the client's problem.

Identification begins the working phase. The nurse-client relationship develops and strengthens as initial attitudes of client and nurse are explored. Their perceptions and expectations of each other are clarified. A trusting relationship may develop if they openly share their thoughts and feelings. During this phase they work to identify the client's problems or difficulties.

Exploitation refers to the discussion of solutions after mutual identification and understanding of the client's problems. The client's and nurse's roles and responsibilities in resolving the problem are clarified, with the client gradually assuming responsibility for control of the problem and decision-making. Progressive independence and self-reliance occurs. During this phase the client may test the relationship and experience dependent and independent feelings that need to be discussed.

Resolution refers to the final phase, when the client and nurse collaborate to resolve the problem; they also must work through their psychological dependency needs. They should discuss termination before the last meeting because this prepares them for the final separation. Successful resolution occurs when both summarize the relationship, its meaning, and accomplishments. Such resolution promotes the growth and maturity of both individuals.

Peplau's model describes nursing as a therapeutic, growth-producing relationship that proceeds through the four phases just mentioned. The nurse and client explore their relationship, the client's problems, and potential solutions. This model is a useful guide to plan implementation strategies or to cite as scientific rationale. It also may serve as a supporting approach to assess and analyze the nurse-client relationships and can be applied to both individual and family clients.

Rogers' Science of Unitary Human Beings

Martha Rogers first described her science of unitary man in 1970. This model was designed to stimulate development of nursing theories rather than to be used for direct application in practice. Rogers' conceptual system focuses on understanding the interaction between human beings and their environment. She views this interaction as the central focus of nursing, as shown in Fig. 2-11. Since 1970 Rogers has further refined her model and presented it at numerous conferences and in various journals (Rogers, 1980, 1990; Cerilli and Burd, 1989; Manhart, 1989; Joseph, 1990).

In Rogers' model, unitary human beings and envi-

◆

Rogers' Beliefs

Nursing: science and art to facilitate and promote symphonic interaction between human beings and their environment

Client: human being or individual and his or her environment

Health: expression of the life process characterized by behaviors emerging from mutual, simultaneous interaction between human beings and their environment; a continuum based on value judgments

Environment: four-dimensional negentropic energy field identified by pattern and organization and encompassing all that is outside any given human field; any setting worldwide where nurse and client meet

---

ronment are interrelated and continually and simultaneously evolving. Both human beings and environment have four major concepts: energy fields, open system, pattern, and four-dimensionality. The nature and direction of the relationship between human beings and their environment are shown through three principles: resonancy, helicy, and integrality.

Unitary human beings are irreducible wholes, different from the sum of their parts, and cannot be understood by reducing them to their parts. Human beings are four-dimensional energy fields characterized by pattern, integral with their own unique environmental fields, and continuously, creatively evolving.

Environment is an irreducible, four-dimensional energy field with pattern and characteristics different from those of its parts. An environmental field is unique to its specific human field, yet both fields continuously change and creatively evolve together.

Energy fields are the fundamental units of humans and the environment. Both humans and the environment are infinite, irreducible fields that evolve together. *Energy* refers to the dynamic nature and *field* is the unifying concept. Human beings and environment are energy fields that cannot be examined separately; they are irreducible, continuously open, and integral to each other.

Open system refers to the continuous, infinite, unbounded exchange between human beings and environmental energy fields. The closed system model of equilibrium, adaptation, and homeostasis is no longer acceptable; causality is invalid in a theory of accelerating evolution.

Pattern is the distinguishing characteristic of the energy fields. Human and environmental energy fields are single wave patterns with changing rhythms and intensity. Each human energy field pattern is unique yet integral with its own unique environmental energy field, with evolving diversity and complexity.

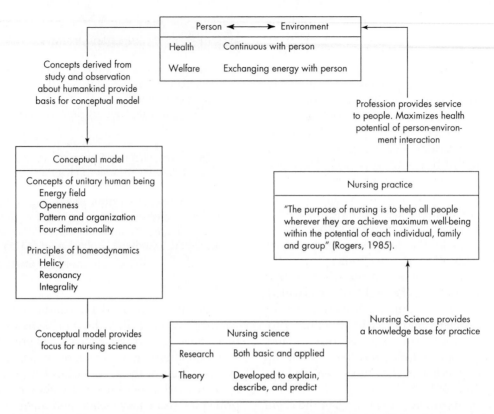

Figure 2-11 Interpretation of Rogers' view of nursing, including interrelationship among person, environment, health, and nursing. (From Fitzpatrick JJ and Whall AL: Conceptual models in nursing: analysis and application, ed 2, Bowie, Md., 1989, Robert J Brady, p. 287.)

Four-dimensionality refers to "a non-linear domain without spatial or temporal attributes" (Rogers, 1984). The "relative present" or the "infinite now" for an individual represents the four-dimensional human field.

Nursing is a learned profession based on application of a science ("an organized body of abstract knowledge derived from scientific research and logical analysis") and an art ("the imaginative and creative use of this knowledge in human service") (1984). The focus of nursing's concern is unitary human beings as a synergistic phenomenon interacting with their environment. Rogers views nursing as concerned with "the nature and direction of unitary human development integral with the environment" (1980:330), to promote symphonic interaction and integrity of the human energy field. Nurses recognize and assist human beings to establish patterns associated with their maximum health potential. *Health* is viewed as a continuous interchange and repatterning toward maximum health potential, with the emphasis on promotion.

Three principles of homeodynamics were postulated by Rogers to describe the nature and direction of change, as derived from the conceptual system just described:

- *Principle of resonancy.* Continuous change from lower to higher frequency wave patterns in human and environmental fields
- *Principle of helicy.* Continuous, innovative, probabilistic increasing diversity of human and environmental field patterns characterized by nonrepeating rhythmicities
- *Principle of integrality.* Continuous mutual human field and environmental field process (formerly titled *complementarity*)

Rogers' concepts and principles are unique to her conceptual system of unitary human beings, although other nurse theorists have adopted some of them. This conceptual system is brought together in Rogers' statement that, "Unitary man (human being) and . . . environment are in continuous, mutual, and simultaneous interaction, evolving toward increased differentiation and diversity of field pattern. . . . Change is always innovative. There is no going back, no repetition. Causality is contraindicated" (1980:333). Application of Rogers' conceptual system in the nursing process requires advanced knowledge and study of the meaning and interrelationship of her concepts and principles.

◆

| *Roy's Beliefs* |

Nursing: promotion of the client's adaptation in the four modes to enhance health using the nursing process

Client: person, family, group, or community with unusual stresses or ineffective coping mechanisms

Health: state and process of being and becoming an integrated and whole person

Environment: all conditions, circumstances, and influences surrounding and affecting the development and behavior of persons or groups; any health-related situation is implied as the setting

Roy's Adaptation Model

Sister Callista Roy first published her conceptual model of adaptation in the 1970s and has continued to refine and further develop her model in subsequent publications (Roy, 1980, 1981, 1984). Roy's model is based on general systems theory as applied to the individual and Helson's view of adaptation as related to focal, contextual, and residual stimuli.

The focus of Roy's model is the set of processes by which a person adapts to environmental stressors. Each person is a unified biopsychosocial system in constant interaction with a changing environment. When the demands of environmental stimuli are too great or the person's adaptive mechanisms are too low, the person's behavioral responses are ineffective for coping.

Roy (1984) views the *person* as an adaptive system that functions as a whole through interdependence of its parts. The system consists of input, control processes, output, and feedback. Input are stimuli from the external environment and the internal self, including information (stimuli) from the cognator and regulator mechanisms. The control processes include both biological and psychological coping mechanisms of the person, as well as cognator and regulator responses. Output is the adaptive and ineffective behavioral responses of the person. Feedback is information regarding the behavioral responses that is conveyed as input in the system (Figs. 2-12 and 2-13).

Each person is affected by stressors called *stimuli.* The *focal stimuli* are a change immediately confronting the person; these require an adaptive response. *Contextual stimuli* (all other stimuli present in the person or environment) and *residual stimuli* (those beliefs, attitudes, or traits that affect the person's present situation) mediate and contribute to the effect of the focal stimuli/stressor and determine the level of stress or adaptation.

Each person's ability to adapt to changing stimuli is determined by the person's *adaptation level,* which is a constantly changing point determined by the collective effect of the focal, contextual, and residual range of stimuli that can be tolerated at a given point in time. Roy describes two basic internal processes used in adaptation, the *regulator subsystem* and the *cognator subsystem.* The regulator subsystem receives and processes changing stimuli from the external environment and the internal self through neural-chemical-endocrine channels. It produces automatic, unconscious reactions on target organs or tissues, which then affect body responses that serve as feedback (additional stimuli) for input. The cognator subsystem receives varying internal and external stimuli involving psychological and social factors. Physical and physiological factors, including bodily responses from the system, are also included. These changing stimuli are processed/controlled through various cognitive/emotive pathways, which include perception/information processing, learning, judgment, and emotion. The regulator and cognator subsystems produce behavioral responses in four effector modes: physiological, self-concept, role function, and interdependence. The person's behavioral responses in these four modes determine whether the adaptation is an effective or ineffective response to stimuli. Adaptive responses promote the integrity of the individual by conserving energy and promoting the survival, growth, reproduction, and mastery of the human system.

Health is defined as "a state or a process of being and becoming an integrated and whole person" (Roy, 1984:39). Through adaptation the person's energy is freed from ineffective coping attempts and can be used to promote integrity, healing, and enhance health. Integrity implies soundness leading to completeness or unity.

Nursing is considered the science and practice of promoting adaptation for holistic functioning of persons through application of the nursing process to affect health positively. Nursing aims to increase the person's adaptive responses by decreasing the energy needed to cope in a given situation so there is more energy for other human processes. Nursing promotes adaptation in the four modes, which contribute to health, quality of life, and dying with dignity.

Roy's model of the nursing process has two levels of assessment. In *first-level assessment* the nurse assesses the person's adaptive and ineffective behaviors in each of the four modes. The *physiological* mode includes oxygenation, nutrition, elimination, activity and rest, skin integrity, the senses, fluids and electrolytes, and neurological and endocrine function. There are three psychosocial adaptive modes: self-concept, role function, and interdependence. The *self-*

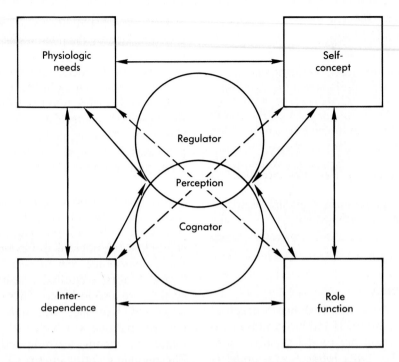

Figure 2-12 Interpretation of Roy's adaptation model, showing relationships among the subsystems of the person. There is direct interaction between all of the adaptive modes and between each adaptive mode and the regulator and the cognator. (From Fitzpatrick JJ and Whall AL: Conceptual models in nursing: analysis and application, Bowie, Md., 1983, Robert J Brady, p. 166.)

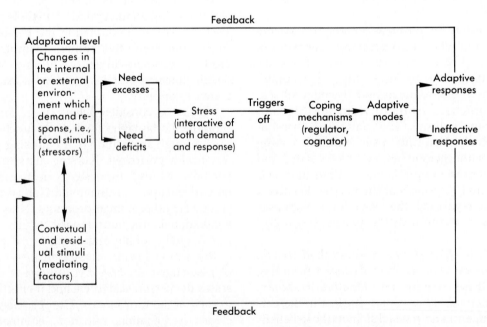

Figure 2-13 Interpretation of Roy's process of stress adaptation. (From Fitzpatrick JJ and Whall AL: Conceptual models in nursing: analysis and application, Bowie, Md., 1983, Robert J Brady, p. 167.)

concept mode consists of the individual's feelings and beliefs at a given point in time that influence behavior. This mode includes psychic integrity, physical self, personal self, self-consistency, self-ideal/self-expectancy, moral-ethical-spiritual self, learning, inner self-concept, and self-esteem. The third mode, *role function,* includes role, position, role performance, role mastery, social integrity, primary role, secondary role, tertiary role, and instrumental and expressive behaviors. *Interdependence,* the fourth mode, addresses the ability to love, respect, and value others and to respond to others in this manner. This mode includes affectional adequacy, nurturing, significant others, support systems, receptive behaviors, and contributing behaviors.

Each of these four modes has specific problems that may be identified. After assessing the adaptive and ineffective behaviors in each mode, the nurse proceeds to *second-level assessment* by determining the focal, contextual, and residual stimuli that contribute to each ineffective behavior or adaptive behavior needing reinforcement. The *focal stimuli* are those immediately confronting the person. *Contextual stimuli* are all other stimuli present within the person or from the environment. *Residual stimuli* are beliefs, attitudes, or traits that have an effect on the person's present situation.

The nursing diagnosis, derived from the two assessment levels, is a statement of the behaviors and stimuli that are ineffective or require reinforcement. Nursing goals are identification of those adaptive behavioral outcomes that are mutually agreed on by the person and the nurse. Nursing interventions to accomplish the goals aim to manage the focal, contextual, or residual stimuli by removing, increasing, decreasing, or altering these stimuli so that they fall within the person's "adaptation level." Evaluation is a reassessment of attainment of the goal of adaptive behavior.

Environment is defined as internal and external stimuli, including focal, contextual, and residual stimuli, which collectively constitute the person's "adaptation level" or zone of coping ability. Environmental stimuli include all the conditions, circumstances, and influences surrounding and affecting the development and behavior of the person or group. The person's stage of development, family, and culture are significant stimuli affecting all human adaptation.

Roy's model views the person as an adaptive system that responds to internal and external environmental stimuli in four adaptive modes, namely physiological, self-concept, role function, and interdependence. The person's adaptation level is determined by the intensity and variety of focal, contextual, and residual stimuli. Nursing promotes the person's adaptation level by manipulating the environmental stimuli to reduce ineffective responses or to reinforce adaptive behaviors. Roy's model includes biopsychosocial factors and is broad enough to use with individuals in all components of the nursing process. It is an excellent tool for assessing and analyzing the client's health patterns and for identifying nursing diagnoses. When nursing implementation strategies are directed at changing focal, contextual, or residual stimuli, Roy's model can serve as a useful theoretical approach.

Watson's Theory of Human Caring

Jean Watson began working on her transpersonal, metaphysical theory of human caring in the 1970s and published her first book, *Nursing: The Philosophy and Science of Caring,* in 1979. She continues to develop her theory, which reflects the new human science paradigm, and has refined it in subsequent publications (Watson, 1985, 1988, 1990). Watson believes nursing goes beyond existential-phenomenological approaches to incorporate concepts of soul and transcendence. The soul is the essence of the person, consisting of the *geist* (spirit or higher sense of self), which possesses self-awareness, a higher degree of consciousness, an inner strength, and a power that can expand human capacities and allow a person to transcend his or her usual self (1989:224). Transcendence refers to the capacity to coexist with the past, present, and future all at once in the here and now.

Transpersonal human caring is viewed as both a moral ideal of nursing and a caring process. The moral ideal consists of transpersonal and intersubjective interactions with persons. The caring process encompasses a commitment to protect, enhance, and preserve humanity by restoring dignity, inner har-

◆

Watson's Beliefs

Nursing: application of the art and human science through transpersonal caring transactions to help persons achieve mind-body-soul harmony, which generates self-knowledge, self-control, self-care, and self-healing

Client: person or group experiencing mind-body-soul disharmony who needs assistance with health-illness decisions to promote harmony, self-control, choice, and self-determination

Health: unity and harmony within the mind-body-soul between self and others and self and nature.

Environment: wherever transpersonal caring interactions transpire between client and nurse

mony, and facilitating healing. The nurse helps others to acquire self-knowledge, self-control, and readiness for self-healing, thus enabling them to regain their sense of inner harmony.

Underlying Watson's (1989) theory are her values and a deep respect for the wonders and mysteries of life, an acknowledgement of life's spiritual dimensions and belief in the internal power of the caring and healing process. This value system is blended with ten carative factors (1979) that include human altruism, sensitivity to oneself and others, and love for and trust of life and other humans and our own inner power.

Watson identifies many assumptions and several holographic principles of transpersonal caring. She believes that one's soul possesses a body that is not confined by space or time. Some of Watson's (1985:32-33) assumptions underlying her human care values in nursing are:

1. Care and love are the most universal and mysterious of cosmic forces and are composed of primal and universal psychic energy.
2. To survive, persons must become more caring and loving to nourish their humanity.
3. Caring and loving oneself is necessary before one can respect and care for others with gentleness and dignity.
4. Caring is the essence of nursing and the most central and unifying focus for nursing practice.
5. The caring role is deemphasized in the health care system and threatened by increased use of medical technology and bureaucratic-managerial institutional constraints.
6. Nursing's social, moral, and scientific contributions to humankind and society lie in its commitment to human care ideals in theory, practice, and research.

Some basic holographic principles that Watson (1990:284) applies to transpersonal caring are:

- The whole caring-healing consciousness is contained in a single caring moment.
- Caring and healing are interconnected and connected to other humans, the environment, and to the higher energy of the universe.
- The human caring-healing (or noncaring-nonhealing) consciousness of the nurse is communicated to the one receiving care.
- Caring-healing consciousness is temporally and spatially extended; such consciousness exists through time and space.

Nursing is defined as "a human science of health-illness-healing experiences that are mediated by pro-fessional, personal, scientific, aesthetic, and ethical human care transactions" (1989:221). Nursing is an art and science based on an underlying knowledge along with clinical and technical competencies and directed toward the protection, enhancement, and preservation of human dignity, health, healing and transcendence. The general goal of nursing is to enhance mental-spiritual growth for self and others as well to discover one's inner power and self-control. More specifically, nursing's goal is "to help persons gain a higher degree of harmony within the mind, body, and soul, which generates self-knowledge, self-reverence, self-healing, and self-care processes while allowing increasing diversity" (Watson, 1989:226).

Through dynamic interpersonal caring transactions, the nurse responds to the person's subjective world to assist clients to find meaning in their existence through exploring the meaning of their disharmony, suffering, and turmoil. These transactions illuminate the mystery of humanity and the higher power of energy in the universe that can facilitate self-knowledge, self-reverence, self-control, and self-care and potentiate the self-healing process. Nurses are co-participants in the transpersonal process: they use their intuitive and aesthetic skills, along with their feelings (including their "geist") and behaviors in relating to others.

Within transpersonal human interactions, the nurse uses ten caring factors (Watson, 1989:227-228) as guidelines for nurse-client interactions that are based on sensitivity to self and others. These primary caring factors are:

1. Formation of a humanistic-altruistic system of values
2. Nurturing of faith and hope
3. Cultivation of sensitivity to self and others
4. Development of a helping-trusting, human caring relationship
5. Promotion and acceptance of the expression of positive and negative feelings
6. Use of creative problem-solving processes
7. Promotion of transpersonal teaching-learning
8. Provision for a supportive, protective, or corrective mental, physical, sociocultural, and spiritual environment
9. Assistance with gratification of human needs
10. Allowance for existential-phenomenological-spiritual forces.

Watson (1989:225) believes that "A *person* exists as a living, growing gestalt, possessing three spheres of being—mind, body, and soul—that are influenced by the concept of self." A client is a person or group needing assistance with health-illness decisions to promote harmony, self-control, choice, and self-determination.

The client determines health or illness in response to the harmony or disharmony that exists within. Watson (1989:226) also believes that people are their own change agents through their own internal, mental-spiritual powers, which allow themselves to be healed. This is reflected in the inner power of the self, choice, inner healing potential, and preservation of harmony with mind-body-soul. These actions seek to maintain and preserve human dignity and integrity. Humans progress to higher levels of consciousness by finding meaning and harmony in their existence through the use of the mind. They can "transcend their physical world by controlling it, subduing it, changing it, or living in harmony with it" (1989:225).

Health involves the "unity and harmony within the mind, body, and soul—harmony between self and others, and between self and nature. Health is also associated with the degree of congruence between the self as perceived and the self as experienced" (1989:226). This is an eudaimonistic view of health, which incorporates many mind-body-spirit aspects. Illness is a disharmony within a person's inner self (mind, body or soul) that may or may not be a disease. "Illness connotes a felt incongruence between the self as perceived and the self as experienced" (1989:225).

Environment reflects occurances or occasions that involve caring interactions and choice by the nurse and individual. If the caring occasion is transpersonal, the capacities of both client and nurse are expanded, leading to personal growth, maturation, and development of the self.

Transpersonal caring in nursing is a moral ideal, a means of communication and intersubjective contact through the coparticipation of one's entire self with another. It is a process whereby each individual moves toward a higher sense of self and harmony in mind, body, and soul with self, others, and nature. It incorporates all the caring factors that occur between the nurse and the one being cared for (the client). Intersubjectivity occurs as the nurse enters into the experience of another person and that person enters into the nurse's experience. The values and views of the nurse are as relevant as those of the client (1989:234).

During caring transactions, the nurse and client are both in a process of being and becoming. Maintaining the client's dignity is an important part of the transaction. During transactions, the nurse's unique self is conveyed through movement, sense, touch, sound, words, colors, and forms that transmit and reflect the client's condition back to him or her. Intersubjective feelings, thoughts, and pent-up energy are released and flow, promoting congruence between the person's perception and experience and helping to release the person's inner power and strength, restore inner harmony, and develop self-knowledge and self-control.

Watson's transpersonal caring values are critical to preserving humanity and promoting client's health and healing in nursing practice. Although caring is emphasized in a few other models, Watson's theory of human caring reflects the new perspective in the human science of nursing. It encompasses relevant caring values and factors to guide application of the nursing process through transactional caring. The client and nurse explore the meanings of the client's disharmony to discover and use an inner power to reach toward self-knowledge, self-control, self-care, and self-healing. This transpersonal caring theory is useful in all components of the nursing process. Other complementary models may also be useful to guide the nursing process. Watson's theory is a valuable contribution to the human science of nursing.

Family Models

The use of a specific family model provides a perspective or focus for understanding the family. Family models have been categorized according to their basic focus as developmental, interactional, structural-functional, and systems models. First, two family developmental models, Duvall's and Stevenson's, are presented. Next, Satir's Family Interactional Model is described. Friedman's Structural-Functional Family Model illustrates the structural-functional focus, as does Calgary's Family Model, which also includes the systems approach. Many other family models are available and relevant in nursing; however, these models serve as a reference and guide for application in the nursing process as described in this book. Application of these models in the nursing process is shown in Sections II and III.

Duvall's Family Developmental Model

Evelyn Duvall's (1977) family developmental framework provides a guide to examine and analyze the basic changes and developmental tasks common to most families during their life cycle. Although each family has unique characteristics, normative patterns of sequential development have been described by Duvall. These stages and developmental tasks (see Table 2-5) illustrate common family behaviors that may be expected at specific times in the family life cycle. The stages of family development are marked by the age of the oldest child, although there is some overlapping of stages when there are several children in the family.

Stage I (*beginning families*) begins with the married couple as they establish a mutually satisfying relationship. The couple's tasks center on forming an intimate relationship and balance in their lives together, family planning, and establishing a harmonious relationship with in-laws and new friends. Adjusting to pregnancy

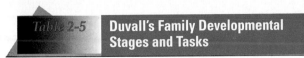

Table 2-5	Duvall's Family Developmental Stages and Tasks

Stages of development	Basic family tasks
I Beginning families	Physical maintenance
II Early childbearing	Allocation of resources
III Families with preschoolers	Division of labor
IV Families with school children	Socialization of members
V Families with teenagers	Reproduction, recruitment, and release of member
VI Launching center families	Maintenance of order
VII Middle-aged families	Placement of members in the larger society
VIII Aging families	Maintenance of motivation and morale

and planning for parenthood are also critical tasks during this stage.

Stage II *(early childbearing)* begins when the first child is between birth and 30 months; at this time the family tasks involve adjusting to the critical needs and demands of an infant while continuing to establish a satisfying home environment. Changes in roles and responsibilities with parenthood are critical tasks.

Stage III *(families with preschoolers)* begins as the parents adapt to the challenging needs and interests of the preschool child in a way to promote the child's growth. In adapting to the preschooler's needs, the parents may find their energy and privacy reduced. With the addition of another infant, parents may experience increased child-rearing responsibilities and the need for more living space in the home and more personal time to maintain intimacy and communication.

Stage IV *(families with school children)* begins as the oldest child enters school; the family tasks revolve around adjusting to community activities involving the child, encouraging the child's educational achievement, and maintaining a satisfying marital relationship. Critical tasks include balancing time and energy to meet the demands of work, the children's needs and activities, adult social interests, and the requirements of open communication and harmony in the marital and in-law relationships.

Stage V *(families with teenagers)* begins when the oldest child becomes a teenager; a gradual emancipation commences as the child develops increasing independence and autonomy. Families with teenagers must adapt to balancing freedom for growth with meeting family responsibilities. Critical tasks during this period are maintaining open communication between parents and teenagers, continuing intimacy in the marital relationship, and establishing outside interests and careers as teenagers leave the home.

Stage VI *(launching center families)* begins when the first child leaves the home and lasts until the last child has left. Parents must both prepare their children to live independently and accept the departure of the children. After the children have left, the parents must reorganize to reestablish the family unit. The roles and responsibilities of husband and wife will shift during this period if the wife returns to work. With the birth of grandchildren, parental roles and self-images require some family accommodation.

Stage VII *(middle-aged families)* begins after the children have left the home, when middle-aged parents have more time and freedom to cultivate their social and leisure interests. This may also be a period for rebuilding the marriage and maintaining satisfying relationships both with aging parents and with the children and their families. Planning for retirement while maintaining physical and emotional health and careers are major family concerns.

Stage VIII *(aging families)* begins with the retirement of one or both spouses and continues until the deaths of both marital partners. Critical tasks focus on finding sufficient energy and motivation to seek and engage in pleasurable leisure activities within financial and health limitations. Major tasks are adjusting to retirement with changing lifestyles and accepting the deaths of friends and spouse. Within this period the family may also close the home and move into a retirement community, thus having to establish ties with new friends in a new community and to find new leisure activities.

Within each of the successive stages of family development, Duvall identified eight basic tasks, shown in Table 2-5, that lead to successful family life within society. These tasks promote family adjustment and adaptation of the individual members. When families fail to accomplish these tasks, the family collectively or its members individually may experience unhappiness, societal disapproval, and difficulty in achieving harmony and self-actualization. The family tasks involve responsibilities to satisfy the biological, cultural, and personal needs and aspirations of the members at each stage of family development. These eight basic tasks include the following:

1. *Physical maintenance.* The family is responsible for providing shelter, appropriate clothing, sufficient nourishing food, and adequate health care.
2. *Allocation of resources.* Resources include finances, personal time, energy, and relationships. Family members' needs are met through division of cost and labor to provide material goods, space, and facilities, and through interpersonal relations to share authority, respect, and affection.
3. *Division of labor.* Family members decide who

will assume what responsibilities, such as providing income, managing the household tasks, maintaining the home and car, caring for young, old, or incapacited family members, and other designated tasks.

4. *Socialization of family members.* The family assumes responsibility for guiding development of mature and acceptable patterns of socially acceptable behavior in eating, elimination, sleeping, sexuality, aggression, and interaction with others.

5. *Reproduction, recruitment, and release of family members.* Childbearing, adoption, and rearing children are family responsibilities, along with incorporating new members through marriage. Policies are established for including others in the family, such as in-laws, relatives, stepparents, guests, and friends.

6. *Maintenance of order.* Order is maintained by the communication of acceptable behavior. The types of intensity of interactions, patterns of affection, and sexual expression are sanctioned by parental behavior to ensure acceptance in society.

7. *Placement of members in the larger society.* Family members establish roots in society through relationships in the church, school, political and economic system, and other organizations. The family also assumes responsibility for protecting family members from undesirable outside influences and may prohibit membership in objectionable groups.

8. *Maintenance of motivation and morale.* Family members reward each other for their achievements and provide for an individual's needs of acceptance, encouragement, and affection. The family develops a philosophy of life and sense of family unity and loyalty, thereby enabling members to adapt to both personal and family crises.

Duvall's developmental model is an excellent guide for assessing, analyzing, and planning around basic family tasks at a specific developmental stage. The nurse must first determine the family's stage of development, then examine the tasks that are appropriate for the respective stage.

However, this model does not include the family structure or physiological aspects, which should be considered for a comprehensive view of the family. The model is applicable for nuclear families with growing children, and families who are experiencing health-related problems.

Stevenson's Family Developmental Model

Joanne Stevenson (1977) describes the basic tasks and responsibilities of families in four stages:

- Emerging family (from marriage for 7 to 10 years)
- Crystallizing family (with teenage children)
- Interacting family (children grown and small grandchildren)
- Actualizing family (aging couple alone again)

She views family tasks as maintaining a common household, rearing children, and finding satisfying work and leisure. These tasks also include sustaining appropriate health patterns and providing mutual support and acculturation of family members. The four stages are delineated by the number of years the couple are married and their approximate age. Tasks for each stage are in the following text.

The Emerging Family

There are two major family tasks in the first 7 to 10 years of marriage. First, the couple strives for independence from their parents. Second, they develop a sense of responsibility for family life, including economic, emotional, and sociocultural responsibilities. Independence and responsibility are accomplished in the following ways:

- Advancing self-development and the enactment of appropriate roles and positions in society
- Initiating the development of a personal style of life
- Adjusting to a heterosexual marital relationship or to a variant companionship style
- Developing parenting behaviors for biological offspring or in the broader framework of social parenting
- Integrating personal values with career development and socioeconomic constraints (Stevenson, 1977:15)

The Crystallizing Family

When families reach the early middle years with teenage children, different responsibilities emerge. The family assumes responsibility for growth and development of individual members and outside organizations. The parents provide assistance to both the younger and older generations without exerting control over them. These tasks are accomplished by the following:

- Developing socioeconomic consolidation
- Evaluating one's occupation or career in light of a personal value system
- Helping younger persons become integrated human beings
- Enhancing or redeveloping intimacy with spouse or significant other
- Assuming responsible positions in occupational, social, and civic activities, organizations, and communities

- Maintaining and improving the home or other forms of property
- Using leisure time in satisfying and creative ways
- Adjusting to biological or personal system changes that occur (Stevenson, 1977:18)

The Interacting Family

In the later middle years most of the children leave the home but return periodically with their own children. The older family members absorb the small children into the home. Relationships between work and leisure change. The older family now assumes responsibility for "continued survival and enhancement of the nation." To accomplish these responsibilities, the adult members are involved in the following activities:

- Maintaining flexible views in occupational, civic, political, religious, and social positions
- Keeping current on relevant scientific, political, and cultural changes
- Developing mutually supportive (interdependent) relationships with grown offspring and other members of the younger generations
- Reevaluating and enhancing the relationship with spouse or significant other or adjusting to their loss
- Helping aged parents or other relatives progress through the last stage of life
- Deriving satisfaction from increased availability of leisure time
- Preparing for retirement and planning another career when feasible
- Adapting self and behavior to signals of accelerated aging processes (Stevenson, 1977:25).

The Actualizing Family

In late adulthood the aging couple are engaged in discovering meaning in their lives. They accept the process of grief and dying. They "assume responsibility for sharing the wisdom of age, reviewing life, and putting [their] affairs in order" (Stevenson, 1977:28). This task is accomplished by:

- Pursuing a second or third career, new interests, hobbies, or community activities
- Learning new skills that are well removed from previous learnings
- Sharing wisdom accrued from the past with individuals, groups, communities, and nations
- Evaluating the totality of past life and putting successes and failures into perspective
- Progressing through the stages of grief, death, and dying with significant others and with self (Stevenson, 1977:29)

Stevenson's developmental model describes family tasks and responsibilities over four stages. The stages encompass child rearing, spouse relationships, and interaction with community organizations. The model is useful with nuclear families because it examines psychosocial patterns at a specific stage of development. However, the model does not include family structure, nor does it address health promotion and health-related concerns that the family may face.

Satir's Interactional Family Model

Virginia Satir (1972) believes that the family's interactional health depends on its ability to share and understand the members' feelings, needs, and behavior patterns. She thinks that healthy, nurturing families help their members know themselves through communication of everyday events. This communication promotes each individual's self-confidence and self-worth. Satir views the healthy family as hopeful, trusting of others, and curious about what society has to offer. The family operates on a growth-producing, reality-oriented basis. This promotes intimacy among its members. Family rules about money, chores, and power are explicit and understood by everyone. Also, the healthy family establishes links with society. These links are established through membership in various groups.

Satir's model of the healthy family consists of four concepts: self-worth, communication, rules, and links to society.

Each member and the family unit demonstrate feelings of high esteem and *self-worth*. These attitudes are conveyed by behaviors showing integrity, honesty, responsibility, compassion, and love. These attitudes flow outward from each individual and all members radiate a sense of trust. They accept their own strengths and inadequacies as well as those of others. Family members who lack self-worth build walls of distrust, isolation, and loneliness. They fear others will cheat them, use them, or step on them. Such fear leads to unhealthy family interaction.

Communication directly influences the relationships among family members. Patterns of communication include body movements, posture, tone of voice, and spoken words. In healthy families communication is open, direct, clear, and honest. The members are receptive and encourage open, honest sharing of feelings and needs. They value what others have to say, supporting each member's attempts in both verbal and physical communication. Unhealthy families block communication among members; they may give ambiguous messages or not listen at all, which leads to distrust and low self-worth among the family members.

Each family has a set of *rules* it lives by. These rules may be explicit or implicit. Most families assume that everyone knows and understands the rules, but this is not always true. Families have rules about money, responsibilities, activities, special privileges, privacy, sexual expression, language, territoriality, and authority. In many situations, rules define what actions are appropriate; they may also guide how feelings are expressed and may help achieve goals or impede goal achievement. Some rules may be outdated, unfair, unclear, or inappropriate. In healthy families the rules are known to all members, allow for freedom, and encourage discussion among the members. Unhealthy families may have implicit rules that restrict family members. These rules may be inflexible and inhibit the growth of the members.

The family unit and individual members have *links to society* through organizations and friends. The organizational links include schools, churches, political groups, recreational groups, and clubs. Links with friends are usually formed through common interests. With these links the family and its members keep actively involved in the community and relate to the world around them. Healthy families have many links with society, believing society has much to offer and trusting their selection of groups to be a positive influence and interaction. They believe society offers opportunities for choices and change, growth, and development. These opportunities are welcomed, desirable, and normal. Unhealthy families view society with distrust and fear exposure to others' values. They avoid involvement in organizations, preferring to remain isolated, and do not welcome experiences outside the family.

Satir's interactional family model addresses four major psychosocial concepts considered important in a healthy family. The model is limited because it does not include family structure, functions, and developmental level. It can be applied to any type of family, but additional models may be necessary for a comprehensive approach in the nursing process.

Friedman's Structural-Functional Family Model

Friedman's (1992) family model was developed from sociological frameworks and systems theory. The family is the focus of the model, as it interacts with suprasystems in the community and with individual family members in the subsystem. The model is composed of two components—structural and functional—as shown in Table 2-6. The structural component examines the family unit, how it is organized, and how members relate to one another in terms of their values, communication network, role systems, and power. The functional component refers to the interactional outcomes resulting from the family organizational structure. There are six parts to family functions. The structural-functional components and parts all intimately interrelate and interact: each component and part is affected by the others.

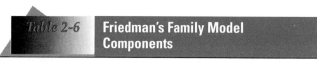

Table 2-6	Friedman's Family Model Components

Structural components	Functional components
Family composition	Affective
Value systems	Physical necessities and care
Communication patterns	Economic
Role structure	Reproductive
Power structure	Socialization and social placement
	Family coping

Structural Components
Value Systems

Values develop over time by exposure to and experience with influential groups and individuals, such as parents, culture, religion, and ethnic groups. Values lead to chosen behaviors, which are reinforced by others, and are expressed by family members' behaviors—how they allocate resources and where time and energy are invested. Some of these values are related to health care, materialism, education, independence, productivity, and cleanliness.

Communication Patterns

As families evolve they develop communication patterns, ways of relating to each other that may be functional or dysfunctional. Communication involves verbal and nonverbal behaviors, including tone, intent, and message. Communication patterns include who talks with whom, who listens, who seeks feedback, and who validates the message. Are family members able to share feelings and needs with others? What are the quality, quantity, and topics of conversation? What topics or types of communication are denied or avoided among the family?

Role Structure

In a family, members adopt varying roles that may change over time. Roles can be formal or informal, adopted or assigned. What are the formal and informal roles of family members? What roles are expected in the family, and which are assigned or adopted by whom? Are there conflicts between role expectations of others and the roles adopted by members? How flexible are family members in changing roles as needed?

Power Structure

The family power structure is determined by various influencing factors. Some factors include the social and ethnic class, family communication patterns, interpersonal and financial resources, family coalitions, and implementation of decisions. To identify the family power structure, consider who is really in charge of the family and why. Who makes the major decisions or has the last word? Who is consulted about family plans or changes? Who makes the rules? Who enforces discipline? The family power structure may be authoritarian, democratic, laissez-faire, paternalistic, maternalistic, or egalitarian, or it may vary with the issue at hand.

Functional Components
Affective

The social and emotional developmental needs of family members must be recognized and met by family members. These functions include reducing tension, maintaining morale, and conveying esteem and love for family members.

Physical Necessities and Care

The adult family members are responsible for providing food, clothing, shelter, health care, and protection from danger for family members.

Economic

The adult family members are responsible for obtaining sufficient resources, including financial, space, and material goods, and allocating these resources appropriately to family members. Both family values and power structure have an impact on allocation of resources.

Reproductive

The adult family members assume responsibility for conception and contraception.

Socialization and Social Placement

The adult family members determine appropriate social roles for children, instill family values and expectations, and confer their socioethnic status on the children. These things are accomplished by providing and sharing experiences with others in the family, schools, community organizations, and religious groups.

Family Coping

For family stability and growth, the members need adaptive patterns and problem-solving abilities to respond to demands and expectations outside the family that create change within the family.

Friedman's structural-functional family model provides a broad framework for examining the interactions among family members and within the community. This model incorporates physical, psychosocial, and cultural aspects of the family along with interacting relationships. The family's developmental stage and additional structural aspects could be added. This model is very applicable in the nursing process to any type of family and its health-related problems.

Calgary's Family Model

Calgary's family model is an integrated conceptual framework of several theorists' work that was adapted for nurses at the University of Calgary (Wright and Leahey, 1994). The model combines three major categories: family structure, function, and development. Each of the three categories is further subdivided, as shown in Table 2-7. Although the family may be examined by looking at specific parts, each part interacts with others and changes the whole family configuration.

Family Internal Structure

Family composition refers to all members living in the home. This definition includes nuclear families, single-parent families, homosexual couples, boarders, grandparents, stepparents, and children. The *family* is defined as a social system of individuals related through bonds of affection, loyalty, and durability that persist over time.

Gender is the "set of beliefs about or expectations of male and female behavior and experiences" (Wright and Leahey, 1994:41) that each family member holds. These beliefs are formed from interactions with family members and society, and influence how individuals feel, think, and behave in all situations.

Rank order refers to the children's ages and birth order. It is believed that birth order influences levels of motivation and achievement, along with vocational choices.

Subsystems in a family are delineated by generation,

Table 2-7	Calgary Family Model	
Family structure	**Family development**	**Family functions**
Internal		**Instrumental**
Family composition	Developmental stage	Daily living activities
Rank order of	Developmental tasks	Gender
members	Attachments	
Subsystems in family		
Boundaries of family		
External		**Expressive**
Larger systems		Communication
Extended family		(emotional, verbal,
		nonverbal, circular)
Context		Problem-solving
Ethnicity		Roles
Race		Influence
Social class		Beliefs
Religion		Alliances/coalitions
Environment		

Adapted from Calgary Family Assessment Model. In Wright LM and Leahey M: Nurses and families: a guide to family assessment and intervention, ed 2, Philadelphia, 1994, FA Davis.

sex, interests, and function, according to Minuchin (1974). Each family member belongs to several subsystems that differentiate the level of power and skills. Examples include a stepparent who lacks power over the children or acts like a child, while a child may have the power of a parent.

Boundary refers to which family member(s) participates in what functions and how. Boundaries protect the family members by obtaining, containing, retaining, and disposing of information, products, or people. For example, a family may prevent members from bringing in drugs or using vulgar language, or it may prevent members from divulging family information to outsiders. Boundaries can be diffuse, rigid, or permeable and may change over time.

Family External Structure

Extended family includes grandparents, aunts, uncles, and cousins along with steprelatives. These family members may live nearby or far away from those in the household.

Larger systems refers to community social agencies and personnel with whom the family members have meaningful interactions. These agencies may include employment places, schools, public and child welfare agencies, recreation agencies, health services, and government agencies. The family's relationship and interactions with these agencies may be positive, neutral, or negative.

Contextual Structure

Ethnicity is a combination of cultural history, race, and religious processes that are consciously and unconsciously transmitted by the family and reinforced by the surrounding community (Wright and Leahey, 1994). Some cultures are highly family-oriented, whereas others maintain a distinct distance between members and generations.

Race influences the individual's and family's core identification and intersects with class, religious, and ethnic variables. "Racial attitudes, stereotyping, and discrimination are powerful influences on family interaction" (Wright and Leahey, 1994:47).

Social class status strongly influences the family value system. The adults' educational attainment, income, and occupation usually determine their values, which influence their lifestyles and behavior patterns.

Religion refers to the family values, size, health care practices, and socialization patterns. It includes level of community involvement and maintainance of certain traditions, both religious and hygienic.

Environment refers to both the general neighborhood and the home. The type of neighborhood (commercial or residential) and proximity to stores, transportation, recreation, and health facilities are considered. In the home the amount of space and privacy, along with access, safety, security, kitchen utilities, and bathrooms, are important factors.

Family Development

Family development is based on the length of marriage and the child-rearing stages. Theorists such as Duvall (1977) have identified eight stages, with eight tasks in each stage. Most other developmental theorists identify fewer stages and tasks. In this model three major areas are defined; these can be further subdivided by referring to other developmental theorists.

Stages refers to the length of the marriage and the age of the eldest child. Families move through normal transitions in child-rearing, although with additional children some stages overlap. Ethnic and cultural differences also should be considered.

Tasks can be considered either general maintenance types of responsibilities, such as employment, spending, health, education, and socialization (which may be defined in a general way), or specifically defined, depending on the family's developmental stage.

Attachments are the unique and relatively enduring emotional ties between two family members. This bond may be between mother and daughter, child and grandparent, or brother and sister. The reciprocal nature of this bond and the quality of the relationship are considered.

Family Functions

Family functions include instrumental and expressive issues and are mainly focused on patterns of responsibility for tasks and interactions among family members.

Instrumental

Activities of daily living are the patterns of working, eating, sleeping, exercise, recreation, and socialization. Which family members take on or are assigned specific tasks, such as grocery shopping, preparing meals, cleaning house, paying bills, and maintaining health? Which activities do family members do together and which are done alone?

Expressive

Communication includes emotional, verbal, nonverbal, and circular forms. *Emotional* communication refers to the range and types of emotions and feelings expressed by members during interactions, including joy, anger, happiness, and sadness. *Verbal* communication focuses on the relationship expressed between the sender and receiver and the meaning of the words. *Nonverbal* communication focuses on the body posture, eye contact, expressions, touch, and gestures as individuals communicate. *Circular* communication refers to the reciprocal pattern of behaviors and inferences between two family members during communication—how their communication is interpreted and the reactions elicited by each person based on that interpretation.

Problem-solving refers to the family's method of identifying and solving problems. Who in the family recognizes and identifies problems? How does the family handle problems? Is one person the decision-maker or do members share the problems and solutions? Are outside family members, friends, or professionals sought for council or assistance? Is there one pattern of problem-solving in the family, or does the manner of problem-solving depend on the type of problem?

Roles are the established patterns of behavior as family members interact with another member. Each member has several overlapping roles that are unique in each dyad but change over time. For example, a woman may be a wife, mother, daughter, employee, student, sister, and friend. Roles may be assumed or assigned, complementary or conflicting. How each member feels about and copes with his or her roles is important.

Influence refers to the methods that family members use to affect each other's behavior. Parents influence their children through rewards such as praise, special privileges, toys, and hugs, or punishment such as criticism, spanking, or denial of rewards. Adults often use words, affection, and gifts or the withholding of these to influence other adult family members. What are the family members' patterns of influencing other members? Are these behaviors normal and healthy, or are they disruptive and dysfunctional?

Beliefs are the fundamental ideas, opinions, and assumptions that the family holds. Beliefs are constructed from interactional, social, and cultural contexts. Family members' beliefs shape the pattern of their choices, actions, and behavior. Are members expected to achieve, excel, save face, or be honest, trustworthy, and reliable? Some families place importance on materialistic status symbols whereas others emphasize altruism, the work ethic, and religious beliefs. The family's values and beliefs influence their lifestyle and behavior patterns, along with how their time and money are spent.

Alliances/coalitions refers to the direction, balance, and intensity of relationships among family members. These relationships may include two or three family members and may change over time. In healthy families, three-member coalitions provide a flexibility for change in the intensity of the relationship among the members.

The Calgary family model is comprehensive and incorporates three major areas, namely, the structure, function, and development of the family. This model is complex, with too many subconcepts for the nurse to fully explore each area. When using this model, the nurse must determine which areas are most important and focus on those, while acquiring some general information in other areas. This is a good model for assessing family data; however, additional knowledge of sociological theories are necessary to analyze and interpret the data and to develop plans for the family. The Calgary family model can be applied to any type of family with any health-related concern.

Summary

This chapter presented an overview of several general, nursing, and family models that can be applied in the nursing process. Major concepts and subconcepts were described and illustrated, and the strengths, limitations, and possible applications of each model were briefly discussed. In any nursing process, a holistic view of the client is desired; however, some models may not include areas that are particularly relevant to the client's health situation. Therefore it is acceptable for the nurse to include another model or certain aspects of another model to supplement the central model. The synthesis of models is part of the creative art of nursing practice. For example, Roy's Adaptation Model may be very appropriate for a specific client situation, but a developmental viewpoint would also be relevant, so Erikson's Stages of Development could be a supplemental model. In a family nursing process Friedman's model may be appropriate, but it lacks specific guides for health care. Therefore Orem's Self-Care Model may provide an appropriate supplement.

Section II describes each component of the nursing process in detail, with examples of how to apply different models in each component. Section III provides case studies for individual, family, and community clients and illustrates application of selected models in a complete nursing process.

Critical Thinking Exercises BY ELIZABETH S. FAYRAM

1. a. Compare and contrast two nursing models in terms of the concepts of nursing, client, health, and environment.
   b. Explain which model is closest to your own philosophy of nursing and the reasons why.
2. Select a specific model described in this chapter. Identify how this model would influence your nursing practice.
3. Identify models that would be appropriate when working with clients with mental health concerns. Provide rationale for your selections.
4. Describe how values and beliefs of a specific population (e.g. Native Americans, Hispanics) would influence the selection of a model guiding your nursing practice.

REFERENCES AND READINGS

Aguilera DC and Messick JM: *Crisis intervention: theory and methodology*, ed 6, St. Louis, 1990, Mosby.

Bishop AH and Scudder JR: *Nursing: the practice of caring*, New York, 1991, National League for Nursing.

Blake M: The Peplau developmental model for nursing practice. In Reihl JP and Roy C, eds: *Conceptual models for nursing practice*, ed 2, New York, 1980, Appleton-Century-Crofts.

Botha ME: Theory development in perspective: the role of conceptual frameworks and models in theory development, *J Adv Nurs* 14:49, 1989.

Bottorff JL: Nursing: a practical science of caring, *Adv Nurs Sci*. 14:26, 1991.

Buchanan BF: Conceptual models: an assessment framework, *JONA* 17:22, 1987.

Campbell V and Keller K: The Betty Neuman health care systems model: an analysis. In Reihl-Sisca JP, ed: *Conceptual models for nursing practice*, ed 3, New York, 1989, Appleton & Lange.

Cerilli K and Burd S: An analysis of Martha Rogers' nursing as a science of unitary human beings. In Reihl-Sisca JP, ed: *Conceptual models for nursing practice*, ed 3, New York, 1989, Appleton & Lange.

Capers DF and Kelly R: Neuman nursing process: a model of holistic care, *Holistic Nurs Pract* 1:19, 1987.

Chinn PL and Kramer MK: *Theory and nursing: a systematic approach*, ed 3, St. Louis, 1991, Mosby.

Clements IW and Roberts FB, eds: *Family health: a theoretical approach to nursing care*, New York, 1983, John Wiley & Sons.

Coker EB and Schreiber R: Implementing King's conceptual framework at the bedside. In Parker ME, ed: *Nursing theories in practice*, New York, 1990, National League for Nursing.

Cuff-Carney D: Holistic family therapy: individuals or families? A therapist's perspective, *Holistic Nurs Pract* 2:45, 1987.

Duvall EM: *Marriage and family development*, ed 5, Philadelphia, 1977, JB Lippincott.

Erikson E: *Childhood and society*, ed 2, New York, 1963, Norton.

Fawcett J: *Analysis and evaluation of conceptual models of nursing*, ed 2, Philadelphia, 1989, FA Davis.

Feathers RL: Orem's self-care nursing theory. In Reihl-Sisca JP, ed: *Conceptual models for nursing practice*, ed 3, New York, 1989, Appleton & Lange.

Fitch M, Rogers M, Ross E, Shea H, Smith I, and Tucker D: Developing a plan to evaluate the use of nursing conceptual frameworks, *CJNA* 4:22, 1991.

Fitzpatrick JJ and Whall AL: *Conceptual models of nursing: analysis and application*, ed 2, Norwalk, Conn., 1989, Appleton & Lange.

Forchuk C: Peplau's theory: concepts and their relations, *Nurs Sci Q* 4:54, 1992.

Friedman MM: *Family nursing: theory and practice*, ed 3, New York, 1992, Appleton & Lange.

Gast HL, et al.: Self-care agency: conceptualizations and operations, *Adv Nurs Sci* 12:26, 1989.

Gaut DA, ed: *The presence of caring in nursing*, New York, 1992, National League for Nursing.

Gaut DA: *A global agenda for caring*, New York, 1993, National League for Nursing.

George J, ed: *Nursing theories: the base for professional nursing practice*, Norwalk, Conn., 1990, Appleton & Lange.

Grubbs J: An interpretation of the Johnson behavioral systems model for nursing practice. In Reihl JP and Roy C, eds: *Conceptual models for nursing practice*, ed 2, New York, 1980, Appleton-Century-Crofts.

Henderson V: *The nature of nursing: reflections after 25 years*, New York, 1991, National League for Nursing.

Huch MH: Theory-based practice: structuring nursing care, *Nurs Sci Q* 1:6, 1988.

Huckabey L: The role of conceptual frameworks in nursing practice, administration, education, and research, *Nurs Admin Q* 15:17, 1991.

Johnson DE: The behavioral systems model for nursing. In Reihl JP and Roy C, eds: *Conceptual models for nursing practice*, ed 2, New York, 1980, Appleton-Century-Crofts.

Johnson DE: The behavioral system model for nursing. In Parker ME, ed: *Nursing theories in practice*, New York, 1990, National League for Nursing.

Joseph L: Practical application of Rogers' theoretical framework for nursing. In Parker ME, ed: *Nursing theories in practice*, New York, 1990, National League for Nursing.

Kalb KA: The gift: applying Newman's theory of health in nursing practice. In Parker ME, ed: *Nursing theories in practice*, New York, 1990, National League for Nursing.

Kane CF: Family social support: toward a conceptual model, *Adv Nurs Sci* 10:18, 1988.

King I: Toward a theory for nursing: general concepts of human behavior, New York, 1971, John Wiley & Sons.

King I: *A theory for nursing: systems, concepts, process*, New York, 1981, John Wiley & Sons.

King IM: King's conceptual framework and theory of goal attainment. In Parker ME, ed: *Nursing theories in practice*, New York, 1990, National League for Nursing.

Leininger M: *Transcultural nursing: concepts, theories and practices*, New York, 1978, John Wiley & Sons.

Leininger MM: Caring: a central focus of nursing and health care services, *Nurs & Health Care* 1:135, 1980.

Leininger M: *Caring: an essential human need*, Thorofare, N.J., 1981, Charles B Slack.

Leininger M: *Care: the essence of nursing and health*, Thorofare, N.J., 1984, Charles B Slack.

Leininger MM, ed: *Culture care diversity and universality: a theory of nursing*, New York, 1991, National League for Nursing.

Manhart EA, ed: *Visions of Rogers' science-based nursing*, New York, 1989, National League for Nursing.

Maslow A: *Motivation and personality*, ed 2, New York, 1970, Harper & Row.

Mayberry A: Merging nursing theories, models, and nursing practice: more than an administrative challenge, *Nurs Admin Q* 15:44, 1991.

Meleis AI: *Theoretical nursing: development and process,* ed 2, Philadelphia, 1991, JB Lippincott.

Morales-Mann ET and Jiang SL: Applicability of Orem's conceptual framework: a cross-cultural point of view, *Adv Nurs* 18:737, 1993.

Moynihan MM: Implementation of the Neuman systems model in an acute care nursing department. In Parker ME, ed: *Nursing theories in practice,* New York, 1990, National League for Nursing.

Neil RM: Watson's theory of caring in nursing: the rainbow of and for people living with AIDS. In Parker ME, ed: *Nursing theories in practice,* New York, 1990, National League for Nursing.

Neil RM and Watts R, eds: *Caring and nursing: explorations in feminist perspectives,* New York, 1990, National League for Nursing.

Neuman B: *The Neuman systems model,* ed 2, Norwalk, Conn., 1989, Appleton & Lange.

Neuman B: The Neuman nursing process format: family case study. In Reihl-Sisca JP, ed: *Conceptual models for nursing practice,* ed 3, New York, 1989, Appleton & Lange.

Neuman BM: The Neuman systems model: a theory for practice. In Parker ME, ed: *Nursing theories in practice,* New York, 1990, National League for Nursing.

Newman MA: Shifting to higher consciousness. In Parker ME, ed: *Nursing theories in practice,* New York, 1990, National League for Nursing.

Nordal D and Sato A: Peplau's model applied to primary nursing in clinical practice. In Reihl JP and Roy C, eds: *Conceptual models for nursing practice,* ed 2, New York, 1980, Appleton-Century-Crofts.

Orem DE: *Nursing: concepts and practice,* ed 2, New York, 1980, McGraw-Hill.

Orem DE: *Nursing: concepts and practice,* ed 3, New York, 1985, McGraw-Hill.

Orem DE: *Nursing: concepts and practice,* ed 4, St. Louis, 1991, Mosby.

Orem DE: A nursing practice theory in three parts, 1956-1989. In Parker ME, ed: *Nursing theories in practice,* New York, 1990, National League for Nursing.

Orlando IJ: *The dynamic nurse-patient relationship: function, process, and principles,* New York, 1990, National League for Nursing.

Parker ME, ed: *Patterns of nursing theory in practice,* New York, 1990, National League for Nursing.

Parse RR: *Man-living-health: a theory of nursing,* New York, 1981, John Wiley & Sons.

Parse RR: *Nursing science: major paradigms, theories, and critiques,* Philadelphia, 1987, Saunders.

Parse RR: Man-Living-Health: a theory of nursing. In Reihl-Sisca JP, ed: *Conceptual models for nursing practice,* ed 3, New York, 1989, Appleton & Lange.

Paterson JG and Zderad LT: *Humanistic nursing,* New York, 1988, National League for Nursing.

Peplau HE: *Interpersonal relations in nursing,* New York, 1952, Putnam.

Pioli C and Sandor J: The Roy adaptation model: an analysis. In Reihl-Sisca JP, ed: *Conceptual models for nursing practice,* ed 3, New York, 1989, Appleton & Lange.

Riehl J and Roy Sr, eds: *Conceptual models for nursing practice,* ed 2, New York, 1980, Appleton-Century-Crofts.

Riehl-Sisca JP, ed: *Conceptual models for nursing practice,* ed 3, Norwalk, Conn., 1989, Appleton & Lange.

Riehl-Sisca JP: Orem's self-care nursing theory. In Reihl-Sisca JP, ed: *Conceptual models for nursing practice,* ed 3, New York, 1989, Appleton & Lange.

Rogers ME: *Theoretical basis of nursing,* Philadelphia, 1970, FA Davis.

Rogers ME: Science of unitary human man. In Reihl JP and Roy C, eds: *Conceptual models for nursing practice,* ed 2, New York, 1980, Appleton-Century-Crofts.

Rogers ME: Space-age paradigm for new frontiers in nursing. In Parker ME, ed: *Nursing theories in practice,* New York, 1990, National League for Nursing.

Rogers ME: Creating a climate for the implementation of a nursing conceptual framework, *J Contin Ed Nurs* 20:112, 1989.

Roy Sr C: The Roy adaptation model. In Reihl JP and Roy C, eds: *Conceptual models for nursing practice,* ed 2, New York, 1980, Appleton-Century-Crofts.

Roy Sr C and Roberts SL: Theory construction in nursing—an adaptation model, Englewood Cliffs, NJ, 1981, Prentice-Hall.

Roy Sr C: *Introduction to nursing: an adaptation model,* ed 2, Englewood Cliffs, NJ, 1984, Prentice-Hall.

Roy Sr C and Andrews HA: *The Roy adaptation model: the definitive statement,* Norwalk, Conn., 1991, Appleton & Lange.

Ryan LG: A critique of nursing: human science and human care. In Reihl-Sisca JP, ed: *Conceptual models for nursing practice,* ed 3, New York, 1989, Appleton & Lange.

Satir V: *Peoplemaking,* Palo Alto, Calif., 1972, Science and Behavior Books.

Schultz PR and Meleis A: Nursing epistemology: traditions, insights, questions, *Image: J Nurs Scholar* 20:217, 1989.

Shea H, Rogers M, Ross E, et al.: Implementation of nursing conceptual models, *CJNA* 2:15, 1989.

Smith MJ: Research and practice related to Man-Living-Health. In Reihl-Sisca JP, ed: *Conceptual models for nursing practice,* ed 3, New York, 1989, Appleton & Lange.

Sohn KS: One method for comparing different nursing models, *Nurs Health Care* 12:410, 1992.

Stevenson JS: *Issues and crises during middlescence,* New York, 1977, Appleton-Century-Crofts.

Swanson KM: Empirical development of a middle range theory of caring, *Nurs Research* 40:161, 1991.

Taylor SG: Practical applications of Orem's self-care deficit nursing theory. In Parker ME, ed: *Nursing theories in practice,* New York, 1990, National League for Nursing.

Tettero I, Jackson S, and Wilson S: Theory to practice: developing a Rogerian-based assessment tool, *J Adv Nurs* 18:776, 1993.

von Bertalanffy L: *General systems theory: foundation, development, and applications,* New York, 1968, George Braziller.

Walker L: The future of theory development: commentary and response, *Nurs Sci Q* 2:118, 1989.

Watson J: *Nursing: the philosophy and science of caring,* Boston, 1979, Little, Brown.

Watson J: *Nursing: human science and human care,* Norwalk, Conn., 1985, Appleton-Century-Crofts.

Watson J: New dimensions of human caring theory, *Nurs Sci Q* 1:175, 1988.

Watson MJ: Transpersonal caring: a transcendent view of person, health, and healing. In Parker ME, ed: *Nursing theories in practice,* New York, 1990, National League for Nursing.

Wright LM and Leahey M: *Nurses and families: a guide to family assessment and intervention,* ed 2, Philadelphia, 1994, FA Davis.

Components of the Nursing Process

CHAPTER 3

ASSESSMENT
Overview
of Data Collection

Paula J. Christensen

General Considerations

Assessment is the foundation of the nursing process. Accurate data collection leads to identi-fication of the client's health status, strengths, and concerns for nursing diagnoses, which provides direction for nursing implementation and alleviation of client concerns. The purpose of assessment is to identify and obtain pertinent data about the client. The American Nurses Association (1980) states that nursing is the diagnosis and treatment of human responses to actual or potential health problems. Therefore the main focus of data collection is the client's *response* to health concerns or problems. These responses can be biophysical, sociocultural, psychological, or spiritual in nature. In other words, nurses consider clients in a multifocal way. Individuals, families, and communities have multiple aspects that are interrelated and influence each other. All these aspects or potential response areas are considered to ensure a comprehensive and accurate assessment. To accomplish this the nurse needs a strong knowledge base in a variety of disciplines. Knowledge of the theories, norms, and standards of behavior and functioning provides a foundation to collect pertinent information from clients, critically analyze the data, and make sound judgments about their health.

This chapter begins with a brief historical overview of data collection. Factors influencing data collection, characteristics of the nurse-client relationship, phases of assessment, and patterns of behavior and functioning are then discussed. Three major methods for data collection and specific examples of each are given. The application of models to data collection is provided. The most important points for assessment are given in the following list and are summarized at the end of the chapter as guidlines.

1. A systematic format is used for data collection.
2. The data are comprehensive and multifocal.
3. A variety of sources is used for data collection.
4. Appropriate methods are used for data collection.
5. The data are verifiable.
6. The data reflect updating of information.
7. The data are recorded and communicated appropriately.

The assessment process is applicable to all clients: individuals, families, and communities. Specific examples of data collection for each type of client are provided in the next three chapters.

Historical Perspectives

Nursing care has frequently included a limited assessment of clients' health-related concerns. Traditionally the nurse depended on medical diagnoses to give direction to nursing care. Nurses also used intuition during contact with their clients, for example, "I just have the feeling that Mr. Polaski is going downhill," or "Something tells me I had better check Ms. Armond's blood pressure more frequently." These intuitions were based on an important form of data collection that still exists today—subjective impression—one that cannot be refuted yet also cannot be the sole source of data obtained. Behavioral, social, nursing, and medical sciences have developed to the point of providing certain concrete indicators of health, cited within theories, norms, and standards. These health indicators provide nurses with a basis for collecting data, analyzing and synthesizing the data, and making judgments.

Nurses have become increasingly accountable and responsible for making sound nursing assessments and clinical judgments on which to base implementation. Medical diagnoses and intuitions now serve as cues for further data collection. Because nursing practice focuses on maintenance, restoration, and promotion of health, the nurse must conduct a comprehensive and valid nursing assessment to meet those goals.

Factors Influencing Data Collection

Several factors influence the process of data collection, including how the data are presented by the client and how they are perceived by the nurse. Both the client and the nurse enter a situation with previous experiences and knowledge that influence their perceptions and interpretations. More specifically, the nurse and the client are influenced by their respective (1) physical, mental, and emotional states and needs; (2) cultural, social, and philosophical backgrounds; (3) spiritual and religious practices; (4) number and functional ability of senses; (5) past experiences associated with the present situation; (6) meaning of the event; (7) interests, preoccupations, preconceptions, and motivational levels; (8) knowledge or familiarity with the situation; (9) environmental conditions and distractions; and (10) presence, attitudes, and reactions of others. These factors create a situation in which both client and nurse may automatically assign personal meanings or interpretations to the situation. Difficulty arises when the nurse's perception or interpretation is used as fact. The nurse can develop the ability to differentiate actual data from personal interpretation through an adequate knowledge base, self-awareness, and conscious attention to potential misinterpretations.

The nurse's level of proficiency also plays a role during the assessment of a client's health status. The novice or beginning nurse relies on more structured guidelines for assessment, ensuring that specific data are obtained in a deliberate and conscious manner. Nurses with more experience develop a perceptual awareness that can begin with vague hunches and intuitive assessments. The process for data collection is internalized and accurate conclusions are made from inadequate information as expert nurses perceive "wholes" rather than "bits and pieces" of information

(Rew and Borrow, 1987). Highly proficient nurses learn to trust their intuitive hunches and follow up on them to find confirming data. Their personal knowledge and experience along with their empirical knowledge provide the basis for transformation of their skills and understanding that leads to expert performance (Benner, 1984).

Nurse-Client Relationship

The nurse-client relationship is the means for applying the nursing process. This relationship is the vehicle by which the nurse works mutually with the client to facilitate the client's optimal level of health. Carl Rogers (1961) identified three aspects that facilitate personal growth in a relationship: (1) genuineness—the ability to be aware of one's own feelings, or being real; (2) respect for the separateness of another—accepting the other unconditionally; and (3) a continuing desire to understand or empathize with the other. These aspects are applicable to all human relationships, especially the nurse-client relationship.

Trust, empathy, caring, autonomy, and mutuality are also important characteristics basic to the development of a nurse-client relationship (Sundeen et al, 1989). These concepts are reciprocal during nurse-client interactions, but the nurse is responsible for their initiation. Therefore the nurse needs to identify specific actions and attributes that communicate trust (consistency, honesty), empathy (touch, sincerity), caring (genuineness, eye contact), autonomy (nonjudgmental and nonthreatening attitude), and mutuality (inclusion of the client in decision-making).

Effective nurse-client relationships can be attained when nurses are willing to look at their own values, beliefs, behaviors, prejudices, strengths, and limitations. Exploration of these aspects of "self" creates an awareness where nurses can consciously use the self during interactions with others. This awareness cannot be achieved through intellectual development alone; nurses must be open to the discovery of their own motivations and feelings through experience and relationships with others.

Communication

Communication skills are necessary for developing relationships. Knowledge of communication theory is essential for acquiring expertise in the ability to understand and be understood by others. Communication is a two-way process that occurs between individuals or groups of people and consists of verbal and nonverbal messages. Verbal messages are communicated through words in a given language. Words are labels placed on an object or event. Our previous experiences with an object or event influence what we perceive when we hear or see a given word.

Therefore, the more abstract the word, the more likely we are to personalize its meaning and misinterpret what another is saying. For example, the word "anxiety" may be interpreted in many different ways, whereas "chair" has a more specific connotation. Nonverbal messages are conveyed through vocal cues, action cues, object cues, use of space, and touch (Stuart and Sundeen, 1990). In many situations nonverbal communication reveals the true, often unacceptable message. These messages may be conscious or unconscious, intended or unintended. The nurse's goal is to communicate verbal and nonverbal messages that are conscious, intended, and congruent. In other words, the verbal and nonverbal messages should be saying the same thing.

Messages are encoded and sent by the sender and decoded by the receiver. The receiver in turn encodes feedback to the sender, and the sender decodes the feedback (Fig. 3-1). The sender and receiver may exchange roles several times during an interaction. This is the dynamic nature of communication: we are always exchanging messages and feedback. Our knowledge of the language, previous experiences, age, cultural background, the situation, anxiety levels, and functional ability of senses influence how we encode and decode the messages and feedback.

Communication occurs on two levels: thoughts and feelings. Thoughts consist of ideas, opinions, beliefs, and facts. Feelings are our emotions. The five basic emotions are happiness, sadness, fear, anxiety, and anger. Many people communicate on the level of thought most of the time. Feelings tend to be buried or hidden in order to protect ourselves from being vulnerable. The nurse's role is to help the client communicate on both levels when appropriate. During times of increased stress or crisis, in particular, clients need assistance in expressing feelings regarding the situation. When feelings are expressed along with thoughts, the client's anxiety level usually decreases and effective problem-solving can occur.

The appropriate and effective use of facilitative communication techniques fosters the development of the nurse-client relationship (Table 3-1). These techniques are useful as enabling methods that should be incorporated naturally into any nurse-client interaction. The techniques chosen are based on the nurse's comfort with them. As with any newly learned skill, the techniques may seem artificial and awkward until they are practiced and mastered. The use of these techniques does not guarantee a meaningful relationship. All aspects of the situation must be taken into account, including the client's health status, environmental influences, and the nurse's knowledge and use of self.

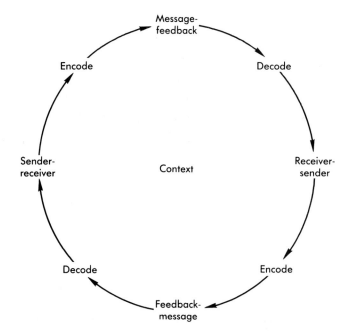

Figure 3-1 Communication model.

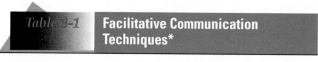

Verbal	Nonverbal
Open-ended statements and questions	Thoughtful silence
Related questions	Touch
Verbalization of the implied	Active listening
Clarification of statements	Watching and eye contact
Consensual validation	Open body language
Sharing of perceptions	
Restatement, repetition of main idea	
Reflection of feelings and content	
Focus	
Summary	

*Definitions of techniques are in the glossary.

Phases of Assessment

The nature and amount of data required and secured for an adequate assessment are determined by the client's health concerns and strengths, type of setting or agency, purpose of the interaction, data sources, nurse's experience and skills, and available resources. The nurse considers all of these variables, using personal, empirical, esthetic, and ethical knowledge, in order to determine what data is appropriate to the situation. For example, data that a nurse obtains when caring for a new young mother and sick child in a walk-in clinic differ greatly in type, depth, and breadth from data obtained when working with an elderly group of clients in a residential facility. In the first situation the nurse has limited time with the client, senses the mother's anxiety over the child's illness, and focuses the assessment on immediate concerns. When assessing the elderly client group, the nurse has ongoing contact and, perhaps, less urgency, thus allowing the nurse to obtain a greater scope of information. Both approaches are considered comprehensive because the nurse collects data regarding multifocal aspects of clients that influence their health.

The client (individual, family, or community group) is the primary source for data collection. Thus the data should reflect the client's perception of the health concern or situation as accurately as possible. The nurse determines the reasons why the client is initiating health care or, if the nurse initiates the contact, the client's perceptions of health concerns. In addition, the nurse should ascertain the client's desires, wishes, hopes, and expectations for achieving optimum health.

The first phase of assessment, then, is to gather preliminary information from the client regarding immediate health concerns, demographic information such as age and lifestyle, and activities of daily living. This database helps the nurse to understand the client's perceptions of health, what factors influence the client's health, and what nursing can do to facilitate the client's achievement of optimum health. Preliminary information is obtained during the initial interview with a client, review of records from the client's previous encounters with the health system, and documentation from other health personnel, if applicable.

The second phase of assessment is to determine which model to use to guide further data collection and provide direction for the remainder of the nursing process components with the client. As indicated in Chapter 1, the nurse considers the major concepts of the model and their interrelationships, the focus and assumptions of the model, and, finally, whether the model gives direction for a plan that is appropriate to the client's health concerns. Thinking through how the model fits the client situation and the nurse's beliefs leads to choosing a model that is congruent with the client, as well as with the nurse's view of health and nursing.

The third phase of assessment is either a more focused or a general assessment of the client's health status. If the client expressed a specific health concern related to pain during the preliminary information phase, the nurse then focuses on determining the exact nature of that concern first. Next, if appropriate, the nurse conducts a general assessment of other aspects of the client's life. The breadth of this type of as-

| Table 3-2 | **Patterns of Behavior and Functioning** |

Individual	Family	Community
Exercise	Communication	Socialization
Circulation	Roles	Power
Self-concept	Physical maintenance	System linkage
Valuing	Decision making	Boundary maintenance

sessment allows for an in-depth understanding of the biophysical, sociocultural, psychological, and spiritual influences on the client's health. Using the chosen model as a guide, the nurse determines the nature and scope of any additional information that is needed to facilitate the identification of concerns and strengths within the context of the situation.

Patterns of Behavior and Functioning

The process of data collection results in obtaining data that may or may not be significant to the client's health concerns. Judgments about a client's health status cannot be made from isolated data alone. Therefore the nurse needs to look for traits or behaviors that relate to each other, occur repeatedly over time, and are pertinent to the client's health status. These reoccurring traits and behaviors are called patterns of data and form the foundation on which the data are analyzed and synthesized and nursing diagnoses are identified.

All clients have common patterns of behavior and functioning. A *pattern* is viewed as a composite sample of traits or behaviors characterized by rate, rhythm, intensity, duration, and amount. The individual is a combination of biophysical, psychological, sociocultural, and spiritual aspects. The family has a certain definable structure and process. The community is made up of systems and subsystems that influence its functions. The patterns given in Table 3-2 are examples of similar characteristics each client group possesses.

Theories, norms, and standards describe the healthy aspects of clients' patterns of behavior and functioning. These patterns can serve as guidelines for data collection. All clients possess certain basic patterns, yet each client may exhibit or combine patterns in a different way. Looking for differences and similarities among clients helps the nurse avoid using personal interpretation of data during the data collection process.

Methods for Data Collection

Data are collected by means of three methods: interaction, observation, and measurement. Interaction data are obtained by means of relevant verbal communication with the client, health care personnel, or significant others. Interactions, including interviews, yield subjective data that represent the client's personal perceptions, feelings, and thoughts. Observation data are gathered by means of the senses and include written documents. Measurement data are obtained by means of instruments that quantify information. Observations and measurements, then, yield objective data that can be verified by others.

When deciding which methods to use, the nurse considers the factors influencing data collection mentioned earlier and is sensitive to the various aspects of the client's situation. In addition, the nurse uses different ways of knowing to help determine what data collection methods are most appropriate. For example, a nurse working with a community group of young women may observe nonverbal communication indicating discomfort when assessing their sexual behavior, birth control practices, and knowledge of the threat of communicable diseases. Because of this the nurse may choose to continue building rapport with the group, perhaps using humor or relaxation techniques while discussing other topics, before approaching the subject again. This decision could be based upon the nurse's (1) empirical knowledge of teaching principles regarding the importance of assessing readiness to learn; (2) ethical knowledge of respecting clients' discomfort and their right to determine their own health care; (3) personal knowledge from experience that young women have difficulty sharing intimate information in groups; and (4) esthetic knowledge that the use of humor and relaxation help decrease anxiety and increase relatedness.

All methods of data collection have strengths and limitations and thus should not be used in isolation. Valid assessments are rarely made by using one method alone. In some situations two methods dominate, depending on the age and health status of the client, the nurse's expertise, and the given situation. Generally, nurses use at least two of the three methods for data collection.

Both subjective and objective data obtained from all methods must be accurate. That is, data needs to be impartial and unbiased by the nurse's personal interpretations of the client's situation. To prevent use of his or her own perceptions, the nurse states or records the information as factually as possible.

Interaction

Interaction is defined as a mutual or reciprocal exchange of verbal information between the nurse and the client. Interactions serve many purposes throughout the nursing process, such as obtaining subjective information regarding the major health concern, patterns of living, and function of systems; building rap-

port; assessing learning needs and providing information; establishing mutual plans to reach expected outcomes; giving directions, explanations, support, and encouragement; and evaluating progress. Our focus here is to discuss interactions in the data collection component. The main purposes, then, are to develop rapport and obtain subjective data. Nursing today is often based on a series of intermittent interactions with clients rather than on sustained relationships. The same characteristics discussed previously about growth-producing relationships also apply to isolated nurse-client interactions.

Interviews or transitory relationships between two people can be classified as directive-interrogative, rapport-building, or open-ended (Enelow and Swisher, 1985). The *directive-interrogative interview* involves asking for specific information; the purpose is primarily to get data. The nurse maintains control of the direction of the interview and the client is a passive participant. This type of interviewing is advantageous when a specific amount of data is needed in a short time. A disadvantage is that the client is passive and may not be able to discuss concerns. History-taking is an example of a directive-interrogative interview. The *rapport-building interview* focuses on building a relationship, not on obtaining information. Open, empathic responses are used by the interviewer to facilitate the client's control of the interview. Data emerge and a relationship develops, but building rapport takes time, and specific data may not be obtained. The *open-ended interview* is a combination of the first two types; the goals are to obtain information from the client and to build rapport. The client's concerns emerge through the use of a variety of communication techniques. The interviewer starts with the least amount of authority (open-ended statements and questions) to encourage the client to direct the topics of discussion. Gradually the interviewer uses increasing authority to provide more specific focus and obtain needed information that has not surfaced.

All three types of interviews have a place in nurse-client interactions. In general the nurse should use the least amount of authority necessary to obtain the information needed within the time allotted.

The nurse enters each client interview with a purpose. Is the interaction primarily to obtain information? If so, what information? What type of interview will facilitate meeting the purpose? The time allotted also affects the method used. If the purpose is to build rapport, what topics and communication techniques promote rapport with this client? The data obtained will be more relevant and meaningful if the nurse is purposeful during an interaction. The client probably will be more cooperative and open when the nurse provides some direction as well.

Subjective data are obtained through effective com-

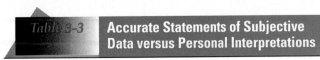

Table 3-3   Accurate Statements of Subjective Data versus Personal Interpretations

Accurate subjective data	Personal interpretations
Individual client	
"I'd rather be left alone now."	Client is angry
"I'm afraid of what they will find during surgery"	Client is afraid of surgery
Family client	
"My mother is hardly ever at home."	Mother does not care about time spent with child
"I'm expected to do all the housework around here with no help."	Family expects mother/wife to do all the work around the home
Community client	
"The city council meets once a month."	City council meetings are held infrequently
"A lot of teenagers in this part of town are pregnant."	Teenage pregnancies are epidemic

munication and interviewing skills. The outcome of interactions is data that reflect what the client said and what the nurse observed. Statements by the client should be noted as direct quotations. Paraphrasing what someone says tends to increase the probability of interpreting or placing one's own meaning to the data. Table 3-3 provides examples of accurate statements of subjective data versus personal interpretations of them. These personal interpretations may or may not be accurate; insufficient data is given to be able to make conclusive judgments. The interpretations need to be used as cues for further data collection. Through the use of communication techniques such as reflection, validation, and clarification, the nurse determines the most accurate meaning of the data presented.

Observation

Observation is a process of objectively noting data or cues through the use of the senses (sight, touch, hearing, smell, and taste). Nurses use these senses in a variety of ways to observe the client's (1) characteristics of appearance and function, (2) content and process of interactions and relationships, and (3) environment. Each sense is discussed in relation to these three categories.

The sense of sight is used to identify visual cues that clients and data sources project. Examples of objective data collected through the use of *sight* include the following:

- Characteristics of appearance and function: posture, gait, balance; dress; color, shape, amount, approximate size of visible elements; prostheses; data from written records about characteristics (such as nurses' notes).
- Content and process of interactions: nonverbal communication such as body movements, gestures, eye contact, personal space, use of touch, seating arrangements, patterns of communication.
- Environment: client's room (home or agency), personal belongings present, space available, cleanliness, and furniture; neighborhood characteristics, such as number of houses and cleanliness; data from written sources about client's environment.

The sense of *touch* is used to determine qualities of an object or person. Through simple touch or the use of palpation* and percussion*, the following data can be obtained:

- Characteristics of appearance and function: texture, moisture, temperature, density, and muscle and skin tone.
- Content and process of interactions: comfort with touch.
- Environment: temperature of air, moisture (humidity), and furniture.

Hearing is primarily used to actively listen to clients' verbal messages or to note subjective data. Other important uses of hearing are:

- Characteristics of appearance and function: auscultation* of lung, heart, and bowel sounds; percussion (along with touch) of tissue; ability to speak
- Content and process of interactions: amount of interaction with others, tone of voice(s), interruptions in conversations, and specific content of what is said
- Environment: client's room (home or agency), auditory stimuli; house/neighborhood noise levels; usual sounds in home or community

The senses of *smell* and *taste* are used less frequently. The odors of the client, room, home, and environment are detected through smell. Local foods and, in some environments, chemicals in the air can be detected through taste.

Maintaining accuracy in observing clients is an important element of data collection. Examples of observation data that are accurate versus notations of personal interpretations are given in Table 3-4. Recording

*The terms *palpation, percussion,* and *auscultation* are specific to the individual client. Refer to physical examination texts for an in-depth explanation of these concepts.

Table 3-4 **Accurate Objective (Observation) Data versus Personal Interpretations**

Accurate objective data	Personal interpretations
Individual client	
Shoulder-length, dark brown hair with dull sheen	Long, dirty brown hair
Smiles frequently	Appears to be happy
Nail beds pink, rapid capillary refill of toes and fingers	Good circulation of extremities
Family client	
Mother does not look at son when he speaks	Mother angry at son
Parents laugh when speaking about sexual history	Parents pleased with sex life
Articles of clothing lying on floor and furniture	Messy house
Community client	
Sounds of two local factories present	Noisy environment
Garbage cans standing upright with lids on	Neat neighborhood
All board members present at meeting	Active and interested people on board

Table 3-5 **Accurate Objective (Measurement) Data versus Personal Interpretations**

Accurate measurement data	Personal interpretations
Individual client	
Blood pressure 130/76	Normal blood pressure
Smoked 10 cigarettes in 1-hour interview	Smokes a lot
Height 5'4", weight 120 lb	Average height and weight
Family client	
Four rooms in house with six family members	Inadequate space for family
Sisters interrupted brother five times in 30 minutes	Sister doesn't respect brother's right to talk
Mother's age, 40 yr; father's age, 40 yr; child's age, 2 yr	Late starting childbearing; didn't want child earlier or infertility problem
Community client	
Fifteen homes located in one city block	Crowded neighborhood
Population 3000	Small town

specifically what is seen, felt, heard, smelled, or tasted is more accurate than recording an interpretation of it.

Measurement

Measurement is a form of observation, a means of obtaining objective data that are conducive to numerical description. Measurement is used to ascertain the extent, dimensions, rate, rhythm, quantity, or size, frequently through the use of instruments in addition to the senses. Some forms of measurement data are laboratory values, vital signs, and height and weight for the individual client; number and ages of family members and number of rooms in dwelling for the family client; and population, number of blocks in a district, and epidemiological data for the community client. General observation data that can be quantified are also considered measurement date (for example, observation datum: smoked cigarettes during interview; measurement datum: smoked five cigarettes during 30 minute interview). Table 3-5 gives examples of accurate measurement data in contrast to personal interpretations of measurement data.

Again, stating or recording measurement data precisely is more accurate than recording a personal in-

terpretation. Only after data are clustered, validated, and analyzed (compared with theories, norms, and standards) should inferences be made.

Use of Models for Data Collection

Nursing and related models provide systematic direction for data collection. The major concepts provide categories within which to collect data. The concepts either directly or indirectly suggest what information is relevant and the data that should be collected. The concept categories also help the nurse organize pertinent data meaningfully. Some models are sufficiently comprehensive to use alone; others may need to be supplemented with additional concepts to achieve an individualized and multifocal assessment of the client situation. Specific examples of models relevant to data collection of individual, family, and community clients are given in subsequent chapters.

Documenting Data

The recording of subjective and objective data is facilitated by the use of a columnar approach for educational purposes (see Table 3-6). This format allows the nurse to note the sequence and methods (interaction, observation, or measurement) used to collect data. Depending on the client situation, two of the three methods are used predominantly. The width of the data collection columns can vary accordingly. For ex-

Table 3-6	Example of a Data Collection Format		

Subjective data	Objective data	
Interactions	**Observations**	**Measurements**
Statements from client/parent/staff	Observations of client/record	Measurements of client

ample, an infant client can provide only minimal, if any, verbal data. Some subjective data may, however, be obtained from the parent or staff. Therefore the subjective data column would be the smallest.

When recording data in the client's record, the nurse notes appropriate data from all three methods of data collection, usually within subjective and objective categories of notations. The data may be organized in a variety of ways. The initial entries are made on the nursing database, health history, or client assessment forms designated by the agency, institution, or practice. Subsequent data entries are made according to the expected documentation procedure. The data may be clustered according to major concepts of a model, nursing diagnoses, problems, goals, or systems. A combination of these approaches also could be used.

Guidelines for Data Collection

The American Nurses Association (1991) standards for nursing practice are the basis for most of the following guidelines for data collection. These guidelines are appropriate for data collection regarding all clients.

1. *A systematic format is used for data collection.* Data collection is systematic. Specific nursing and related models provide guides for data collection. Other, more eclectic approaches are useful as well. The nurse begins data collection by assessing the client's major concern first, including multifocal influences related to the concern. Next, a more general assessment of the client's health status is included, if appropriate. The general assessment is based on the selected model, the client situation, and the practice setting.

2. *The data are comprehensive and multifocal.* The data reflect the life experiences of the client. Whatever the type of client (individual, family, or community), the nurse considers socioeconomic, political, biophysical, developmental, cultural, psychological, and spiritual influences. Given the amount of potential data that can be obtained from or about any client, totally comprehensive data collection is unlikely. Yet the data must represent a variety of factors that influence the client's patterns of living. The nurse uses judgment in focusing data collection on areas most pertinent to the client's health situation.

3. *A variety of sources is used for data collection.* The client is usually the primary source for data collection, but inasmuch as perceptions of events and circumstances vary, other sources are also necessary. Validation of data through a variety of sources strengthens the nurse's assessment. Specific examples of sources are given in the following chapters on the data collection of individual, family, and community clients. Some general examples of data sources include the client, family, and significant others; health care personnel; printed documents concerning the client; and written records.

4. *Appropriate methods are used for data collection.* At least two data collection methods are used to ensure validity of subjective and objective data obtained. The appropriateness of the methods depends on the client's situation, including age, health status, and sources used, as well as on the nurse's knowledge and abilities.

5. *The data are verifiable.* The data gathered through the use of interaction, observation, and measurement can be substantiated. The nurse's personal interpretations or perceptions of a situation may lead to further data collection but should not be stated as data themselves. Subjective and objective data are confirmed by obtaining additional information from the client or other sources. Interaction, observation, and measurement skills are used to validate and clarify the client's (or other's) statements, nurse's observations, and any incongruencies in the data.

6. *The data reflect updating of information.* Data collection is continuous. The data reflect appropriate updating of information from the variety of sources used. As new data are obtained, any changes in the health concerns or status of the client also should be noted.

7. *The data are recorded and communicated appropriately.* Data collection is virtually useless unless it is communicated appropriately in the client's record. To increase nurses' accountability and responsibility for data collection, information is written and kept in a retrievable record-keeping system.

Summary

A variety of factors influencing the process of data collection are discussed, along with the importance of the nurse-client relationship. Interaction, observation, and measurement are the three methods used for collecting subjective and objective data. General guidelines are identified to facilitate application and an accurate assessment of the client's health status, strengths, and concerns. Chapters 4 through 6 provide specific examples of these guidelines as applied to data collection for individual, family, and community clients.

Critical Thinking Exercises BY ELIZABETH S. FAYRAM

1. Explain why assessment is the foundation for the other components of the nursing process.
2. Describe the importance of the nurse-client relationship to the nursing process.
3. Identify nurse behaviors that convey trust, empathy, caring, autonomy, and mutuality toward clients.
4. Identify whether each of the following is accurate data or a personal interpretation:
   a. IV is infusing on time
   b. Client slept well
   c. Pulse is 72 and regular
   d. Parents interacted nonverbally with each other using direct eye contact and smiles
5. Explain the results if a systematic format is *not* used for data collection.
6. Identify how the nurse ensures that data are comprehensive and multifocal.
7. Compare and contrast *sources of data* available for use when an individual client is hospitalized versus an individual receiving nursing care at home.

REFERENCES AND READINGS

American Nurses Association: *Standards: nursing practice,* Kansas City, Mo., 1991, The Association.

American Nurses Association: *Nursing: a social policy statement,* Kansas City, Mo., 1980, The Association.

Arnold E and Boggs K: *Interpersonal relationships: professional communication skills for nurses,* Philadelphia, 1989, WB Saunders.

Atkinson LD and Murray ME: *Understanding the nursing process,* ed 4, New York, 1990, Macmillan.

Bates B: *A guide to physical examination and history taking,* ed 5, Philadelphia, 1990, Lippincott.

Benner P: *From novice to expert: excellence and power in clinical nursing practice,* Menlo Park, Calif., 1984, Addison-Wesley Co.

Enelow AJ and Swisher SN: *Interviewing and patient care,* ed 3, New York, 1985, Oxford University Press.

Grimes J and Burns E: *Health assessment in nursing practice,* ed 3, Boston, 1992, Jones and Bartlett.

Malasanos L, Barkauskas V, Moss M, and Stoltenberg-Allen K: *Health assessment,* ed 5, St. Louis, 1989, Mosby.

Murray RB and Zentner JP: *Nursing assessment and health promotion strategies through the life span,* ed 5, Norwalk, Conn., 1993, Appleton & Lange.

Rew L and Borrow EM: Intuition: a neglected hallmark of nursing knowledge, *Adv Nurs Sci* 10:49, 1987.

Pinnell NN and deMenses M: *The nursing process: theory, application, and related processes,* Norwalk, Conn., 1987, Appleton-Century-Crofts.

Rogers C: *On becoming a person,* Boston, 1961, Houghton Mifflin.

Stuart GW and Sundeen SJ: *Principles and practice of psychiatric nursing,* ed 4, St. Louis, 1990, Mosby.

Sundeen SJ, Stuart GW, Rankin ED, and Cohen SA: *Nurse-client interaction: implementing the nursing process,* ed 4, St Louis, 1989, Mosby.

CHAPTER 4

ASSESSMENT *Data Collection* *of the Individual Client*

Paula J. Christensen

General Considerations

Historically the individual client has been the main focus of nursing care. Nurses now realize that caring for the individual involves working with more than the client and his or her isolated health concerns. The client's family and significant others, beliefs, and background all influence the client and subsequent care. A *client database* is essential to identify the client's responses to health concerns. Thus the way in which nurses collect and organize data is important so that appropriate nursing diagnoses are identified. The *client's perceptions* of health concerns and related responses, reasons for seeking health care, and expectations for achieving optimum health are essential data in the nursing assessment. Data reflecting the client's biographical status and biophysical, psychological, sociocultural, and spiritual health are needed to ensure a multifocal approach to care. All three methods for data collection—interaction, observation, and measurement—are used to obtain a comprehensive and accurate set of subjective and objective data.

Nurses use their empirical, personal, esthetic, and ethical knowledge to determine the methods to use and the type of data to obtain during the assessment. Data should be collected that are relevant to generating nursing diagnoses for independent nursing actions (health promotion, maintenance, and restoration or referral), as well as collaborative biomedical health concerns (pathological condition or medical treatment). Ongoing assessment and monitoring of both the nursing and biomedical domains are important to the professional nurse.

This chapter describes the phases of assessment applied to the individual client. A discussion of the types of biographical data needed and the sources of information is included. Examples of selected models used to guide data collection for the individual client are also provided. Some sample methods and questions are given to facilitate the nurse's use of models during assessment.

Preliminary Information

Preliminary biographical information is obtained during the initial interview with the client. Most agencies have a specific form indicating what information is needed. The box on p. 69 provides an example of important biographical data. A directive-interrogative interview approach is frequently used to complete the data form. Ideally, much of the information could be obtained during an open-ended discussion.

Other preliminary information for the individual client includes a brief assessment of the client's health concerns and strengths. Many health care agencies provide a guideline, such as a nursing history form, for obtaining these data. Often the forms are organized according to patterns of biophysical health such as nutrition, elimination, rest/sleep, activity/exercise, and hygiene; psychological health such as coping, interaction, and self-concept; sociocultural health such as cultural practices, recreation, and significant relationships; and spiritual health such as religious beliefs and values. Appendix C includes a selected number of nursing history forms or guides that have been

---

Biographical Data

Name _____

Address _____

Age _____

Date of birth _____

Place of birth _____

Gender _____

Ethnic group _____

Religious preference _____

Primary language spoken _____

Marital status _____

Education _____

Occupation _____

Health insurance _____

Income _____

---

used in different settings. Modifications of these forms are made to individualize data collection for clients representing different age groups (children, elderly) or for clients experiencing similar health concerns (pregnancy, chronic illness).

It is important for the nurse to ascertain the client's responses to the health concern and how the concern affects the client's lifestyle. Additional data are obtained to ensure a multifocal and comprehensive database after the nursing model is chosen to guide further data collection.

Sources of Data

The individual client is usually the primary source of data. Other sources used to collect data are:

Family and significant others	Nursing care conferences
	Nursing notes
Survey of client's physical environment	Nursing rounds
	Change of shift reports
Medical records	Progress notes
Social service records	Kardex
Developmental records	Health team members
Results of diagnostic tests	

Models for Data Collection

Nursing and other models provide useful approaches to data collection. They give direction to obtaining systematic and purposeful data. The nurse decides which model or combination of models is appropriate for the client's age, health status, and situation. The nurse's knowledge of various models and the client situation determine the choice. For example, if a nurse is working in an emergency room or on a telephone hotline, a crisis-oriented model is most appropriate. If the client population requires long-

term care, a model addressing promotion of self-care and optimum independence is the choice. The chosen model is considered a *general guide* for data collection, not a rigid tool.

Initial data collection focuses on the client's primary expressed concerns and how the concerns affect or are affected by other patterns of living. Additional data are obtained using the major concept categories of the chosen nursing model, along with any other supplemental concepts that facilitate a multifocal view of the client's health situation. For example, if the client's expressed concern is psychological, related to coping with stress, the nurse begins by assessing psychological coping and health. To obtain multifocal data, the nurse uses the nursing model and related psychological concepts to determine the nature and scope of additional information needed as to how the client's stress affects or is affected by other patterns of living.

Nursing Models

A number of nursing models assist with systematic data collection of individuals. Chapter 2 provides examples of current nursing models. Also, several nursing textbooks provide an overview of nursing models, for example, Riehl-Sisca (1989), George (1990), and Fitzpatrick and Whall (1989). Besides the examples of forms based on nursing models in Appendix C, Chapters 13 and 14 provide two case studies of individual clients using Orem's (1991) and Roy's (1991) frameworks, respectively. The ensuing discussion focuses on the use of the model developed by Sr. Callista Roy as a systematic format for data collection.

Roy's Model

Roy provides a multifocal approach in her first-level assessment of the client's four modes of adaptation. The adaptive or effector modes are identified as physiological, self-concept, role function, and interdependence. The *physiological mode* includes activity and rest, nutrition, elimination, oxygenation, fluids and electrolytes, endocrine function, skin integrity, the senses, and neurological function. The *self-concept mode* incorporates the physical self and personal self. *Role function* involves role performance and role mastery as well as primary, secondary, and tertiary roles. The need for affectional adequacy and support systems of family, friends, and community are all parts of the *interdependence mode*.

During first-level assessment the nurse determines the client's adaptive and ineffective behaviors in each of the four modes. Examples of methods (and questions) for data collection using this model are shown in Table 4-1. The methods are arranged according to interactions, observations, and measurements, which will yield subjective and objective data. After the first-

Table 4-1	Data Collection of Individual Client Based on Roy's Model

Area of data collection	Interactions	Observations	Measurements
A. Physiological mode*			
1. Activity and rest	What kinds of physical activity do you engage in? How long has it been since you've exercised? What type of work do you do for a living? Are you satisfied with the amount of exercise you get each week? How much sleep and rest do you get each 24 hours? Do you take naps? Do you feel rested with the amount of sleep you get? What helps you sleep (e.g., backrubs, music)? How often do you wake up during the night?	What is the tone of the client's muscles? Is weight appropriate for height? Is any atrophy present? Observe motor function: Muscle masses Joint mobility Posture and gait Coordination What is the client's nonverbal language? Yawning Circles under eyes Concentration on discussion	Frequency and regularity of exercise Duration of physical exercise Length of time since client has exercised Height and weight Usual number of hours of sleep and rest Number of hours sleep and rest needed to feel rested Medications and dose used for sleep
2. Nutrition	How many meals do you eat per day? How much and what types of liquid do you drink each day? What is your knowledge of the basic food groups? With whom do you eat? Where do you eat your meals? How often do you eat at home? In restaurants? Do you take daily vitamins? With iron? With minerals? Any recent changes in diet or weight? Any increase or decrease in appetite? What kind of foods can and do you eat?	What are the tone, texture, and coloring of skin and mucous membranes? Is weight appropriate for height? What is the texture of hair? Condition of scalp? What is the condition of nails?	Three-day recall: specific food and fluid intake for 3 days Height and weight Fat caliper reading Lab results: CBC, electrolytes
3. Elimination	How often do you urinate and have a bowel movement? What do your bowel movements look like (consistency, color)? What does your urine look like (clarity, color)? Do you have any burning or foul smell of your urine? Do you need laxatives to have a bowel movement? Enemas? Do you experience any pain during a bowel movement?	What are the color and odor of the urine? What are the consistency and color of stools?	Frequency and amount of urination Frequency of bowel movement Amount and kind of laxative, bulk agent, or enemas Lab results: urine and feces
4. Oxygenation	Do you smoke cigarettes? Cigars? A pipe? Do you inhale the smoke? What do you understand about the effects of smoking? Are your arms or legs unusually cool to the touch? Do you have any bleeding problems? Do you have high blood pressure? Do you experience chest pains, shortness of breath, or "fluttering" in your chest? Any cough?	What are the color and temperature of extremities? Face? Note characteristics of respirations, use of accessory muscles, cough. Is there rapid capillary refill when toenails and fingernails are pinched? What is the color of mucous membranes? Are pedal pulses palpable?	Number of cigarettes, cigars, or pipes smoked per day Number of seconds it takes for capillary refill Blood pressure, pulses, respirations, temperature ECG Lab results: CBC, prothrombin time

Table 4-1 **Data Collection of Individual Client Based on Roy's Model—cont'd**

Area of data collection	Interactions	Observations	Measurements
5. Fluid and electrolytes	How much fluid do you drink per day? Are you unusually thirsty? Do you have a history of high blood pressure? Are you receiving any medication to regulate your blood pressure or "water" in your body? Do you add salt to food while cooking? At the table? Do you take any potassium supplements?	What is the client's skin turgor? What is the condition of the mucous membranes? Is dependent edema present? Note signs of fatigue, restlessness, level of consciousness.	Amount of fluid drunk per day Blood pressure, pulse, respiration, temperature Medication and dose Measurement of ankles ECG Lab results: CBC, electrolytes, urinalysis
6. Endocrine function	Are you cold or hot most of the time? Do you have a history of diabetes? Thyroid problems? If so, what medications are you taking? Women: Have you ever had any difficulty with hormones? When was onset of secondary sex characteristics? Are you taking birth control pills? How old were you when your first period started? When was your last period? How often do you get your period? Do you know how to examine your breasts? Do you have regular Pap smears?	Are height and weight proportional? What are the texture and appearance of body hair? Skin?	Temperature Names and doses of medications Blood pressure, pulse, respirations, temperature Lab results: thyroid function, hormone levels Date of last menstrual period Number of days in usual cycle Frequency of self-examination of breasts
7. Skin integrity	Describe your skin condition. Is it dry, oily, itchy? Do you have any rashes or cuts? Are you able to sense pain and change in temperature?	What is the condition of the skin? Temperature Turgor Pigmentation Character Perspiration	Size of areas affected by dryness, rash Length of break in integument
8. Senses	Do you have difficulty with your sight? Hearing? Touch? Taste? Smell? How long have you had the difficulty? How has this affected your lifestyle? What have you done to compensate for this change? Are you experiencing any pain? When did it start? Is it constant, or does it come and go? Describe the pain.	Are there any physical defects in the client's eyes, ears, nose, tongue, hands, or skin? Note nonverbal indications of sensory impairment: Difficulty seeing or hearing Pain	Number of impairments Duration of time affected by the difficulty
9. Neurological function	Have you noticed any changes in your attention span? Alertness? Memory? Do you have any difficulty swallowing? Eating? Walking? Have you ever experienced a seizure? When? How many? Do you have tremors? Where? How long?	Note level of consciousness, orientation, gait. Look for changes in facial, mouth, and neck function (cranial nerves). Check for: Pupil reactivity Strength and equality of grip and foot push Sense of pain and light touch	Reflex function EEG Lab results: blood gases, electrolytes Blood pressure, pulse, respiration, temperature
Self-concept mode 1. Physical self	What is your highest and lowest weight? Have you had any physical alterations of your body? Was or is it difficult for you to accept those changes?	What is the nature of the client's clothes? Tight or loose-fitting? Does the client shield or avoid touching or looking at certain areas of the body?	Height and weight

Table 4-1 | **Data Collection of Individual Client Based on Roy's Model—cont'd**

Area of data collection	Interactions	Observations	Measurements
	How have those changes affected your relationship with others? How do you feel about your weight and appearance?	What is the nature of scars, deformed body parts, and alterations in function? Whom does the client interact with? What is the client's affect?	
2. Personal self	What religion and values were you raised with? Do you practice them now? What kind of involvement do you have with your church? Are you comfortable with that? How do you usually express your feelings and thoughts to others? Are there some times when you don't? When are they? Describe some characteristics of the type of person you'd most like to be. Do you see yourself as that person? Is your description realistic to you? What do you do when you have a problem? How do you see yourself in relation to other people? Better than? Equal to? Less than equal to?	Note nonverbal communication: Body language Eye contact Gestures Affect Tone of voice How is the client groomed? Hair Clothes Nails Teeth Skin	Frequency of attendance at church-related or spiritual activities
C. Role function mode	What is your family's expectations of you? Significant others' expectations of you? Are these people clear in expressing their expectations? Are they expressed verbally, through actions, or hints? What do you think others expect of you? What are your expectations of yourself? How do they fit with what others expect of you? What do you do for a living? Are you meeting your own and others' expectations at work? Are they compatible? If not, do you talk with those concerned? Do you feel overextended? Underachieving?	Note activities of the client: Parenting Studying Reading Cooking Cleaning Leisure Being sick Occupation Gender	How much time per day or week the client spends in various activities listed Age
D. Interdependence mode	Who are the people in your family? To whom do you feel closest? For what reasons? Who are other people important to you? Who do you socialize with other than your family? How often? Are you satisfied with this contact? What activities in and outside the home are you involved with? How do you see yourself fitting into your family? Your group of friends? Do you feel in competition with family or friends (for example, material goods or status)? How do you show affection and caring for others? How do others show affection and love toward you? Are you satisfied with the amount of affection you show others? They show you? Do you have any pets? What are their names?	Note nonverbal signs while interacting with others (such as family, friends, interviewer, pets). Observe nurturing behaviors: care and attention, protection, recognition, offering help, signs of love/respect/value, touch. Observe client's ability to receive nurturing from others.	How often the client interacts with family Number of people or activities the client interacts with outside work and family Number of pets

*Physical examination: inspection, auscultation, palpation, and percussion of all physiological patterns.

level assessment, the nurse then determines the focal, contextual, and residual stimuli that contribute to each ineffective or adaptive behavior needing reinforcement. This second-level assessment focuses on the factors that influence the behaviors of concern. They are directly related to the etiological clause in the nursing diagnosis statement.

Eclectic Nursing Model

Specific assessment data to determine patterns of health can be obtained using a variety of general concepts in an eclectic multifocal model. Viewing the individual client as a biopsychosociospiritual being provides a basis for data collection. The concepts within this model are compatible with most nursing models. The eclectic model is particularly useful in combination with a nursing model because many nursing models are limited in their scope. Therefore the nurse can use these concepts as a guide for a nursing database along with the major concepts of a nursing model to obtain comprehensive and multifocal data. The box on p. 74 shows a format based on this model. The sequence of these concepts and patterns listed provides an order that the nurse may use throughout the interview and examination process. This order provides a systematic and purposeful approach to data collection. The nature and amount of data obtained vary, depending on the client's health status, type of setting, purpose of interaction, data sources, the nurse's skills and knowledge, and the resources available.

The nurse begins with a discussion of the *major concern* and *history of the major concern,* allowing the client to express the primary issues that initiated the need for health care services. By doing this the nurse reinforces interest in the client's situation.

The *current health status* is addressed next. Most of these data are obtained through interaction and observation. Because the *biophysical health* of the individual includes numerous facets, assessing each is an overwhelming task. However, some general patterns of biophysical health serve as a starting point for data collection. Assessing the client's mental status is usually done within the context of the interview. Observations regarding the client's appearance and behavior; speech and language; mood; thought processes, thought content, and perceptions; and cognitive functions (Bates, 1987) are elicited as the nurse interacts with the client. More specific mental status examinations are indicated for clients exhibiting alterations in this function. Daily patterns of nutrition, elimination, exercise, hygiene, substance use, sleep and rest, and sexual activity provide an understanding of the client's biophysical capabilities and limitations. Anatomy and physiology texts, as well as sources on health maintenance and promotion, give

norms of physical appearance and function to guide data collection. Past biophysical health data are important to gain a perspective on the client's current health status. Restorative interventions, such as surgeries, major treatments, allergies, and immunizations, should be known. Important past health data also include the presence or absence of alterations in growth and development, foreign travel, and family health history, including genetic and familial physical and emotional illnesses.

Psychological health is assessed through data collection related to patterns of interaction, cognition, emotions, coping, self-concept, sexuality, and family coping. Texts on mental health, psychology, family theory, sexuality, and communication provide norms of psychological health that guide data collection.

Sociocultural health patterns that are important to discover during assessment are cultural background, significant relationships, and recreation. Data concerning the client's environment and economic situation also are included. Social patterns are found in sources describing specific cultures, social influences, leisure theory, personal space, and interpersonal relationships, and provide a base for data collection regarding sociological health.

Spiritual health includes religious beliefs and practices, and values and valuing practices. The congruence of beliefs, values, and their practices is often important in maintaining spiritual health. References that deal with "meaning of life" issues, specific religious practices, and valuing help the nurse collect data about spiritual health patterns.

The *review of systems* data are obtained primarily through the interaction method. The nurse interviews the client regarding the function and suspected dysfunction of the major systems of the body. Some systems are addressed in the aforementioned daily activity patterns of biophysical health and so do not need to be repeated. The focus is on other systems, such as skin, eyes, cardiac, respiratory, and musculoskeletal. Refer to texts regarding health history and physical assessment for in-depth guidance in obtaining these data.

A *physical examination* or assessment is needed to validate data obtained during interviews and to obtain new data. Whether the nurse conducts the initial complete physical examination is determined by the accepted procedure of the agency, institution, or practice. Ongoing physical assessment is done by the nurse to assess the client's functional abilities and behaviors, to monitor the client's condition to detect changes or trends, and to determine need for consultation or referral to other health care professionals. Observation and measurement methods are used through the skills of inspection, auscultation, palpation, and percussion to perform physical assessments. The nature and amount of physical assessment data

Format for Data Collection Using Biopsychosociospiritual Model

Informant _____
Major concern _____
History of major concern _____
Current health status
  Biophysical health
    Mental status _____
    Daily activity patterns
      Nutrition _____
      Elimination _____
      Exercise _____
      Hygiene _____
      Substance use _____
      Sleep and rest _____
      Sexual activity _____
    Past biophysical health
      Restorative interventions _____
      Allergies _____
      Immunizations _____
      Growth and development _____
      Foreign travel _____
      Family health history _____
  Psychological health
    Coping patterns _____
    Interaction patterns _____
    Cognitive patterns _____
    Self-concept _____
    Emotional patterns _____
    Sexuality patterns _____
    Family coping patterns _____
  Sociocultural health
    Cultural patterns _____
    Significant relationships _____
    Recreation/leisure patterns _____
    Environment _____
    Economic _____
  Spiritual health
    Religious beliefs and practices _____
    Values and valuing practices _____
Review of systems
Physical examination

obtained is dependent on the situation. Whatever the scope of data, a systematic approach should be used. In general, a cephalocaudal/regional format is usually appropriate. Components of a complete physical examination include observation and pertinent measurement of the major body systems and functions. Physical examination and health assessment texts provide norms for the anatomy and physiology of systems and functions and examination techniques.

Gordon's Framework

Gordon (1994) presents an eclectic multifocal model for data collection based on 11 functional health patterns. This assessment structure can be ap-

plied to many of the nursing models as well. She recommends that the nurse obtain the history of the patterns during the interview and then examine the client for indicators of patterns. The functional health patterns identified by Gordon are (1) health perception–health management, (2) nutritional-metabolic, (3) elimination, (4) activity-exercise, (5) cognitive-perceptual, (6) sleep-rest, (7) self-perception–self-concept, (8) role-relationship, (9) sexuality-reproductive, (10) coping–stress tolerance, and (11) value-belief.

In her work, Gordon defines each pattern and gives questions and direction to guide the nursing history and client examination. A sample history form based on Gordon's model is located in Appendix C.

Other Models and Theories

Models from other disciplines are useful in providing a systematic approach to data collection. A more general or multifocal model is Maslow's (1968) work on hierarchy of needs.

Theories from other disciplines are more specific and limited in scope. They are quite useful in conjunction with nursing models, by providing a description of key concepts and their interrelatedness. Theories give direction to nursing assessment, as well as to the other components of the nursing process. For example, Erikson (1963) discusses psychosocial development throughout the life span for persons in a traditional family. Piaget (1951) provides a model for assessing cognitive development of children and adolescents. Selye's (1976) stress theory is useful in looking at physiological and psychological coping. Aguilera and Messick (1989) provide a model to work with individuals in crisis.

Some models are very limited in scope, too. The more limited in scope the approach is, the greater the need to combine it with other models and theories to provide a multifocal data collection of the client.

Summary

Nursing models are used as overall guides for data collection. Data collection begins with a database of preliminary biographical information and discussion of the major concerns and current health status. Additional focused or general information is obtained after selection of a nursing model to guide further assessment. A review of systems and a physical examination are completed to ensure a multifocal and comprehensive assessment. The nature and amount of data obtained depend on the client's health status, type of setting, purpose of interaction, data sources, nurse's skills and knowledge, and resources available. The general guidelines for data collection apply to nursing assessment of the individual client.

Critical Thinking Exercises BY ELIZABETH S. FAYRAM

1. You have selected Roy's Adaptation Model to incorporate into the nursing process with a 56-year-old man adapting to chronic obstructive pulmonary disease.
   a. Identify how this model influences the format for data collection.
   b. List three questions that would elicit the client's perception of his health concern.
   c. Explain how you verify the client's perceptions of his health concerns.
2. Ms. Gonzalez is a 20-year-old victim of a hit-and-run accident. She is comatose when she is admitted to the neurological ICU. Identify *sources of data* for both preliminary and general information.

3. Identify possible results when client information is *not* documented for other health team members.
4. You are working with two clients today. Mrs. Lee is a client you worked with previously. Mr. Jackson is a new client with whom you will be working.
   a. Identify how your assessments would be influenced by whether you have worked with a client previously.
   b. Identify the benefits to assessment when the same nurse cares for a particular client.
   c. Describe how assessment can be consistent when different nurses care for a particular client.

REFERENCES AND READINGS

Aguilera DC and Messick JM: *Crisis intervention: theory and methodology,* ed 7, St. Louis, 1994, Mosby.

Barkauskas VH, Stoltenberg-Allen K, Baumann LC, and Darling-Fisher C: *Health and physical assessment,* St. Louis, 1994, Mosby.

Bates B: *A guide to physical examination,* ed 5, Philadelphia, 1990, Lippincott.

Block GJ, Nolan JW: *Health assessment for professional nursing: a developmental approach,* ed 2, Norwalk, Conn., 1986, Appleton-Century-Crofts.

Eliopoulos C: *Health assessment of the older adult,* ed 2, Redwood City, Calif., 1990, Addison-Wesley Nursing.

Erikson EH: *Childhood and society,* ed 2, New York, 1963, Norton.

Fitzpatrick JJ and Whall AL, eds: *Conceptual models of nursing: analysis and application,* ed 2, Norwalk, Conn., 1989, Appleton & Lange.

George J: *Nursing theories: the base for professional nursing practice,* ed 3, Englewood Cliffs, N.J., 1990, Prentice-Hall.

Gordon M: *Nursing diagnosis: process and application,* ed 3, St. Louis, 1994, Mosby.

Guzzetta CE, Bunton SD, Prinkey LA, et al: *Clinical assessment tools for use with nursing diagnoses,* St. Louis, 1989, Mosby.

King IM: *A theory for nursing: systems, concepts, and process,* New York, 1981, Wiley.

Maslow A: *Toward a psychology of being,* New York, 1968, Van Nostrand.

Orem D: *Nursing: concepts of practice,* ed 4, St. Louis, 1991, Mosby.

Piaget J: *The psychology of intelligence,* ed 2, London, 1951, Routledge & Kegan Paul.

Riehl-Sisca JP, ed: *Conceptual models for nursing practice,* ed 3, Norwalk, Conn., 1989, Appleton & Lange.

Rogers ME: *The theoretical basis of nursing,* Philadelphia, 1970, FA Davis.

Roy Sr C: *Introduction to nursing: an adaptation model,* ed 2, Englewood Cliffs, N.J., 1984, Prentice-Hall.

Roy Sr C and Andrews HA: *The Roy adaptation model: the definitive statement,* Norwalk, Conn., 1991, Appleton & Lange.

Selye H: *Stress without distress,* New York, 1974, Lippincott and Crowell.

Selye H: *The stress of life,* New York, 1976, McGraw-Hill.

CHAPTER 5

ASSESSMENT
Data Collection
of the Family Client

Janet W. Kenney*

The Family

A paradigm shift is evolving in family nursing practice. Previously, family-centered nursing viewed the family as the contextual background of the individual client, who was the focus of care. In 1984 Wright and Leahey introduced family systems nursing, in which the whole family was viewed as the client and the focus of care. Although some authors distinguish between the family as context and the family as client, many do not. In addition, the term *family health* is often used interchangably with the concepts of family functioning, healthy family, or health of family members. Since the concept of family health lacks clarity and concensus, considerable confusion arises when defining family health and implementing family nursing practice. Therefore nursing is challenged to integrate family health models and assessment tools in the nursing process. Use of critical thinking skills is essential to meet this challenge.

There are many definitions of family. Traditionally the nuclear family, composed of a married couple and their children by birth or adoption, was the accepted definition. This limited definition of the family is no longer acceptable because, the nuclear family no longer represents the majority of families in the United States. Changes in family structure are reflected in the facts that nearly half of all marriages end in divorce and that one in three marriages is a re-marriage. As a result of divorce or unmarried parenting, 20% of all families are headed by single parents; of those who remarry, many become stepparents.

Also, the number of cohabitating couples, including gays and lesbians, has nearly doubled in the last decade. These trends reflect a shift in family structure from the nuclear family toward multiple variations of alternative lifestyles. To reflect these changes in family composition and structure, most authors use broad criteria to define the family. A *structural* definition of family includes kinship members with differentiated positions in a family system, such as grandparents, aunts, uncles, cousins, and any genetic relatives. A *functional* definition of family is any social group engaged in certain family activities, such as child-rearing, nurturing, socializing, and so forth.

In this book a *family* is a group of two or more people living together who are committed to each other. These people may or may not be related by genetics or marriage, but they care about each other. This definition encompasses diverse groups, including single-parent families, extended families, nuclear families, married and unmarried couples, homosexual couples, aging couples, and even communes, convents, and monasteries.

In today's society the family is the basic biological, psychological, and sociological unit, which is affected by economic, cultural, and environmental factors. Sometimes legal implications are also considered important in looking at a family. As a *biological* unit, the family produces children who may inherit genetic

*Parts of this chapter were written by Linda L. Delaney, author in the first and second editions.

traits or have a predisposition to specific health problems, such as depression, diabetes, or heart disease. As a *psychological* unit, interactions and relationships of members of the nuclear family and often extended family members—such as grandparents, stepparents, aunts, uncles, and cousins—are considered. Family relationships and interactions may profoundly influence each member's values, beliefs, and behaviors.

Sociological aspects of the family include the multiple roles and activities or tasks that members carry out both within the family structure and in the community. Ethnic and cultural values, traditions, and practices are often passed on and guide younger family members' behavior patterns. Roles and activities may be viewed within the context of working, learning, socializing, child-rearing, housekeeping, exercising, community functioning, religion, and so forth. The *legal* aspects of the family are found in definitions of state and local laws that may have an impact on the family. For example, decisions regarding who qualifies to pay child support and who is considered a "family member" with visitation privileges in a hospital are determined by legal interpretations.

Economic factors that affect the family include poverty and financial hardships faced by lower socioeconomic groups, single parent families, and families living on a fixed income. With limited financial resources, these families may focus all their energy on meeting their basic needs in the struggle for survival. *Cultural* factors tremendously influence the family. With the growth of various ethnic populations of Mexican-Americans, Hispanics, African-Americans, and Native Americans, we now celebrate cultural diversity. Each ethnic group has unique and strong family traditions, beliefs, and values that influence their health and family functioning. *Environmental* factors, such as urban or rural living, pollution, sanitation, availability and type of housing, and access to health care services, also influence family health. The nurse must assess all of these factors and consider their impact on the family's health and nursing intervention strategies.

Family Health

Family health has many different dimensions and can be defined within various contexts from both family theory and nursing theoretical models. Several nurses have defined family health in the following ways:

- Family health is characterized by stability and integrity of structure, adaptive rather than maladaptive functioning, and mastery of developmental tasks leading to progressive differentiation and transformation to meet the changing requisites for survival of the system (Wright and Leahey, 1984).
- A healthy family regulates its boundaries, uses

energy, communication, and power, the resources of health service and self-care to achieve the biopsychosocial functioning that enables the family and its members to have reasonable well-being; environmental, genetic, familial, behavior characteristics, the health care system, and self-care practices influence family health (Crayton, 1986).

- The continuing viability of the family unit as a functional and productive network has a sense of togetherness that promotes the capacity for change, a balance between mutual and independent action on the part of the family members and adaptation to life events (Petze, 1984).
- Family health is the family's quality of life as it is affected from a holistic perspective by such variables as nutrition, stress, environment, recreation and exercise, sleep, and sexuality (Bomar, 1989).

In addition to the above definitions, Loveland-Cherry (1989) identified four views of *family health* based on models of individual health:

- *Clinical:* Lack of evidence of physical, mental, social disease or deterioration or dysfunction of family system
- *Role performance:* Ability of the family system to carry on family functions effectively and to achieve family developmental tasks
- *Adaptive:* Family patterns of interaction with the environment characterized by flexible, effective adaptation or ability to change and grow
- *Eudaimonistic:* Ongoing provision of resources, guidance, and support for realization of family's maximum well-being and potential throughout the family life span

Although there are numerous areas of assessment to determine family health, many nurses wonder what are the characteristics of a healthy family. From a survey of professionals who work with families, Curran (1983) identified 15 traits of a healthy family. A healthy family's members:

1. Communicate and listen
2. Affirm and support one another
3. Teach respect for others
4. Develop a sense of trust in members
5. Have a sense of play and humor
6. Exhibit a sense of shared responsibility
7. Teach a sense of right and wrong
8. Have a strong sense of family in which rituals and traditions abound
9. Have a balance of interaction among members
10. Have a shared religious core
11. Respect the privacy of one another
12. Value service to others

13. Foster family table time and conversation
14. Share leisure time
15. Admit to and seek help with problems (pp. 24-25).

Family Stress and Coping

Family health is closely related to the amount and types of stressors family members experience and their coping or adaptive abilities and resources. During the family life cycle, each family experiences change and transitions as members grow, move, seek new opportunities, or become ill. Change may be *situational,* such as job loss or advancement, divorce, death, illness, or poverty, or *maturational,* such as marriage, pregnancy, parenthood, or advanced age. Each change, whether positive or negative, may create stress on family members. The change and resulting stress may alter family members' roles and the way they interact with each other. Nurses work with individual family members and with families as a whole. During a family member's illness, especially if the person is hospitalized or is diagnosed with a chronic disease, family members experience change and, usually, stress.

The family's ability to cope or adapt to stressors is a complex process that usually involves the collective efforts of family members. Factors that may influence the family's coping abilities include their culture, communication patterns, cohesion and flexibility, social support systems, stage of family development, and resources available to the family. Coping resources may include physical, psychological, sociological, or economic assets that can be readily mobilized. Health, family solidarity, open communications, and economic security are some examples of these resources. However, some families do not recognize their strengths or fail to use them during times of stress. Nurses who work with a family as client assess both their sources of stress and their coping abilities and resources. The nurse uses family models to identify patterns and trends of family interactions and behaviors and to assist families to find or develop strengths, resources, and healthy interactions.

Data Collection

The nurse's definition of family guides and influences data collection. Because each nurse grew up and probably lives in some type of family, many nurses have preconceived ideas about how family members "should" interact. Nurses' past and present lived experiences with their own families and others may create personal and emotional biases, which can lead to faulty perceptions of the family and inaccurate data collection. For example, during a teenager's prenatal clinic visit, the girl's mother answered each question that the nurse directed at her daughter. The nurse could mistakenly assume that the mother was overly concerned about the daughter or that the daughter was incompetent. However, the daughter may have been too embarrassed to discuss her problems or may have resented her mother's intrusions and felt she was checking up on her.

Nurses should be careful not to let their personal and emotional biases influence their perceptions of the family. Also, information for data collection cannot be based on inferences from only one family member. The data need to be validated, sometimes with several family members or other health personnel. Although the family members are the primary source of data, other relevant sources for data collection are:

Extended family members	Health team members
Close friends	Nursing notes
Home and community	Nursing rounds
Medical and social records	Shift reports
	Progress notes
	Nursing care conferences

Guidelines for assessment were discussed in Chapter 3 and apply to data collection for the family. Both objective and subjective measures are used to obtain comprehensive and accurate data. Important points to remember in assessment are listed below:

1. A systematic format is used for data collection.
2. The data are comprehensive and multifocal.
3. A variety of sources is used for data collection.
4. Appropriate methods are used for data collection.
5. The data are verifiable.
6. The data reflect updating of information.
7. The data are recorded and communicated appropriately.

Critical thinking skills are used throughout the family assessment. The nurse uses rational and logical thinking to determine what information is relevant and important and when further data should be obtained. Distinguishing relevant and important data from irrelevant data requires logical, reflective thinking and use of knowledge and past experiences. Also, the nurse must decide on the best source of relevant information—a family member, notes in the chart, or another health care provider.

Family Models
Types of Family Models

Family theories and models, primarily developed within the disciplines of psychology or sociology, have provided direction for nursing practice. Each family model has a unique perspective or way of understanding a family. Family models are categorized as developmental, interactional, structural-functional, or systems models. Some theorists' models represent these types, whereas other theorists have combined two or more basic family models into a comprehensive model. For example, the Calgary family model uses the structural-functional and systems models, but also includes a developmental model. Characteristics of the basic four categories of models are shown in Table 5-1.

Nursing Models Applicable to Family

Although most nursing models were originally developed to focus on individual clients, a few are considered applicable to families. King views the family as a social system or group of interacting individuals, and family health as the dynamic life experiences and environmental stressors to which the family adjusts to achieve their maximum potential. Roy views the family as the client's immediate social environment; Neuman's concept of family is harmonious relationships among family members. These theorists focused on the individual client with the family as context. In contrast, Rogers views the family as an irreducible whole with patterns that cannot be predicted by knowledge of family members alone. Rogers' view represents the family as client.

Selection of Family Model

Selection of a model usually occurs during the initial contact with the family, as described in Chapter 1. The nurse gathers preliminary data about the family and identifies its unique and common patterns. Next, the nurse decides whether a model that represents the family as context or the family as client would be more useful. The selection of a family model is based on how the nurse perceives and defines family health. If a family as client model is chosen, the nurse may choose a model based on (1) family development with its stages and tasks, (2) the family as a dynamic interacting group, (3) the family as a system interacting with subsystems and suprasystems, or (4) the family as a structural-functional unit.

Using critical thinking skills, the nurse compares and evaluates the family's situation and health concerns to select a model that best fits the family and will guide appropriate nursing interventions. A family model can be used alone, in combination with a nursing model, or as a supplemental model when working with an individual client. Some nurses are more familiar with and prefer one model; others, with the knowledge of a variety of family models, use an eclectic approach to choose the model they feel best fits or is most appropriate to the family situation.

The nurse also considers potential nursing strategies that may assist the family toward reaching their optimal health. Nurses who are familiar with several different models can compare the family's preliminary data with several models and identify a model with the best "fit." For example, the family with an adolescent diabetic may have difficulty regulating the teenager's activities and food intake. One nurse may choose a developmental model to examine family tasks and responsibilities at this stage; another nurse may believe that an interactional model with a focus on family members' roles would be the best model for the same situation. Each family is unique, as are their health concerns. Therefore different models are useful for different family health situations.

Family Models Applied in Nursing
Developmental Models

Although several family developmental models are available in the literature, Duvall's (1977) model is the most well-known. This model is based on the premise that the life cycle of families follows a universal sequence of development. Although the developmental model emphasizes ongoing stages and changes over time, it shares similarities with a systems model. The family is viewed as a social system characterized by interrelated, interdependent roles and positions, rela-

Table 5-1	Types of Family Models		
Developmental	**Interactional**	**Systems**	**Structural-functional**
Nuclear family	Unity of interacting personalities	Social system with interacting parts	Social system
Sequential family life cycle	Dynamic life process	Structure	Composition
Tasks and responsibilities	Multiple changing roles	Permeable boundaries	Values-beliefs
Goal orientation	Perception of self and other's interactions	Interaction with environment	Daily tasks
			Communication
			Power/influence
			Roles
			Equilibrium

tively semiclosed boundaries, ongoing adaptive processes, and task performance. Each stage represents major developmental tasks and responsibilities for the family to accomplish, as shown in Table 5-2.

Duvall has identified eight basic tasks within each stage. These tasks are performed during each stage but are unique for each family. The eight basic tasks listed below were described in Chapter 2:

1. Provide physical maintenance
2. Allocate or manage resources
3. Determine division of labor
4. Ensure members' socialization
5. Expand and reduce family size
6. Maintain communication/order
7. Establish links with society
8. Maintain motivation and morale

The nurse who is working with a family initially gathers preliminary information about the family members' ages, general patterns of living, and perception of their health concerns. The nurse considers what factors influence this family's health problems and how nursing can best assist them in achieving their health goals. The major developmental stages and the eight basic tasks are compared with the family's health concerns. If the family's health concerns best fit with the developmental model, the nurse selects and uses that model to collect additional data. For example, a middle-aged married woman with grown children is scheduled for a mastectomy. The

woman expresses concern about maintaining her relationship with her spouse and seeking employment to support their children in college. The nurse can use Duvall's model to assess the marital relationship in the middle-age stage and focus on the tasks of establishing communication and managing resources.

Assessment of the family using Duvall's model is illustrated in Table 5-3, with the use of objective and subjective data collection tools. This assessment guide is a representative sample of data and is not intended to be all-inclusive. Additional data can be beneficial. Duvall's model is applicable to traditional families but has limited use with cohabiting couples and communal families.

Interactional Models

Interactional models were first developed by philosophers in the early twentieth century to describe social interaction. These models focused on how individuals define themselves in relation to their situations. Current interactional models view the family as a unity of interacting personalities and focus on the internal family dynamics. These models are based on the premise that individuals selectively note and assess their surroundings through continuous perception and interpretation in which they define the situation and determine their actions. Individuals constantly form and revise their actions through interpretation of each other's actions. Interactions are considered roles that family members carry out; however, environmental interaction is not considered important. Life is viewed as a process rather than a state of equilibrium.

Satir (1972) developed a simple yet broad model to examine family interactions (Table 5-4). This model focuses on how family members' roles are enacted and how role performance is perceived in each family. Four major concepts of family life are addressed: *communication* patterns, *self-worth* of family members, *rules* about how members should feel and act, and the family's *links to society*. Healthy families have open communication patterns among members, hold high views of each other's self-worth, have flexible rules that are clearly defined, and have successful interactions with established networks in society. Satir's major concepts are more fully described in Chapter 2.

Using an interaction model, the nurse initially gathers preliminary information about the family members' ages, general patterns of living, and the family's perception of their health concerns. The nurse then considers what factors influence this family's health problems and how nursing can best assist them to achieve their health goals. The nurse who decides that the family's health concerns best fit Satir's model would apply it throughout the nursing

Table 5-2	Major Developmental Tasks for Family

Life cycle stage	Major developmental tasks
1. Married couple	Establish a mutually satisfying marriage.
2. Childbearing	Adapt to parenthood; establish a satisfying home.
3. Preschool age	Adapt to child's needs and interests; cope with diminished energy and privacy.
4. School age	Encourage children's educational achievements; fit into community of school-age families.
5. Teenage	Balance teenage responsibility and freedom; establish mutual parental interests.
6. Launching	Release young adults while maintaining supportive home base.
7. Middle age	Rebuild marital relationships; maintain ties with other generations.
8. Aging	Adjust to retirement, loneliness, and bereavement.

Modified from Duvall E: *Marriage and family development,* ed 5, Philadelphia, 1977, JB Lippincott.

Table 5-3	**Data Collection of the Family Client Based on Duvall's Model**		
Task	**Interactions**	**Observations**	**Measurements**
Physical maintenance			
Shelter	Where do you live? What type of community is it? Do you have a stove, refrigerator, washer, dryer? Do you rent or own your home/ apartment? Who lives with you? What are the major problems in your home?	Type of housing (apartment, house) Condition of rooms, furniture and appliances (cluttered, neat) Light and heat sources, odors, noise Safety features—fire/smoke detectors, locks on doors, windows, screens	Number of rooms, bathrooms
Clothing		Type of clothes on family members (suitability to weather, condition of clothes) Compare adults/children's attire	
Food	What does your family eat for breakfast, lunch, dinner, snacks? How often does your family eat out?	Snacks and food visible in kitchen Physical appearance of family members Condition of skin, hair, nails, eyes	Three-day diet recall Height and weight— appropriate
Health care	Do you have a family health care provider? Who? When did you last see the health care provider? Why? What immunizations have your family members had? Do you have a family dentist? When did family members have their last dental check-up? Have your family members had their eyes checked? When?	Condition and color of teeth Presence of eyeglasses	Frequency of visits to health care providers and dentists
Resources			
Financial	Who is employed in your family? What do they do? What are your major regular expenses? How do you make ends meet? What would you like to buy or need that you cannot afford now?		Total amount of family income, regular expenses, debts, family savings
Time	How do family members spend their time in a typical week, weekend? Who has the most free time? The least free time?	In the home, what activities are family members doing?	Number of hours adults are away at work
Energy	What activities of family members regularly take the most energy? What types of activities do family members do for relaxation?	Appearance of family members (energetic, strong, weak, lethargic, happy, depressed)	
Relationships	Which family members are the most helpful? Which members require the most care and time? Describe how. How do family members share authority, respect, and affection?	Who talks to whom in what manner? Who volunteers information, help, affection? Who asks for information, help, affection?	A sociogram of family members' relationships

Continued

Table 5-3	Data Collection of the Family Client Based on Duvall's Model—cont'd

Task	Interactions	Observations	Measurements
Division of labor			
Employment	What types of employment do family members have (accounting, sales, sewing in the home, delivering newspapers)? What hours do family members work outside/inside the home?		
Household responsibilities	Who plans, shops, prepares, and cleans up after meals? Who decides who does household chores? Who cleans, who does the laundry? Who shops for clothing and household goods? Who decides where the money is spent?	What is the condition of the rooms (neat, cluttered, clean, dusty)? Are home chores kept up with, or is there laundry to be done, dishes to wash, mail to sort?	
Care of members	Who takes care of the children, elderly, incapacitated? Who looks for illnesses and seeks health care? Who takes care of pets?	Types of pets	Ages of children and elderly Number of pets
Yard and car	Who maintains the yard, farm? Who handles car maintenance?		Size of yard Number of cars
Socialization			
Eating	What are mealtimes like for your family? How do the children behave during meals? How do family members feel about other members' eating habits?	In the home, are children's manners and interactions appropriate for their age? Do they use knife, fork, and spoon appropriately?	
Interactions	How well do family members get along with each other? To whom is each member closest? Who fights with whom? Verbally or physically? Who comforts whom?	Who sits close together or apart from others? Who talks to whom? Who has eye contact, touch?	Number of times members touch, make eye contact
Sexuality	How do family members express their sexuality (behavior, appearance, verbally)? Are family members comfortable with the way others express their sexuality?	Appearance of family members (hair combed, makeup, jewelry, tight or loose clothing, revealing or concealing clothing, attractive vs disarray)	
Expressing feelings	How do family members express joy, sorrow, anger, frustration? Are other family members comfortable with the ways each member expresses feelings?	Behavior patterns of family members (touch, posture, stance, facial expressions, closeness, or distance)	
Expansion and reproduction	Do you plan to have any (more) children? How do you feel about the number of children you have? Are you using birth control? Which method? Are you satisfied?	Nonverbal expressions between husband and wife (touch, smile, eye contact, distancing)	Number of children desired Ages of children currently at home Number and age of children living outside family home

Table 5-3	Data Collection of the Family Client Based on Duvall's Model—cont'd		
Task	**Interactions**	**Observations**	**Measurements**
	At what age do you feel your children will be on their own? How do you feel about your children leaving? Where will they go? Will your parents or in-laws be living with you in the near future? Will any special accommodations be necessary (diet, avoid stairs, commode)? How will this affect your family lifestyle?		
Order and communication	Who makes decisions about how family members spend their leisure time together and apart (sports, vacations, education)?	Who talks to whom in the family? What tone and attitude are used among members?	
Decision-making	How are decisions communicated to other family members? Who established the family rules? What are the rules (homework, late hours, bedtime, meals, snacks, friends)? Are rules rigid or flexible? How is discipline handled? By whom?	Who answers questions? Who interrupts? Types of discipline (saying "no," spanking, slapping, verbal putdowns, sending child from room)	Number of interruptions
Affection	How do family members show approval and love for each other? What are each member's special needs? Do family members recognize and try to meet other members' needs? What things do members like and dislike about family members?	Ways of touching and expressing affection between family members	
Community/neighbors	Who are the close friends of family members? How often do members get together with friends? Which schools do your children attend? How do you and they feel about their school? What stores and services (post office, library, transportation) are convenient for your family? Do family members regularly use neighborhood recreational areas? How do you monitor family members' activities outside the home (drugs, alcohol, groups, movies, hang-outs)?	Which friends visit home, hospital? Are there cards, pictures, or flowers from friends? Types of neighborhood, stores, services, transportation Facial expressions and gestures	Number of friends Number of hours children spend at school
Organizations	Does your family attend church regularly? Are family members active in any clubs or organizations (scouts, athletic, musical, PTA, civic)?	Religious symbols in home; worn as jewelry Trophies, medals, awards, pictures	Number of hours members spend in clubs/ organizations A sociogram of the family's relationships with community organizations

Continued

Table 5-3	Data Collection of the Family Client Based on Duvall's Model—cont'd		
Task	**Interactions**	**Observations**	**Measurements**
	How do family members feel about participating in local clubs and organizations? What is the relationship between employed family members and their co-workers?		
Motivation and morale	What are the family goals? Individual member's goals? What plans do you have for reaching those goals? Are goals shared by all members? How does the family handle members' achievements/success (promotions, good grades, awards)? How does the family handle a member's failures? How does the family encourage members to do better? What happens in the family when the going gets rough? When there is a crisis? What's special about your family? What special things does your family do together?	Members' tone and affect, posture, and gestures when speaking Who speaks up and how often? Types of punishments (criticism, withholding TV or treats, sent to bedroom) Special projects such as decorations, games, traditions	

Table 5-4	Satir's Concepts as Related to a Healthy Family
Major concepts	**Healthy families**
Communication	Open, direct, clear, honest; share feelings and needs
Self-worth	High self-esteem, integrity, responsibility, compassion, and love
Rules	Known to all members, clear; flexible and allows individual freedom
Links to society	Trust and have many friends; belong to various groups and clubs

process. For example, a family in which the 38-year-old father has had a heart attack seeks the nurse's assistance. The mother and young children are very upset about the father's prognosis and about finances. The nurse believes that if the family members openly discuss these problems (communication), strengthen each member's feelings of self-worth, and identify community resources (links to society) for assistance, their concerns would decrease. Each of these areas requires changes in family members' roles. The nurse first must consider the typical way members relate to

each other in their accustomed roles, listen to their viewpoints yet not take everything at face value, and understand how each member perceives the situation.

Satir's model is sufficiently broad to encompass different types of families, including couples, single-parent families, and small groups. However, the model does not address the family structure and health. Supplemental models that address these aspects can be combined with Satir's model.

Table 5-5 illustrates how the nurse collects data using Satir's model with objective and subjective tools. This assessment guide suggests possible questions but is not all-inclusive.

Structural-Functional Models

In structural-functional models the family is viewed as a social system, with the focus on the family composition (structure) and members' interactions (functions) during socialization and communication. Systems theory is usually integrated within this model; family members are viewed as interacting subsystems and community groups represent suprasystems. Friedman's (1992) family model depicts the typical concepts in a structural-functional model, with some additional concepts included, as shown in Table 5-6 and described in Chapter 2.

Table 5-5 | **Data Collection of the Family Client Based on Satir's Model**

Concept	Interactions	Observations	Measurements
Communication	Which family members talk together regularly? Are there any members who seldom talk? What topics do family members discuss together? What topics are only discussed between certain members? Are family communications superficial or in-depth? Which family members express their feelings about others? Which members seldom express their feelings? How are feelings expressed? How does each member feel about the other family members? What happens when family members disagree? Does anyone feel threatened? How do members communicate their needs?	Who speaks to whom? Who gets involved in discussions and who does not contribute to the conversation? Do family members make eye contact when addressing each other? How often? Is discussion open? Spontaneous? Friendly? Closed? Halting? Are meanings hidden? Do family members sit close or touch each other? Do members show empathy toward each other? Do members feel understood?	Number of times each person speaks Number of times members interrupt each other A sociogram showing family members' relationships
Self-worth	How does each member feel about himself or herself? Do family members trust each other? What is special about this family and each member? Who nurtures the family? Who is the disciplinarian? What is the family emotional climate (happy, angry, exhausted, chaotic, indifferent)?	What words are used to describe family members (sweet, mean, bossy, kind)? What tone is conveyed (authoritative, docile, critical, ingratiating)? What attitude is displayed (caring, responsible, apathetic, passive)? What is the body posture of members (rigid or relaxed)?	
Rules	What family rules are known to all members? What are your family's rules about spending money? Household chores? Discipline? Schoolwork? Television? What activities are members encouraged to participate in or to avoid? Are there rules about privacy or use of words? Who makes the rules in the family? Are family rules firmly adhered to or flexible? How are rules enforced? What happens when a rule is broken? How do members feel about family rules? How do rules get changed?	How do members behave while discussing rules (body posture, eye contact, tone of voice)? Were any rules noticed during interview with family (e.g., children sent to do homework, father expecting dinner at a specified time, mother upset when someone left a room cluttered)?	Number of rules

Continued

Table 5-5	Data Collection of the Family Client Based on Satir's Model—cont'd		
Concept	**Interactions**	**Observations**	**Measurements**
Links to society	To what community organizations or groups do family members belong? How often do members participate in community education, recreational or cultural programs/groups? Would you like the family to be involved more or less in community activities? Why? How do family members contribute to the community? What kinds of support does the family receive from the community?	Were there any signs of family participation in community activities, such as trophies, sports equipment, awards, notices, religious symbols?	A sociogram of the family's links to community agencies

Table 5-6	Friedman's Structural-Functional Family Model	
Structural components		**Functional components**
Family composition		Affective
Value systems		Physical necessities and care
Communication network		Economics
Role system		Reproduction
Power structure		Socialization and placement
		Family coping

The *structure* of the family considers the immediate family members—their names, ages, and the relationship of those who reside together. The family composition includes extended members who are actively involved with the immediate family. Data are collected about the immediate family and relevant extended family members. The extent and depth of data collection about the family structure depend on the purpose of the interview. A genogram is constructed to clarify the relationships and relevant data about each family member. The health, genetic influences, and occupation of the immediate and extended family members are considered very important in the genogram (see Fig. 5-1, p. 87).

The Green's nuclear family, as shown in Fig. 5-1, includes Joe and Jane, who have been married 20 years, and their two children, Josie and Jake. On Joe's side of the family, his father, John, died of emphysema at age 65. Joe's mother, Alice, is 60 years old and has heart disease. John and Alice were divorced after 10 years of marriage. Joe's older brother, Jim, died recently at age 45 in a car accident; his sister, Jean, who was adopted, is alive and well. Joe is 38 years old and has been an alcoholic for 20 years. His wife, Jane, is 38

years old, has diabetes and recently had a mastectomy for breast cancer. On her side of the family, her mother, Carol, died at age 50 of uterine cancer. Her father, Tom, is 62 years old and has diabetes, hypertension, and obesity problems. Jane's younger sister, Julie, age 37, is obese and separated from her husband, Fred, after 17 years of marriage. They have three young children who are alive and well. Joe and Jane have two teenagers, Josie, who is 18 years old and pregnant, and Jake, a 15-year-old with allergies. As can be seen from Fig. 5-1, a three-generational genogram can provide clear information about the age, relationships, and health of family members.

Structural data also include information about (1) family values, (2) communication patterns among members, (3) roles of each member, and (4) power structure patterns. Healthy families work toward specific goals, and the structure serves to facilitate the accomplishment of these goals.

The functions of the family are the activities and interactions of members to achieve their goals. Functions describe the family's purpose or how the family meets individual member's needs and those of society. Friedman (1986) identifies six family functions: (1) affective, (2) physical necessities and care, (3) economic, (4) reproductive, (5) socialization, and (6) coping. These functional components are interrelated in addition to being interactive with the structural components. Change in any one component usually affects other components. (Each component in the structural-functional model is described in Chapter 2.)

In working with a family, the nurse initially gathers preliminary information about the family health situation and compares these data with optimal family health. The nurse considers what factors influence this family's health problems and how nursing can best assist them to achieve their health. Then the

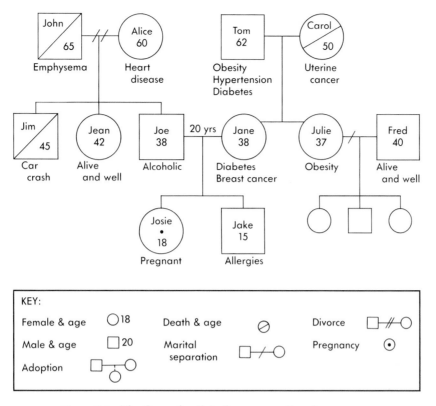

Figure 5-1 The Green family's three-generational genogram.

nurse decides whether the structural-functional model fits this family situation. For example, a young family with two preschoolers, one of whom is slightly retarded, is having difficulty sharing the increased burdens of caring and planning for the handicapped child. Areas of concern that the nurse identifies are family communication patterns, roles, power, economics, physical care, and coping. The nurse thinks that by increasing the parents' communication about handling the problems (including financial) created by the presence of a handicapped child and sharing their roles and power, the family may strengthen their coping abilities. Thus the nurse selects the structural-functional family model to continue gathering assessment data and uses this model for the family nursing process.

The basic structural-functional model provides a broad framework to assess the family. This model can easily be applied to different types of families and is useful to the nurse who is working with a family for an extended period of time. However, the basic structural-functional model is limited to the present view of the family and focuses on family equilibrium and stability. Growth, change, and disequilibrium in the family are minimized. Therefore Friedman incorporates relevant aspects from developmental and systems models into her structural-functional model.

Biological data about individual family members are also needed for a comprehensive view of the family. Data collection based on Friedman's model is shown in Table 5-7. This guide is a representative sample of questions and does not include all possible data. Additional data can be included as needed. A family case study applying Friedman's model is presented in Chapter 16.

An Eclectic Model

The Calgary Family Assessment Model (Wright and Leahey, 1984) was developed at the University of Calgary. This broad comprehensive model incorporates a structural-functional approach with a systems and developmental perspective. The three major concepts—family structure, development, and functions—each have numerous subconcepts, as shown in Table 5-8. The family is viewed as a social system composed of members who interact with each other, with extended family members, and with the community. Boundaries are considered semipermeable and changeable over time; thus information and energy are continuously exchanged. The focus is on how family members interact to achieve instrumental and expressive functions of the family. According to Wright and Leahey, the family tries to create a balance between change and stability rather than trying to main-

Table 5-7	Data Collection of the Family Client Based on Friedman's Structural-Functional Model

Concept	Interactions	Observations	Measurements
Structural			
Family composition	Genogram data		
Value system	What inherent and cultural/ethnic values are important to your family (work/productivity, education, individualism, materialism, cleanliness/ orderliness, achievements health, family, religion)? How are these values conveyed to family members and acted upon? Do any value conflicts currently exist among family members? How do major family values affect the family's health and functioning?	Are value-laden objects in the home (numerous books, expensive home furnishings, framed diplomas/awards, sports equipment/trophies, medicine)?	Number of value-laden objects: type
Communication	How do family members share their needs and feelings? Is communication open, closed, tolerant, or receptive among family members? Who talks with whom and in what manner? Which family/personal issues are open/closed to discussion? What are the emotional issues for the family? How often does the family discuss issues together as a group?	Note degree of functional/ dysfunctional communication among family members (congruence between verbal and nonverbal communication and between content and intended message). Which family members listen, are attentive, receptive, encourage feedback, validate information, share views? What tone/affect is used by each member? Is there eye contact or touch among members?	A sociogram of family members' relationships
Role system	What formal (dyadic) roles does each family member fulfill (husband-wife, father-mother, sister-brother, mother-daugter)? What informal (implicit) roles does each member assume (breadwinner, nurturer, scapegoat, compromiser, negotiator, distractor, dominator)? How does each family member carry out both formal and informal roles? How do family members feel about their own and other members roles? Are there any role conflicts (supermom)? Are members able to change roles?	Who answers what questions? Who cares for children, pets? Who prepares meals, handles bills, purchases household supplies? Who maintains car, yard? Who runs errands, chauffeurs others?	
Power structure	What topics/issues does the family discuss and make decisions on (vacations, education, major purchases, community activities, household chores)? What decision-making processes are used by the family (consensus, bargaining, compromise, coercion)? How does your family make decisions?	What are the nonverbal behaviors of family members during this topic of discussion (voice tone, eye contact, posture, touch)?	

| | **Table 5-7** | **Data Collection of the Family Client Based on Friedman's Structural-Functional Model— cont'd** | |

Concept	Interactions	Observations	Measurements
Power structure	Who makes what decisions? How important are these decisions to the family? Who usually has the "last word"? What types of power does each family member have (authority, seniority, expert/experience, reward, coercive, affectional)? Are there any member coalitions in your family (mother-father, mother-daughter)?		A sociogram depicting power structure
Functional			
Affective	What are the needs of each family member? How does each member express his/her needs? How do members respond to other family members: needs for privacy, recreation, socialization; work pressures, financial burdens; household tasks? With whom does each member share special problems and feelings? Are each member's needs, interests, and unique qualities respected by others? How to family members nurture and support each other? Are your family members close or distant? What makes each member special?	Are members aware of and responsive to the needs and feelings of each other?	
Physical necessities and health care	Where do you live? What type of community is it? Do you have a stove, refrigerator, washer, dryer? Do you rent or own your home/apartment? Who lives with you? What are the major problems in your home?	Type of housing (apartment, house) Condition of rooms, furniture, and appliances (cluttered, tidy) Light and heat sources; odors, noise Safety features: fire/smoke detectors, locks on doors, windows, screens Type of clothes on family members (suitability for weather, condition of clothes) Compare adults'/children's attire	Number of rooms, bathrooms
	What does your family eat for breakfast, lunch, dinner, and snacks? How often does your family eat out?	What snacks and food are visible in kitchen? Physical appearance of family members Condition of skin, hair, nails, eyes	Three-day diet recall Height and weight
	Do you have a family health care provider? Who? When did you last see a health care provider? Why?		Frequency of visits to health care providers and dentist

Continued

Table 5-7	Data Collection of the Family Client Based on Friedman's Structural-Functional Model—cont'd		

Concept	Interactions	Observations	Measurements
Physical necessities and health care	What immunizations have your family members had?		
	Do you have a family dentist? When did family members have their last dental checkup?	Condition and color of teeth	
	Has your family had eye examinations? When?	Presence of eyeglasses	
	How does your family maintain their health (check-ups by nurse practitioner, dentist; nutrition, exercise)?	Condition of family members' skin, eyes, teeth, weight to height appropriate	
	What types of physical activity (work, recreation, exercise) does each member participate in regularly?		
	What drugs (OTC) and prescriptions do family members take regularly?		
	How do you decide a family member is ill?		
Economics	Who is employed in the family? What types of occupations/skills do they have?		
	What are your sources of income (occupation, social security, stocks and bonds, interest from savings, alimony, child support, welfare, aid for dependent children [ADC])?		
	What are your major regular expenses (housing, food, clothes, school, health care, transportation, insurance)?		
	What types of insurance does your family have (life, health, dental, care homeowners)?		
	Are you able to adequately meet your family's needs with your income?		
Reproduction	Do you plan to have any (more) children?	Nonverbal expressions between partners (touch, smile, eye contact, distancing)	Number of children desired
	How do you feel about the number of children you have?		Ages of children currently at home
	Are you using birth control? Which method? Are you satisfied?		Number and age of children living outside family home
	At what age do you feel your children will be on their own?		
	How do you feel about your children leaving? Where will they go?		
	Will your parents or in-laws be living with you in the near future?		
	Will any special accommodations be necessary (diet, avoiding stairs, commode)? How will this affect your family lifestyle?		

	Data Collection of the Family Client Based on Friedman's Structural-Functional Model—cont'd		

Concept	Interactions	Observations	Measurements
Socialization and placement	What are your family's views of such child-rearing practices as discipline, autonomy, dependence, reward and punishment, age-appropriate behaviors, learning, watching TV, friendship? What do you consider appropriate behavior for your children—during mealtimes, at school/nursery, with peers, with personal cleanliness, use of language?	How do children react to a stranger (nurse)? How are children and older family members regarded by the adult members (joy or burden, helper or helpless, with pride or despair)?	
	What community groups/ organizations/services are family members involved in regularly?	Number of community groups/ organizations in which each member participates Sociogram showing family connections with community groups	
	What cultural beliefs or social class factors influence your family members activities?	Are there any visible signs symbols of community involvement, such as trophies, religious symbols, sports equipment, newsletters?	
Family coping	What types of problems has your family experienced recently: death, divorce, job loss/promotion, new member, moves, arrests, health concerns? How does your family usually handle problems and increased stress (coping strategies)? What resources/strengths does your family have or seek (relatives, friends, information, spiritual, community agencies)? What are family members' inner strengths (patience, wisdom, humor, problem-solving, sharing thoughts/feelings, seeking information)?		

tain equilibrium or homeostasis. Families are characterized as evolving toward greater complexity, flexibility, adaptivity, and self-direction. Each subconcept in this model is described in Chapter 2.

As the nurse begins working with a family and gathers preliminary data, the family's health concerns are compared with the nurse's view of family health, factors influencing their health, and nursing. The nurse considers which factors influence this family's health problems and how nursing can best assist the family members in achieving their health goals. If the family concerns are complex and diverse, the nurse may choose the Calgary Family Model to obtain a comprehensive assessment of interacting family components. Then the nurse explores those concepts which seem most relevant to the family's concerns. The breadth and depth of data collection for each concept are based on the family's concerns and priorities. Use of too many concepts may provide irrelevant data, whereas an inadequate amount of data may provide a distorted view of the family. The nurse must obtain sufficient data in the relevant areas

Table 5-8	Calgary Family Model

Family structure	Family development	Family functions
Internal	Developmental stage	**Instrumental**
Family composition	Developmental tasks	Daily living activities
Gender		
Rank order of members	Attachments	Allocation of tasks
Subsystems in family		
Boundaries of family		**Expressive**
		Communication
External		Problem-solving
Extended family		Roles
Larger systems		Influence
		Beliefs
Context		Alliances/coalitions
Ethnicity		
Race		
Social class		
Religion		
Environment		

Adapted from Calgary Family Assessment Model. In Wright LM and Leahey M: *Nurses and families: a guide to family assessment and intervention,* ed 2, Philadelphia, 1994, FA Davis.

and strive to integrate these data within the three major concepts for a holistic assessment. Thus the nurse moves back and forth among the major concepts and subconcepts during data collection to fill in data gaps as additional data are needed. Data collection for each concept in the Calgary Family Model is illustrated in Table 5-9. This guide represents areas of data that can be obtained; however, the examples are not all-inclusive.

The Calgary Family Model is very useful during assessment because it can be applied to various types of families, such as single-parent, blended, and communal families. It also includes extended family members. Another advantage of this model is that it integrates sociocultural, ethnic, and community data. However, family members' biological data and the family's goals and values may need to be added to present a complete holistic view of the family.

Table 5-9	Data Collection of the Family Based on the Calgary Model

Concepts	Interactions	Observations	Measurements
Family structure: internal			
Family composition and rank order	What are the family members' ages, places of birth, relationships (father, mother, sister, uncles, etc), health status, marital status, occupation? (See genogram, Fig. 5-1.)		
Gender	How do you express your femininity or masculinity? What do you feel are acceptable and unacceptable behaviors for males and females	How do family members express their gender in their behaviors and appearance?	
Subsystems	Which family members form subgroups (mother and children, all the children, grandparent and grandchildren)? What effect do these subgroups have on other family members?	Which family members show loyalty to whom? How is this coalition maintained and expressed?	Number of family subgroups
Boundary	In which groups can family members participate? To whom do family members turn with problems? Whom do family members avoid? What problems or secrets can be shared outside the family? Which ones cannot be shared?	Is the family open/receptive to interacting with others? Is the family too enmeshed—emotionally close?	

Table 5-9	Data Collection of the Family Based on the Calgary Model —cont'd		
Concepts	**Interactions**	**Observations**	**Measurements**
Family structure: internal			
Extended family	Where do your parents live? How often do you see and/or talk with them? With which relatives do you have the most contact? The least? Which relatives can you count on for help?	Pictures of relatives in the home	
Larger systems	What social agencies have family members used in the last year? Have these agencies assisted family members? If so, how?	Materials, records, or documents from social agencies	
Family structure: context			
Ethnicity and race	What is the family's racial/ethnic background? What type of racial/ethnic neighborhood are they living in now? How long have they lived in the United States? How does their race/ethnicity influence their daily lives (diet, socialization, work, relationships, power/authority, household responsibilities)? What languages are spoken in the home? How does their race/ethnicity influence their health beliefs and health care services?	Presence of symbols or objects representing race/ethnicity Use of racial/ethnic mannerisms and behavior patterns	
Religious	What is the family's religion and how actively do members engage in religious practices? What religious beliefs or values are important to family members?	Presence of religious symbols or artifacts in home/yard	
Social class	What are the education level and skills of family members? What are family members' occupations? Which members are currently employed? Where, and what type of work? Does the family receive any supplemental income? If so, from where?		
Environment	Where do you live? In what type of community? Do you have a stove, refrigerator, washer, dryer? Do you rent or own your home/apartment? What are the major problems in your home? Community?	Type of housing (apartment, house) Condition of rooms, furniture, appliances Light and heat sources, odors, noise Safety features: fire/smoke detectors; locks on doors, windows, screens	Number of rooms, bathrooms

Continued

Table 5-9	Data Collection of the Family Based on the Calgary Model—cont'd		
Concepts	**Interactions**	**Observations**	**Measurements**
Family development	See Chapter 2 Duvall's Family Developmental Model, p. 49		
Stages	Stages of development: 1. Beginning families 2. Early childbearing 3. Families with preschoolers 4. Families with school children 5. Families with teenagers 6. Launching-center families 7. Middle-age families 8. Aging families		
Tasks	See Duvall's Data Collection, p. 51 Physical maintenance Resources Division of labor Socialization Expansion and reproduction Order and communication Societal links Motivation and morale		
Attachments	How well do family members get along with each other? To whom is each member closest? Who fights with whom? Verbal or physical? Who comforts whom?	Who sits close together or apart from others? Who talks to whom? Who has eye contact, touch?	Number of times members touch, have eye contact
Family functions: instrumental			
Activities of daily living	How do family members spend their time? Weekdays? Weekends? Who works? What hours? Who attends school? What hours? Which members have part-time jobs? Where, doing what, when? Who helps with household chores, pets, child care, yard work? Who runs errands? What recreational/leisure activities do members participate in together? Alone? What times are meals taken? Who eats together? When is bedtime for each member?	What are family members doing during visit (watching TV, eating, homework)?	Number of hours family members spend apart and together
Family functions: expressive			
Communication	Which family members talk together regularly? Do any members seldom talk? What topics do family members discuss together? What topics are only discussed among certain members? Are family communications superficial or in-depth?	Who speaks to whom? Who gets involved in discussions and who does not contribute to the conversation? Do family members make eye contact when addressing each other—how often?	Number of times each person speaks Number of times members interrupt each other A sociogram showing family members relationships

Table 5-9 | **Data Collection of the Family Based on the Calgary Model—cont'd**

Concepts	Interactions	Observations	Measurements
	Which family members express their feelings about others? Which members seldom express their feelings? How are feelings expressed? How does each member feel about the other family members? What happens when family members disagree? Does anyone feel threatened? How do members communicate their needs?	Is discussion open? Spontaneous? Friendly? Closed? Halting? Are meanings hidden? Do family members sit close together or touch each other? Do members show empathy toward each other? Do members feel understood? How do family members react to each other?	
Problem-solving	Who makes decisions about how family members spend their leisure time together and apart (sports, vacations, education)? How are decisions communicated to other family members? Who establishes the family rules? What are the rules (homework, late hours, bedtime, meals, snacks, friends)? Are rules rigid or flexible?	Who talks to whom in the family? What tone and attitude are used between members? Who answers questions? Who interrupts?	Number of interruptions
Roles	What formal (dyadic) roles does each family member fulfill (husband-wife, father-mother, sister-brother, mother-daughter)? What informal (implicit) roles does each member assume (breadwinner, nurturer, scapegoat, compromiser, negotiator, distractor, dominator)? How does each family member carry out both formal and informal roles? How do family members feel about their own and other members' roles? Are there any role conflicts (supermom)? Are members able to change roles?	Who answers what questions? Who cares for children? Pets? Who prepares meals, handles bills, purchases household supplies? Who maintains car? Yard? Who runs errands, chauffeurs others?	
Influence	How do members influence each other (use of objects or privileges such as money, candy, time together, watching TV; or use of communication and feelings such as hugs, praise, spanking, criticism)? What are the major rules in the family? Who enforces the rules? How are rules enforced?	How do members behave during discussion of rules: body posture, eye contact, tone of voice? Were any rules or methods of influence noticed (children praised or scolded, spouse or children reprimanded)?	

Continued

Table 5-9	Data Collection of the Family Based on the Calgary Model—cont'd		
Concepts	**Interactions**	**Observations**	**Measurements**
Beliefs/values	What inherent and cultural/ethnic values are important to your family (work/productivity, education, individualism, materialism, cleanliness/ orderliness, achievements, health, family, religion)? How are these values conveyed to family members and acted upon? Are there any value conflicts currently among family members? How do major family values affect the family's health and functioning?	Are there value-laden objects in the home (numerous books, expensive home furnishings, framed diplomas/awards, sports equipment/trophies, medicine)?	Number of value-laden objects—type
Alliances/coalitions	What is the nature of these relationships: Who holds the power? What roles do members assume? How strong is the relationship?	Which family members hold similar viewpoints or stay in close proximity to other members?	Are there any special coalitions/strong ties among your family members (mother-daughter, brother-sister)?

Family Assessment Tools

Several tools have been developed by sociologists to assess and evaluate various dimensions of family health. Some of these tools are used to determine the level of family functioning and to identify specific problems. The Family Function Index (FFI) by Pless and Satterwhite (1973), the Family Apgar by Smilkstein (1982), the Family Adaptability, Cohesion Evaluation Scales (FACES III) by Olson et al (1989), the Double ABCX of Family Behavior by McCubbin (1983), and the Family Crisis Oriented Personal Scales (F-COPES) by McCubbin et al (1985) are examples of some family assessment tools that may be useful with broader family models.

A few nurses have developed family assessment guides based on their work with families. Friedman's family assessment model and Whall's assessment guideline are in Appendix D, along with McCubbin's family crisis–oriented personal scales.

Summary

Family health is complex and multidimensional. According to Wright and Leahey (1994), the most significant variable that promotes or impedes family-centered care is how a nurse conceptualizes the family health problems. Family health can be viewed as the contextual background of an individual family member or the family as a whole can be viewed as the client. How the nurse views the family determines what data is collected, how it is organized, the nursing diagnoses, and interventions used to promote family functioning. It is essential that both the family and the nurse clarify and share their understanding of family health so that they may develop shared goals and appropriate interventions.

Four models for family assessment have been presented. Each offers a different perspective of the family and focuses on unique family characteristics. Nurses who perform family assessments must be aware of their own personal view of the family to avoid gathering false impressions and inaccurate data. Nurses use critical thinking skills during the assessment to collect relevant and important data, to determine areas for in-depth assessment, and to compare and choose which model best "fits" the family health situation. The model chosen to guide data collection, as well as the depth of assessment, depend on the client-family situation, the health care setting or home, and the purpose of the nurse-client interaction. Comprehensive data collection includes biological, psychological, sociocultural, and spiritual data. Frequently, supplemental data or an additional assessment tool are added to a family model for a more complete family assessment.

Critical Thinking Exercises BY ELIZABETH S. FAYRAM

1. Compare how two different types of family models would influence data collection.
2. List factors to consider when selecting a specific family model.
3. The Morgan family consists of Tom and Mary, both married for the second time, Mary's two children, Tom's two children who visit every other weekend, and a new baby. You are the school nurse at the elementary school Mary's children attend. You are assessing the family since a concern about one of the children's behavior has been brought to your attention by a teacher.

a. Identify which of the four types of family models described in this chapter is most appropriate in this situation. Provide rationale for your selection.
b. Identify the areas you would assess based on the format of this model.
c. Discuss how you would gather data about this family.
4. Discuss your view of "families as clients," as individuals within the context of a family, or the family as a whole. Explain how your view of families influences your nursing practice.

REFERENCES AND READINGS

Anderson KH and Tomlinson PS: The family health system as an emerging paradigmatic view for nursing, *Image* 24:57, 1992.

Baranowski T and Nader P: *Family involvement in health behavior change programs,* New York, 1985, Wiley.

Beavers WR: *Psychotherapy and growth: a family systems perspective,* New York, 1977, Brunner/Mazel.

Beavers WR and Voeller M: Family models: comparing and contrasting the Olson circumplex model with the Beavers systems model, *Family Process* 22(1):85, 1983.

Bell J, Watson W, and Wright L, eds: *The cutting edge of family nursing,* Calgary, Canada, 1990, University of Calgary.

Bomar PJ, ed: *Nurses and family health promotion: concepts, assessment and interventions,* Baltimore, 1989, Williams & Wilkins.

Burr W, Hill R, Nye FI, and Reiss I, eds: *Contemporary theories about the family,* vol 2, New York, 1979, Free Press.

Campbell T: The family's impact on health: a critical review, *Family Systems Medicine* 4:135, 1986.

Carden ML: The women's movement and the family: a socio-historical analysis of constraints on social change, *Marriage and family review* 7(3/4):7, 1984.

Clements IW and Roberts FB: *Family health: a theoretical approach to nursing care,* New York, 1983, Wiley.

Crayton J: Family and community health. In Logan B and Dawkins C, eds: *Family-centered nursing in the community,* Menlo Park, Calif. 1986, Addison-Wesley.

Curran D: *Traits of the healthy family,* Minneapolis, 1983, Winston Press.

Curran D: *Stress and the healthy family,* Minneapolis, 1985, Winston Press.

Department of Health and Human Services: *Identifying successful families: an overview of constructs and selected measures,* Washington, D.C., 1990, Government Printing Office.

Doherty W and Campbell T: *Families and health,* Newbury Park, Calif., 1988, Sage Publications.

Duvall EM and Miller BC: *Marriage and family development,* ed 6, New York, 1985, Harper & Row.

Epstein NB, Bishop DS, and Baldwin LM: McMaster model of family functioning: a view of the normal family, *Family Studies Review Yearbook* 2:75, 1984.

Fawcett J and Whall AL: Family theory development in nursing: state of the art and science. In Bell JM, Watson WL, Wright LM, eds: *The cutting edge of family nursing,* Calgery, 1990, University of Calgary.

Fife BL: A model for predicting the adaptation of families to medical crises: an analysis of role integration, *Image* 17(4):108, 1985.

Fine M, Schwebel AI, and Myers LJ: Family stability in black families: values underlying three different perspectives, *J Comparative Family Studies* 18(1):1, 1987.

Fisher BL, Giblin PR, and Hoopes MH: Healthy family functioning: what therapists say and what families want, *Family Studies Review Yearbook* 2:563, 1984.

Forman BD and Hagan BJ: Measures for evaluating total family functioning, *Family Therapy* 11(1):1, 1984.

Friedman MM: *Family nursing: theory and practice,* ed 3, Norwalk, Conn., 1992, Appleton & Lange.

Getty C and Humphreys W: *Understanding the family: stress and change in American family life,* New York, 1981, Appleton-Century-Crofts.

Gilliss CL: Family nursing research, theory, and practice, *Image* 23:19, 1991.

Gilliss CL, Highley BL, Roberts BM, and Martinson IM, eds: *Toward a science of family nursing,* Menlo Park, Calif., 1989, Addison-Wesley.

Humenick SS: *Analysis of current assessment strategies in the health of young children and childbearing families,* Norwalk, Conn., 1982, Appleton-Century-Crofts.

Johnson S: *Nursing assessment and strategies for the family at risk,* ed 2, Philadelphia, Penn., 1986, JB Lippincott.

Kane CF: Family social support: toward a conceptual model, *Adv Nurs Sci* 10:18, 1988.

Kinston W, Loader P and Miller L: Quantifying the clinical assessment of family health, *J Marital Family Therapy* 13:49, 1987.

Krentz L, ed: *Nursing and the promotion/protection of family health,* Portland, 1988, Oregon Health Sciences University.

Lansberry CR and Richards E: Family nursing practice paradigm perspectives and diagnostic approaches, *Adv Nurs Sci* 15(2):66, 1992.

Leahey M and Wright LM: *Families and psychosocial problems,* Springhouse, Penn., 1987, Springhouse Publications.

Leahey M and Wright LM: *Families and life-threatening illness,* Springhouse, Penn., 1987, Springhouse Publications.

Levitt MB: *Families at risk: primary prevention in nursing practice,* Boston, 1982, Little, Brown.

Logan BB and Dawkins CE, eds: *Family-centered nursing in the community,* Menlo Park, Calif., 1986, Addison-Wesley.

Loveland-Cherry C: Family health promotion and protection. In Bomar PJ, ed: *Nurses and family health promotion: concepts, assessments, and interventions,* Baltimore, Md., 1989, Williams & Wilkins.

Loveland-Cherry C: Issues in family health promotion. In Stanhope M and Lancaster J, eds: *Community health nursing: process and practice for promotion health,* ed 2, St. Louis, 1988, Mosby.

Marchione J: *Pattern as methodology for assessing family health: Newman's health theory,* New York, 1986, NLN Publication (15-2152).

McCubbin HI and Patterson JM: The family stress process: the double ABCX model of adjustment and adaptation, *Marriage Family Review* 6:7, 1983.

McCubbin HI and Figley CR, eds: *Stress and the family: coping with normative transitions,* vol 1, New York, 1983, Brunner/Mazel.

McCubbin HI and Thompson AI, eds: *Family assessment inventories for research and practice,* Madison, Wisc., 1987, University of Wisconsin—Madison.

Mercer RT: Theoretical perspectives on the family. In Gilliss CL, Highely BL, Roberts BM, and Martinson IM, eds: *Toward a science of family nursing,* Menlo Park, Calif., 1989, Addison-Wesley.

Miller JR and Janosik EH: *Family-focused care,* New York, 1980, McGraw-Hill.

Miller SR and Winstead-Fry P: Family systems theory in nursing practice, Reston, Va., 1982, Reston Publishing.

Murphy S: Family study and family science, *Image* 18:170, 1986.

Neuman B: Family intervention using the Betty Neuman health-care system model. In Clements IW and Roberts FB, eds: *Family health: a theoretical approach to nursing care,* New York, 1983, Wiley.

Olson DH et al: *Families: what makes them work,* Beverly Hills, Calif, 1983, Sage Publications.

Olson DH: Circumplex model and family health. In Ramsey CN, ed: *The science of family medicine,* New York, 1989, Guilford Press.

Petze CF: Health promotion for the well family, *Nurs Clinics N Amer* 19:229, 1984.

Phillips CA: Vulnerability in family systems: application to antepartum, *J Perinat Neonatal Nurs* 6(3):26-36, 1992.

Ross B and Cobb K: *Family nursing: a nursing process approach,* Menlo Park, Calif., 1990, Addison-Wesley.

Satir V: *Peoplemaking,* Palo Alto, Calif., 1972, Science and Behavior Books.

Smilkstein G, Ashworth C, and Montano D: Validity and reliability of the family APGAR as a test of family functioning, *J Family Practice* 15:303, 1982.

Speer JJ and Sachs B: Selecting the appropriate family assessment tool, *Pediatric Nurs* 11:349, 1985.

Stenvig TE: External family structure and cohesion, *Pub Hl Nurs* 7(3):161, 1990.

Stevenson JS: *Issues and crises during middlescence,* New York, 1977, Appleton-Century-Crofts.

Szinovacz ME: Changing family roles and interactions, *Marriage Family Review* 7:163, 1984.

Tanner EKW: Assessment of a health-promotive lifestyle, *Nurs Clin N Amer* 26(4):845, 1991.

Thomsom B and Vaux A: The importation, transmission, and moderation of stress in the family system, *Amer J Comm Psych* 14(1):39, 1986.

Turk D and Kerns R: *Health, illness, and families,* New York, 1985, Wiley.

Vosburgh D and Simpson P: Linking family theory and practice: a family nursing program, *Image: J Nurs Scholar* 25(3):231, 1993.

Walker LO: *Parent-infant nursing science: paradigms, phenomena, methods,* Philadelphia, Penn., 1992, F.A. Davis.

Walsh F, ed: *Normal family processes,* New York, 1982, Guilford Press.

Whall AL: Family system theory: relationship to nursing conceptual models. In Fitzpatrick J and Whall A, eds: Conceptual models of nursing: analysis and application, 1983, Bowie, Md., Robert J Brady.

Whall AL: Family therapy theory for nursing, Norwalk, Conn., 1986, Appleton-Century-Crofts.

Woods N, Yates B, and Primono J: Supporting families during chronic illness, *Image* 21:46, 1989.

Wright LM and Leahey M: *Nurses and families: a guide to family assessment and intervention,* Philadelphia, 1984, FA Davis.

Wright LM and Leahey M: *Nurses and families: a guide to family assessment and intervention,* ed 2, Philadelphia, 1994, FA Davis.

Wright L and Leahey M: Trends in nursing of families. In Bell J, Watson W, and Wright L, eds: *The cutting edge of family nursing,* Calgary, Canada, 1990, University of Calgary.

CHAPTER 6

ASSESSMENT
Data Collection of the Community Client

Karen Saucier Lundy
Judith A. Barton

Community nurses have traditionally included nursing assessments of whole communities. The focus of the nursing assessment is on the community's health status rather than the individual's health status. Historically, community assessment was first seen as a nursing practice role by Florence Nightingale. Nightingale was concerned with assessing the physical and social environment as a possible cause of illness. Nightingale's own community assessments included an analysis of the 1861 census data of England, which served as the foundation of England's sanitary reform acts (Kopf, 1986). She also included community assessment as a nursing role for district nurses. District nurses, as conceived by Nightingale, were to visit families within a certain geographical district for the purpose of improving the health status of that particular community. These nurses were to assess both the physical and social environments of the community in order to determine what health teaching and social reform programs were needed by the community (Montero, 1985). From its earliest history, the nursing profession has viewed community assessment as an important nursing role directed toward improving the health of whole communities.

Today, recommitment toward community assessment is a vital nursing practice role (APHA, 1980; ANA, 1980; AACN, 1986). This recommitment coincides with research findings that demonstrate the important role that physical and social environments play in health and disease (Lalonde, 1974; Cassel, 1976; Rodgers, 1984). Nursing can make an important contribution to community health by considering the current ecological perspective on health and disease. Knowledge of community assessment is now considered essential for the baccalaureate nurse (Ruth, Eliason, and Schultz, 1992).

The purpose of this chapter is to provide basic frameworks for conducting community assessments. In the following section, multiple definitions of community are discussed as the target or unit for nursing assessment.

Definitions of Community as Target of Assessment

The first step in designing a community assessment is to define the community to be assessed. This step is necessary because of the many definitions applied to the concept of community. Goeppinger (1982) discusses how nursing tends to use the term *community* to mean a *geopolitical community* (a geographical area with boundaries such as city limits and a political structure for managing the area), as well as a *community of shared functions* requiring interaction (a community whose members share functions such as the growing and distribution of food, which in turn require interactions among members of the community).

Shamansky and Pesznecker (1981) incorporated the geopolitical aspects of community with the shared functional aspects in a nursing model that included three interdependent factors: (1) *people factors* (persons who constitute a community), (2) *space and time factors* (the history and geographical/environmental features of a community), and (3) *for what purpose factors* (the functional processes carried out in the community, such as lines of communication, government policies, and educational services).

Public health officials responsible for protecting the health of persons who reside within a given geopolitical area prefer to define community as a *population* or an *aggregate group*. An *aggregate group* is defined as a group of individuals who share common personal or environmental characteristics, but who may or may not interact with one another (Williams and Highriter, 1978). An aggregate group that shares a personal characteristic but different environments is the entire group of unemployed persons in the United States. An example of an aggregate group that shares a common environmental characteristic is all persons who live in a particular neighborhood. By defining community as an aggregate of individuals, the public health official can target subgroups within the greater geopolitical community for clinical or environmental services.

McKay and Segall (1983) incorporated the concept of the aggregate as a community for assessment in a nursing model. The purpose of the model is to compare "community" as the *target* of assessment and diagnosis with "community" as the *environment* for intervention and evaluation. In this model illustrated in Fig. 6-1, the aggregate is viewed as a subsystem of the geopolitical community. In other words, the aggregate should never be considered in isolation. Aggregates are always a part of, are affected by, and affect the greater geopolitical community. This model includes all but the planning components of the nursing process, and moves from assessment on the community level to intervention within community organizations and families and government.

When the focus is on assessment and diagnosis, the aggregate within the context of the greater community is considered the target system. When the focus is on intervention and evaluation, the concept of community is defined as the environment for the target system. For example, the nurse may target high school seniors as an aggregate within the context of the greater community. Therefore, a thorough assessment of this group within the context of the greater community is conducted. A primary diagnosis emerging from this assessment is that high school seniors have a serious drug abuse problem. As interventions concerned with this identified problem are planned, carried out, and evaluated, the concept of community is defined as the environment for the target system of high school seniors. The emphasis in the McKay and Segall model is that community assessment involves knowing how the aggregate and greater geopolitical

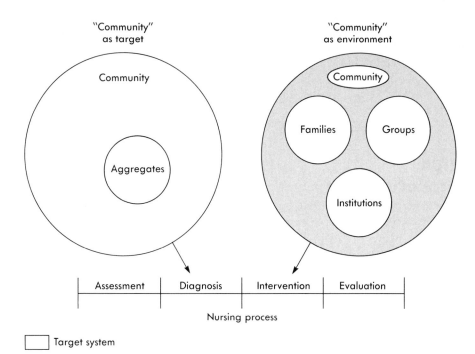

Figure 6-1 Comparison of "community" as target or environment. (From McKay R and Segall M: Methods and models for the aggregate. Copyright 1983 American Journal of Nursing Company. Reprinted from *Nurs Outlook* 31(6):329, 1993. Used with permission. All rights reserved.)

community are interrelated. This knowledge is needed to diagnose and intervene on the community level.

Rodgers (1984) agrees with McKay and Segall's definition of community as both a target and an environment. Rodgers further points out that the problems of aggregates overlap with those of the greater geopolitical community. In other words, if the aggregate at risk within a geopolitical community is pregnant teenagers, interventions must be directed toward both the aggregate and the geopolitical community. Perhaps an intervention with the teenagers involves a class on labor and delivery. On the geopolitical community level, an intervention may involve instituting a teen pregnancy prevention program. In conclusion, Rodgers points out that aggregate health assessments require a shorter time frame for analysis and intervention and are less complex than greater community health problems. Greater community health problems require regional and national level analysis and intervention, which in turn require a longer time frame.

This chapter focuses on the aggregate within the context of a geopolitical environment. Nursing and general models serve as guides to the community client assessments. General data collection considerations, techniques, and sources for community data collection are described. Three conceptual models for aggregate assessment within the context of a geopolitical environment are presented. The model that a nurse selects to guide the assessment of the aggregate depends on the type of aggregate, the aggregate characteristics, the model's focus, and the nurse's preference among other factors. One non-nursing model and two nursing models for community assessment are presented. Each model is followed by a chart, with guidelines for data collection based on the model's concepts. These guidelines for data collection focus on the aggregate as the designated community client.

Data Collection

General Data Collection Considerations

The collection of meaningful data about a community depends on the nurse's gaining entry successfully into the community. According to Goeppinger and Schuster (1988:262), "gaining entry or acceptance into the community is perhaps the biggest challenge in assessment." Activities such as participation in community events, demonstration of interest in community leaders, and the use of an assessment guide can be successfully utilized.

The nurse maintains confidentiality after entry into a community has been accomplished. Protecting the identity of community members who provide sensitive or controversial data is a critical issue for the nurse

conducting a community assessment (Goeppinger and Schuster, 1988).

Techniques and Sources for Data Collection

The primary goal of data collection is to acquire meaningful and useful information about the community and its health. A systematic and informed nursing assessment in partnership with the community is obtained by means of a variety of techniques and resources (Smith and Barton, 1992).

There are five methods of collecting community data: informant interviews, participant observation, secondary analysis of existing data, constructed surveys, and windshield surveys. The community health nurse should attempt to collect data using several different methods because no method is without bias. The process of using multiple complementary methods is termed *triangulation*. These five methods and sources are described below and summarized in Table 6-1.

Informant interviews are conducted by directly questioning community residents. The nurse uses appropriate communication techniques in directed conversation with selected members of a community. These interviews can be structured, involving specific questions, or unstructured, in which the informants guide the interviews. Data gathered through informant interviews are considered subjective and can yield valuable information about the resident's perspective of health values and health care. For example, how do the residents perceive their community health care services? Such data are recorded in the resident's own words and noted as direct quotations in the interaction column of the assessment tool.

The nurse uses *participant observation* by observing what is occurring in selected settings. The nurse observer looks and listens for significant events and occurrences that are taking place and systematically records these observations. Relevant conversations of community residents are noted and recorded in the interaction column of the assessment tool. Places where people gather (such as town meetings or bar-

Table 6-1	Methods and Sources for Data Collection

Method	Source of data
Informant interviews	Community or aggregate members
Participant observation	Observations in social setting(s)
Secondary analysis	Census data, historical accounts, diaries, court records, minutes, previous community studies
Constructed surveys	Community or aggregate members
Windshield surveys	Observations of community from automobile

bershops) can be a source of data collection utilizing participant observation.

Secondary analysis used by the nurse is analysis of records, documents, and other previously collected data. The nurse may not have to collect new data when conducting the community assessment. Such data may already exist in the form of census data, historical accounts, diaries, previous studies of the community or aggregate, court records, minutes from community meetings, and research studies of other community workers. These are invaluable sources of information that can reveal the characteristics of the community as well as the attitudes of people in the community and how they cope with their lives on a daily basis.

In *constructed surveys,* community or aggregate members provide answers to specific written or oral questions based on a random sample of the population. This technique is costly and time-consuming and is used only when other resources have been exhausted. For example, if a nurse is interested in abortion attitudes and if very little information is available through other techniques, a survey of community members may provide useful information about this issue.

The nurse can conduct a driving tour of the geopolitical community as a technique for data collection. *Windshield surveys* use observations through the window of an automobile as a way of collecting information about a community's environment. As an initial data collection technique, a windshield survey often reveals common characteristics about the way people live, where they live, and the type of housing they live in. A nurse can observe the presence or absence of street people, where people "hang out," and the social atmosphere of neighborhoods (Goeppinger and Schuster, 1988).

General Systems Assessment Model

The reader is encouraged to review Chapter 2 for a detailed presentation of the basic concepts and tenets of general systems theory. The systems approach can assist the nurse to understand the relationships within a complex system such as a community. Systems theory provides an approach for defining a specific community and for organizing assessment data into a meaningful format for decision-making, priority setting, and program planning (Higgs and Gustafson, 1985). According to Hazzard (1975:384), "one advantage of systems theory is that it puts the total system at the core, and the concern is with the whole and not the parts."

A system has been previously described as a "set of components or unity interacting with each other within a boundary that filters both the kind and the rate of flow of input and output to and from the system" (Von Bertalanffy, 1968). A system has both structure and process, and both must be addressed when conducting the community system assessment.

Structure

The structure of a system can be defined as a static arrangement of a system's parts at any given time. A significant feature of a system is its hierarchical structure. Boundaries are specified, thus determining what is inside the system and what is outside the system. In terms of community assessment, the *system* is considered to be the target community. The target community could be a geopolitical community, such as a town, or a population aggregate, such as adolescent parents. The *subsystem* is a smaller system included within a designated system. An example of a subsystem is a religious group that exists within the designated community system. The *suprasystem* is the larger system of which the system is a part. It is everything that is *not* included within the identified system, such as a state, a country, or a continent. However, the suprasystem has great relevance to the system and to the assessment process.

The identified community system interacts constantly with the suprasystem, while the subsystems exist in dynamic interplay within the system. Relationships among subsystems, system, and the suprasystem must be considered for a full understanding of the dynamics of any given system (Hazzard, 1975). The hierarchy of systems in a typical geopolitical community is illustrated in Fig. 6-2.

Process

Process refers to the dynamic change among and between the components of the system—how the system works to meet goals. This process of responding to internal and external stimuli assists the system to maintain a sense of balance or equilibrium. Fig. 6-3 illustrates the concepts from systems theory that apply to the dynamic processes between and among components of the total system.

Boundaries maintain the integrity of the system. These may be geographical, such as rivers or building walls, or socioeconomic, such as poverty. Cultural boundaries such as language may also exist to define the system's parameters. The boundaries of an aggregate community are common characteristics of the group (such as being an alcoholic or a pregnant adolescent) or a common environmental factor (such as residence in an urban slum).

Boundaries control the exchange of matter, energy, and/or information into and out of the system. When

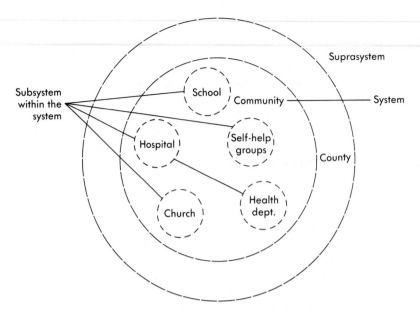

Figure 6-2 Hierarchy of a community system.

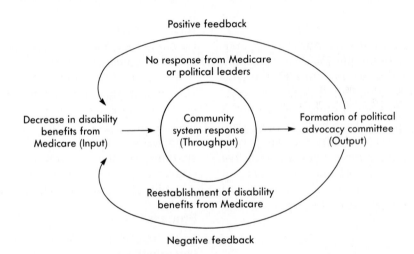

Figure 6-3 Diagram of flow of input, throughput, output, and feedback in a community.

this exchange is directed toward the system from the suprasystem, it is called *input*. An example of input for an aggregate with multiple sclerosis is a decrease in disability benefits from Medicare. The exchange from the system to the suprasystem is termed *output*. An example of output from the multiple sclerosis aggregate is the formation of a political advocacy committee. *Throughput* is formed as the inputs are processed and the output is developed. An example of throughput is the aggregate's initial response, such as letters to the editor in a local newspaper.

Because some portion of the output or results of the throughput is returned to the system, the result is termed *feedback*. Feedback may be positive or negative. Positive feedback maintains disequilibrium within the system, whereas negative feedback tends

to return the system to a state of balance. An example of positive feedback would be no response from Medicare or political leaders after being contacted by the aggregate's political advocacy committee regarding the reduced disability benefits. Negative feedback would be the reestablishment of disability benefits from Medicare based on congressional action. Therefore positive feedback maintains the disequilibrium because of a lack of response, whereas negative feedback implies systemic action that promotes constructive changes.

The processes of throughput, output, and feedback have both beneficial and disruptive effects on the system. However, any action has the potential for both growth-producing and growth-inhibiting effects on the community system (Neuman, 1982). Table 6-2 il-

Structure/process	Interactions	Observations	Measurements
Structure			
Target system	Do members of the aggregate say that they are stigmatized by others because of a shared characteristic such as being overweight?	Are boundaries for the aggregate natural or artificial? For example, does the commonality for the aggregate involve an artificial boundary (high-rise apartment complex for the elderly) or a natural boundary (shared characteristic of being a pregnant teenager)? Within the aggregate's artificial boundary, are fire standards applied to the high-rise complex for the elderly? Is the lighting adequate in the hallways? What is observable about the aggregate's shared characteristic(s)? For example, is the observable characteristic an overweight population?	What is measurable about the aggregate? What are the statistics relating to age distribution, gender ratio, marital status, income level, occupation, educational levels, ethnic background, religion, nationality?
Subsystem	Is there interaction among members of the aggregate? Is this interaction cooperative or conflictive?	Can you actually observe formal or informal subgroups within the target aggregate? For example, can you attend a support group sponsored by the aggregate for the purpose of taking field notes?	
Suprasystem	What is the relationship between the aggregate and the greater community? Is there cooperation? Conflict? Is there an understanding and caring attitude for the aggregate? What agencies best serve the needs of the aggregate? What agencies could assist the aggregate but currently do not do so? What professionals best serve the needs of the aggregate?		What statistical data are available on the number of services designed specifically for the aggregate? For example, are there specific health clinics, how many, what is the utilization rate?
Process			
Input	Is the aggregate open to input from the greater community? Open to assistance and support from the greater community? Is funding available for the aggregate's care? Are protective services available for the aggregate?	Statistically, is there an increase in the number of persons included in the aggregate? For example, are number of persons to be included in the aggregate of homeless persons increasing statistically?	What is the amount of funding available from the greater community for the aggregate? What health and recreational facilities can be found in a particular neighborhood aggregate?
Output	How does the aggregate respond to input from the greater community? Does the aggregate have political power, or is the aggregate low in power? What mechanisms are used by the aggregate in response to input from the greater community (e.g., lobbying groups or self-educational groups)?	Can any political action groups be observed?	

Continued

Table 6-2	Data Collection of the Community Client Based on a General Systems Model—cont'd		
Structure/process	**Interactions**	**Observations**	**Measurements**
Throughput and feedback	Is the aggregate in a state of equilibrium or disequilibrium? (In other words, is the aggregate experiencing stability, or anxiety and disorganization?)		Statistically, do records demonstrate an increase or decrease in services available for the aggregate? Are agencies and professionals responding to the aggregate's output with added services (negative feedback)? Is the aggregate's output being ignored (positive feedback)?

lustrates how the nurse can collect data on an aggregate as the target of community assessment based on the major concepts of general systems framework.

Community-As-Client Assessment Model

Based on nursing theorist Neuman's (1982) systems model, the Community-as-Client Model was developed by Anderson, McFarlane, and Helton (1986). This model was created to illustrate public health nursing as a synthesis of public health and nursing. The model is presented in Fig. 6-4. Concepts from the model guide both the assessment and the analysis. The reader is encouraged to review Neuman's Systems Model in Chapter 2 to assist in understanding the Community-as-Client Model.

The community assessment wheel as depicted in Figs. 6-4 and 6-5 on pp. 109 and 110 guides the assessment phase according to the model. The community core (the aggregate) and the eight subsystems surrounding the core direct the collection of data. Techniques and sources for data collection for the core and the eight subsystems follow.

Aggregate Core

The *core* represents the people who constitute the designated community-based aggregate. It includes the values, beliefs, and history of the aggregate. The people who make up the core are influenced by and in turn influence the eight subsystems of the greater community within which they reside. According to Anderson, McFarlane, and Helton (1986:220), "the people and subsystems in dynamic interaction comprise the whole of the community. As a system this whole represents more than simply the sum of its parts."

Self-concept

In order to assess the core, the community nurse must learn about the people who make up the aggregate core. What makes the identified aggregate different from any other aggregate? Just as an assessment of an individual client includes self-identity, an assessment of an aggregate community is incomplete without the aggregate's "self-concept." How the aggregate views itself is usually based on history and traditions from the past. How does one find out what kind of self-identity the aggregate has of itself? Ask the membership! Each aggregate community often thinks of itself in terms of such descriptors as "we are friendly," or "we just leave each other well-enough alone." These perceptions can reflect whether the members of an aggregate see themselves as being connected to each other. Listen to the aggregate members as they communicate with each other. Are they proud of being a member of the designated aggregate, or are they ashamed of or apathetic about being a member of the aggregate? As Klein (1965:303) states, "it is reasonable to expect that differing community images would lead to quite varied responses" in terms of health care service utilization. In other words, a poor self-image and feelings of shame or apathy could serve as a resistance to health care service utilization.

History

Another area in core assessment concerns the changes that an aggregate has experienced over time and its response to those changes. Understanding the history of the aggregate, such as how and when it was identified as an aggregate, assists the nurse in assessing change and community response over time. Was the aggregate stigmatized early in its history, as was the aggregate of AIDS patients? How has the aggregate responded to system changes such as technical advancements in medicine? How has the aggregate of

Assessment

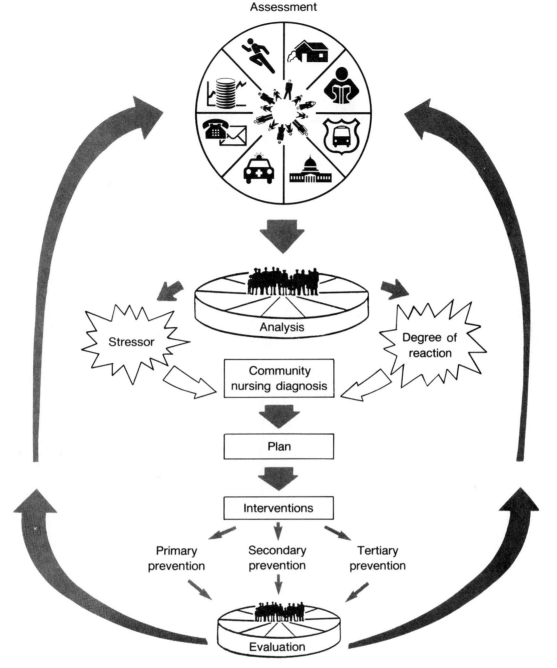

Figure 6-4 Community-as-client model. (From Anderson ET and McFarlane JM: Community as client: application of the nursing process, Philadelphia, 1988, JB Lippincott, p. 158.)

parents of premature babies responded to the "high tech" nursery? Did parents accept turning over their baby to technology, or did they insist on being more involved in the care of their child? An aggregate's ability to mobilize resources in response to problems significantly affects how the aggregate will respond to future interventions. Community nurses can assist an aggregate within the greater community in maintaining its equilibrium. As such, knowledge about the aggregate's past can give perspective to the present and make realistic health planning possible.

Statistics

Indices of the aggregate are somewhat more difficult to obtain than those of the individual client. Indices for the aggregate client are demographics, vital statistics, and health statistics. The assessment includes the morbidity and mortality rates, and distributions of gender, age, ethnicity, and race. Other indices are education, occupation and employment patterns, and socioeconomic standing. Morbidity statistics provide a picture of the aggregate in terms of the incidence and prevalence of specific diseases associated with the aggregate.

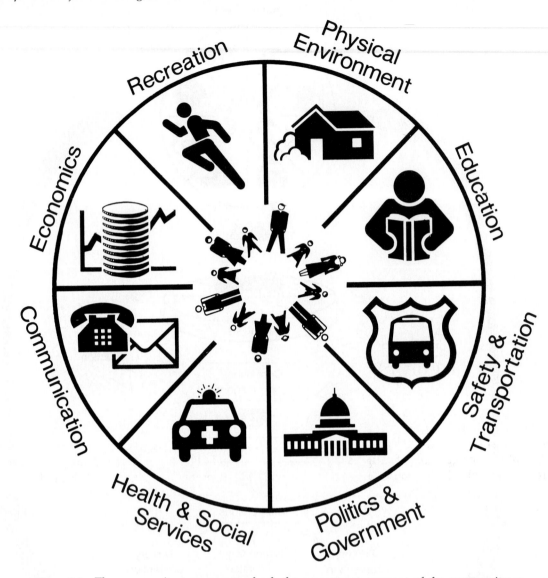

Figure 6-5 The community assessment wheel, the assessment segment of the community-as-client model. (From Anderson ET and McFarlane JM: Community as client: application of the nursing process, Philadelphia, 1988, JB Lippincott, p. 170.)

Indices of the aggregate can be found in the literature associated with the aggregate. Volunteer organizations associated with the aggregate are also a source of indices. For example, the American Heart Association at the local or national level has statistical information on the aggregate of cardiac patients. The nurse determines the aggregate density (number of aggregate members included in the geopolitical space); age, ethnic, race, and gender distribution; socioeconomic characteristics (income, education, employment); and marital status. These demographic data are examined in a historical context. Aggregate communities often experience age-related shifts over time. For example, statistics in Table 6-3 demonstrate a downward shift in the age at which adolescent drug use begins (Clayton and

Table 6-3	Age at Onset of Marijuana Use			
Age at survey (yr)	Birth year	High school class	Percent of users	Median age at first use (yr)
12	1967	1985	4%	11
14	1965	1983	26%	13
16	1963	1981	43%	14
18	1961	1979	60%	15
20	1959	1977	68%	16
25	1954	1972	63%	17
30	1949	1967	51%	20
35	1944	1962	34%	25

This hypothetical table is based on research findings by Clayton and Ritter (1985).

Ritter, 1985). Appropriate planning for an aggregate of adolescent drug abusers would consider the historical shift in beginning age for drug use.

The relationship between aggregate demographic characteristics and the health status of the aggregate has been well established. The links among ethnicity, socioeconomic status, and educational status are of utmost importance if health planning is to be effective. For example, an aggregate of lower socioeconomic persons living near a toxic dump site has less power to clean up their environment than an aggregate of higher socioeconomic persons. The health statistics (morbidity and mortality) for an aggregate located in one region are compared with a similar aggregate located elsewhere to determine the significance of the health statistics. The health statistics for the target aggregate should also be compared with general population health statistics. These comparisons provide clues as to what health problems exist in a particular aggregate and the effectiveness of existing health services.

Culture

The values, beliefs, and religious practices of the aggregate membership comprise another facet of the core. Certain aggregates have a wide range of cultural factors to be considered because culture can influence people's health. The aggregate of drug-abusing adolescents is an example. Drug abuse by adolescents is found in all ethnic, racial, and socioeconomic groups. Some aggregates are more homogeneous in terms of culture. An aggregate of workers, such as migrant farm workers, would be skewed toward the Hispanic culture. It is especially important to determine the aggregate's attitudes toward health in general. Is health care a priority among the members? Is health valued, as evidenced by observations of preventive health practices? An assessment of health values can reveal where health fits into the aggregate's priority structure.

The culture of the aggregate is often difficult to assess during the initial phase. The nurse as a community outsider interacts with members of the aggregate to assess the aggregate culture. Norms and values are intangible and become apparent to the nurse only through direct involvement with the group membership. Each aggregate is unique, with different values, belief systems, and practices rooted in tradition. These characteristics evolve and continue to exist because they meet the needs of a particular community (Anderson and McFarlane, 1987).

Social Networks/Support

Dean (1986:544) contends that "social networks strongly influence people's well-being and should therefore be included in any client assessment." Social networks are identified by examining the degree of social isolation that exists for the aggregate. Aggregates with inadequate social support networks experience more stress and use fewer available resources (McKinley, 1973). Whom do they call when they need health advice or have health problems? Examples of data collection activities associated with social networks include asking members of the aggregate to identify individuals and agencies that give emotional, informational, and material support.

Interacting Subsystems
Physical Environment

The physical geopolitical community has a significant effect on the health status of aggregate members. An aggregate of elderly persons may reside in a high-rise apartment complex. An aggregate of hypertensive black clients may reside in particular neighborhoods. An aggregate of persons with lung disease may reside in a highly polluted urban environment. Factors that may be assessed within *interacting subsystems* are shown in Fig. 6-5 and described in the following sections.

The assessment of the physical environment for the aggregate is similar to the physical examination of the individual client: all five senses are used to collect pertinent data. A physical examination of the environment for the aggregate involves a "hands-on" approach. Perhaps a "feet-on" approach would be more descriptive! Shumway and Wisehart (1969) suggest a walking tour of the environment. They advise that "getting a feel" for a community involves a systematic observation to increase sensitivity to the surrounding ecological elements. For example, one would want to identify through sight and smell the sources of food for a particular aggregate. Does the aggregate prefer fast foods, or ethnic or regional foods?

If the community can be defined by geographical parameters, boundaries are defined and described as clearly as possible. Parameters are defined in several ways: census tracts; natural boundaries, such as rivers or mountains; roads or streets; proximity to needed resources; and isolation or proximity to other communities.

Environmental threats to health, such as air, water, and noise pollution, as well as hazardous wastes, are major detriments to the health status of a community. Environmental factors such as road conditions, the animal population, housing conditions, and general appearance of the community also are noted in the physical assessment of the community.

A community's climate, just like a person's basal temperature, can have a significant effect on health status. A desert or a mountainous climate can affect the lives of the aggregate in dramatic ways. An aggregate of cardiac patients may experience an increased incidence of angina at a high altitude.

Health and Social Services

The health care delivery system has been described as delivering "two-class" health care: one kind to those who can pay and another kind to those who cannot pay. This division between public and private health care has implications for the assessment of health services for the aggregate within the geopolitical community. Services also can be grouped into type of service and number of persons served. Services can be further identified as being extracommunity (outside the geopolitical community) or intracommunity (within the geopolitical community). Table 6-4 describes the major components of the health and social services within a geopolitical community and sources of information for data collection.

In addition to gathering data about the services provided and cost to clients, the nurse also examines the quality and use of the services and the degree of coordination among services. Which health and social services are frequently used by the aggregate? Why are some services not frequently used by the aggregate? Is the aggregate being discriminated against by these resources? Are some resources unknown, inaccessible, or unacceptable services for members of the aggregate?

Some appropriate health care sources may not reflect traditional health care roles. For example, in rural communities the local pharmacist or the lay midwife may be the primary source of health information and therefore would be included in the assessment.

Economics

The assessment of the economic system includes the major businesses and industries within the geopolitical community. In addition, census information on the local unemployment rate, percentage of families living below the poverty level, major occupations, and median family income are included in the assessment. The economic system essentially represents the goods and services available to community members, as well as the patterns of how these resources are distributed (Anderson and McFarlane, 1987). These same indices are assessed within the target aggregate. How does the aggregate compare with the greater geopolitical community in terms of these indices? How does the economic base of the greater geopolitical community affect the health and social well-being of the aggregate? If a community industry that employs primarily males closes, how is the aggregate of female-headed families affected? Is this aggregate now at risk for a higher rate of unemployment?

Safety and Transportation

Community safety includes protective services such as police and fire services. How safe do members of the aggregate feel? If the aggregate is a minority group residing in a particular neighborhood, do members feel they are given the same safety services as in other neighborhoods? Is safety education being provided? Does the police department assist the community in developing neighborhood watch pro-

---

Table 6-4	Health and Social Services

Component	Sources of information
Health services	
Extracommunity *or* intracommunity facilities. Once identified, group into categories (e.g., hospitals and clinics, home health care, extended care facilities, public health services, emergency care)	Chamber of Commerce Planning Board (county, city) Phone directory
For each facility collect data on	Talk to residents
1. Services (fees, hours, new services planned, and those discontinued)	Interview administrator or someone on the staff
2. Resources (personnel, space, budget, record system)	Facility annual report
3. Characteristics of users (geographic distribution, demographic profile, transportation source)	
4. Statistics (number of persons served daily, weekly, monthly)	
5. Adequacy, accessibility, and acceptability of facility according to users and providers	
Social services	
Extracommunity *or* intracommunity facilities. Once identified, group into categories (e.g., counseling and support, clothing, food, shelter, and special needs)	Chamber of Commerce United Way Directory Phone directory
For each facility collect data on the area 1-5 listed above	

From Anderson ET and McFarlar.e JM: *Community as client: application of the nursing process*, Philadelphia, 1988, JB Lippincott, p. 186.

grams? Does the fire department uphold the standards of fire prevention and evacuation for elderly high-rise housing?

Sanitation services, including water treatment and environmental pollution control, are assessed within the subsystem of safety. Are there any special risks involved in living in this particular community?

The assessment of transportation includes the sources of transportation for residents. Is mass transit available, and do these services include special handicapped services? What transportation services are available for traveling outside the community? Are emergency transportation services available to all members inside and outside the geopolitical community? Transportation has a significant influence on the ability of residents to access health care services and is assessed accordingly (Lassiter, 1992).

Politics and Government

The political subsystem of a community can be assessed through a variety of sources: interviews with formal and informal leaders, reading the local newspaper, and observing political action groups. The aggregate may have developed its own political action group. The political values of a community can make a significant difference in health planning and successful health services. If political values lean toward conservatism, the community may have fewer resources for indigent care. The community may value health care as a consumer good rather than a social right (Reinhart, 1984). If the aggregate is a minority group of low socioeconomic status, access to health and social services are affected.

Communication

Communication patterns, both formal and informal, are an integral component of the community's subsystems. Communication is a necessary process by which people exchange information and interact with each other, and is basic to community living. Language is the keystone to cultural beliefs and health concerns of both the geopolitical community and the aggregate (Robertson, 1981). Assessment of formal and informal communication patterns can reveal how linked together the total community is and what is being communicated regarding health needs and services.

Informal communication tends to occur wherever people gather: post offices, local cafes and bars, recreation centers, and barbershops. Key informants may be identified in such gatherings of people and are a source of information regarding community beliefs and needs. Other sources of informal communication patterns are bulletin boards such as those found in local supermarkets.

Formal communication sources include all forms of the media: newspapers, television, radio, telephone services, and the postal system. Is the aggregate ever the focus of these formal communication channels? Is the homeless aggregate being written about in the local newspaper? Are the media accounts sympathetic or nonsympathetic to the conditions of the homeless?

Education

The general educational status of the geopolitical community is assessed by means of census data. Census data includes the number of residents attending school, the average years of education for residents, and the percentage of residents who can read. What are the major educational resources available in the community? Has the community responded to a high rate of illiteracy by providing specialized educational services? The target aggregate may include many illiterate persons who are in need of such services.

Recreation

The recreational resources of a community often reflect the community's interest in relaxation and fitness. An assessment of the community's "fitness" includes exercise and fitness facilities, such as jogging and bicycling trails. In addition, information on the use of these facilities by the general population and the target aggregate is important. Are specialized fitness centers available for the handicapped, such as warm exercise pools? Assessment of the recreation subsystem provides information on the value of health and fitness for the geopolitical community. Does the aggregate share the fitness value of the larger community?

Summary of Community-as-Client Assessment Model

Anderson and McFarlane's (1988) Community-as-Client Model includes concepts from general systems theory. The model describes specific subsystems found within a community as to content and how each is related to the goal of health. The nurse may use this model as a guide for collecting data on the aggregate as the target of community assessment, as illustrated in Table 6-5.

Community Competence Assessment Models

The two preceding models primarily focus on the status of a community (the indicators of the health of a community such as morbidity and mortality rates) and

Table 6-5	Data Collection of the Community Client Based on Community-as-Client Model		
Structure/process	**Interactions**	**Observations**	**Measurements**
Core structures			
Self-concept	How do aggregate members view themselves? (Are there perceptions of feeling good about being a member of the aggregate, or are the perceptions indicative of shameful feelings?)		Does statistical data indicate a trend toward increasing morbidity rates of clinical depression for the aggregate group?
History	How do aggregate members perceive their history as a group with a common personal or environmental characteristic? How do aggregate members perceive changes that have occurred in health and social welfare programs affecting the group? Have the changes had a positive or negative effect? How has the aggregate responded to changes in the health and welfare system? For example, have self-help groups formed in response to inadequate health care?		Statistically, when was the aggregate first considered to be at risk? For example, when did morbidity statistics first indicate that smokers were at risk for lung cancer?
Statistics			What are the current statistics for the aggregate on a. age distribution b. gender distribution c. literacy rate d. educational level e. morbidity and mortality rates f. income levels g. occupational composition h. ethnicity i. nationality Have these statistics changed over time? How do these statistics compare with those of other aggregate groups within the greater community?
Culture	What are the values and beliefs of the aggregate? Is there a common culture shared by the aggregate such as a belief system that values holistic medicine above Western medicine? Is there a special language and tradition for the aggregate? How are health and illness defined by the aggregate?	Can specialized clothing or equipment be observed for the aggregate?	
Social network/support	Do members of the aggregate report a high level of stress? Are there supportive agencies and professionals for the aggregate? What type of support is given by these agencies? Is a strong natural helping network operating for the aggregate?		

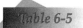

Table 6-5	Data Collection of the Community Client Based on Community-as-Client Model—cont'd		
Structure/process	**Interactions**	**Observations**	**Measurements**
Interacting subsystems			
Physical environment		Are service facilities such as health and social service agencies in close approximation to the target aggregate? Are there smells and sounds in the aggregate's physical environment?	What do you see as you walk or drive through the aggregate's identified geopolitical community? Is the environment in good repair or a state of disrepair?
Health and welfare services	What health and social services are available within the geopolitical community? How do members of the aggregate feel about the acceptability and quality of care given by health and social service agencies? Do members of the aggregate perceive any stigmatization by health and social services staff? How are services between health and social service facilities coordinated for the aggregate? What nontraditional health care does the aggregate utilize? Are there specialized health and social services for the target aggregate?		What statistical data are available on health and social services designed specifically for the aggregate. How many clinics are available? What is the utilization rate?
Economics	How does the economic base affect the health and social well-being of the aggregate?		What is the unemployment rate for the aggregate? How does this rate compare with the unemployment rate for the geopolitical community? What percentage of aggregate members are living under the poverty line? What is the median family income? What is the occupational composition? What is the educational level?
Safety and transportation	How safe do members of the aggregate feel within their environment? Do members of the aggregate feel that they are given the same safety services as other aggregates within the geopolitical community? What safety services are available in the geopolitical community (police, fire protection, sanitation services, environmental controls, emergency services)? Are these same safety services available to the aggregate? What public transportation services are available in the geopolitical community? Are special services available for the handicapped? Do the general and specialized transportation services serve the target aggregate?		What is the crime rate for the geopolitical community? What is the crime rate for the target aggregate?

Continued

Table 6-5	Data Collection of the Community Client Based on Community-as-Client Model—cont'd		
Structure/process	**Interactions**	**Observations**	**Measurements**
Politics	Does the aggregate have a formalized governing body? If so, what is the structure of the formalized governing body (officers and chairpersons, a board of directors)? What are the political values of the aggregate? Is the aggregate more liberal or conservative? How do the political values of the aggregate compare with the greater community's political values. How do the political values of the greater community affect the health and social well-being of the aggregate? Do members of the aggregate feel that they are represented politically within the greater community? Is power equally distributed within the aggregate? Is the aggregate divided as to who has power? Who represents the aggregate in the greater community?	Are there records of organizational charts, minutes of meetings, or newspaper clippings that record events or interactions between the aggregate and the greater community? For example, are there newspaper accounts of the aggregate's struggle in terms of political strength or lack of strength?	
Communication	How is information communicated within and to the aggregate? What newsletters or bulletin boards are available to the aggregate? Are community leaders available to the aggregate? What are the meeting areas for the aggregate (clubroom, school, or other)? Do aggregate members attend community meetings? Do they give information? What is done with this information?		Is the aggregate being focused on within the media? Can members of the aggregate be observed on television or heard on radio? How many times per week?
Education	Do members of the aggregate feel that they need more education or a different type of education? What educational resources are available to the aggregate? Do any of these resources specialize in the education of the aggregate?	What percentage of the aggregate is currently attending school? What is the average number of years in school for aggregate members? What percentage of the aggregate cannot read?	
Recreation	What "fitness" facilities are available in the geopolitical community? Are there biking and walking trails? Is there a system of community-sponsored reactional centers? What special recreational services are accessible to the handicapped? Do the recreational facilities meet the aggregate needs? What is the value toward "fitness" for the aggregate? How does this value compare to other aggregates within the geopolitical community?	What observations can be made about recreational opportunities? Are there parks in the community? What type of equipment is found in these parks? Are people seen using park equipment?	

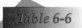 **Table 6-6** | **Data Collection of the Community Client Based on Community Competence Model**

Conditions of competence	Interactions	Observations	Measurements
Commitment	How do members of the aggregate demonstrate a commitment to the welfare of the group? Are there sponsored activities directed toward meeting aggregate needs. (For example, does the aggregate sponsor a program for exchanging material goods needed by members of the aggregate, such as wheelchairs, baby clothes, etc.)		What percentage of the total aggregate attend monthly support meetings?
Self-other awareness	Do members of the aggregate express that they have differing needs from the larger community, or are aggregate members unorganized and passive about their needs? Do members of the aggregate recognize that not all members of the aggregate have the same needs? Are there mechanisms for recognizing differences among aggregate members? For example, are all members included in decision-making? Do some members receive more services than others?		
Articulation	How does the aggregate make their needs known to the greater community? For example, how does an aggregate of homebound, frail elderly organize to obtain homemaking services? Does the aggregate sponsor lobbying activities on behalf of the aggregate?		
Effective communication	How do members of the aggregate demonstrate that they understand the common element that ties the group together? For example, does the aggregate sponsor a newsletter or a bulletin board? What type of information is conveyed?		
Conflict containment and accommodation	How do members of the aggregate express differing opinions? Does the aggregate sponsor a forum for an exchange of ideas on issues affecting the aggregate? How do members of the aggregate work together to settle their differences? Does the aggregate use a competitive model or a consensus model for settling differences?		
Participation	How do members of the aggregate demonstrate participation? Are group activities sponsored? Do members join in group activities?		
Management of relations with larger society	How do members of the aggregate demonstrate that they are aware of the supports available in the greater geopolitical community? What resources are available and how are these resources used by members of the aggregate? How do members of the aggregate negotiate with larger society for needed services? Is there a collective effort to gain the needed services, or is each member on his/her own?		
Machinery for facilitating participant interaction and decision-making	What mechanisms exist (phone calls, personal contacts, membership on boards/committees) for influencing what goes on within the aggregate?		

the structures found within the community (the various subsystems such as health and recreational resources). Although both models address community process or interactions among groups within a community, process is not the emphasis of these assessment models.

Goeppinger, Lassiter, and Wilcox (1982) developed a nursing process–related model for community assessment designed to address the importance of community processes. They recognized that the process perspective of community health is less popular than perspectives that include community status and community structures. The primary focus of the process-related model is community competence. To assess community competencies, the nurse examines the health capabilities and potential health actions of the community. The basic assumption of the community competency model is that health assessments need to include the community's strengths and abilities to improve their own health status.

The model is based on research conducted by Goeppinger and Baglioni (1986) that was designed to discover indices of community competence. These competencies are not considered mutually exclusive but interrelated. The conditions of competence are described as follows:

1. *Commitment.* Community members demonstrate an attachment to the community. For example, if the community assessed is an aggregate of elderly persons, do the aggregate members have a support group that meets on a regular basis? How many members of the aggregate participate in the support group? These behaviors demonstrate attachment and commitment to the group.
2. *Self-other awareness.* Do community members recognize that not all members agree on community issues? Are members of the community with minority views on issues listened to by others in the community?
3. *Articulation.* How well does the community articulate their needs to the greater community (vertical communication)? In other words, is an aggregate group of working mothers able to organize and inform the greater community of their needs for better day care?
4. *Effective communication.* How well do community groups communicate with one another (horizontal communication)? For example, in a community divided by two primary aggregate groups of whites and blacks, do these two groups communicate with one another? Is that communication effective in meeting both groups' needs?
5. *Conflict containment and accommodation.* How does the community deal with conflict? Does the aggregate use a consensus model, or are those of differing opinions expected to conform to the group?
6. *Participation.* Is there evidence of active community-oriented participation? Do members of the community attend the town council meetings? An example of participation would be members of the aggregate organizing a fund-raising event and a majority of aggregate members participating in it.
7. *Management of relations with larger society.* How do members of the community obtain external support for their community? An example of good management of relations with the larger society is found in the chronic kidney failure aggregate community. This aggregate community was able to secure medicare insurance coverage for their medical needs, regardless of age.
8. *Machinery for facilitating participant interaction and decision-making.* What mechanisms exist for facilitating interaction among community members? Does the aggregate community have a network system of phone calls among members to keep all members informed on certain issues? Does the aggregate community have a governing board designed to implement the desires of the aggregate?

Assessing community competencies requires a hands-on experience with members of the community. The nurse cannot rely on others' opinions of the community or on statistical data. The nurse must assess the community by interviewing community members. Members of the community define their own competencies. Table 6-6 proposes assessment questions that the nurse may ask to gather information on community competence. These assessment questions are based on Goeppinger's initial method for measuring each of the eight competencies using the Community Residents Survey (CRS) instrument.

Summary

Three models for community assessment as applied to the aggregate within a geopolitical community have been presented. The reader should note that although different models are used, the data are often similar. Each model addresses both structural and process aspects of the community, with Goeppinger's community competence model emphasizing process aspects. The model that the nurse chooses for the assessment depends on the community setting, the focus, and preference.

Critical Thinking Exercises BY ELIZABETH S. FAYRAM

1. Identify a target aggregate for a community assessment. Explain how you would gain acceptance by this group to assess the aggregate.
2. Using the Community-As-Client Model:
   a. Select one component of the community assessment wheel. Identify sources useful in data collection for this component.
   b. Describe the data you would collect for this component of the community assessment wheel.

3. There has been an increase in the number of homeless families in your community.
   a. Select a model useful in the assessment of this aggregate group. Provide rationale for your selection.
   b. Explain how this model would influence and guide the assessment of this aggregate.

REFERENCES AND READINGS

American Association of Colleges of Nursing (AACN): *Essentials of college and university education for professional nursing: final report,* Washington, DC, 1986, AACN.

American Nurses' Association (ANA), Division of Community Health Nursing Practice: *Conceptual model for community health nursing,* Kansas City, 1980, The Association.

American Public Health Association (APHA), Public Health Nursing Section: *The definition and role of public health nursing in the delivery of health care, a position paper,* Washington, DC, 1980, APHA.

Anderson ET and McFarlane JM: *Community as client: application of the nursing process,* Philadelphia, 1987, JB Lippincott.

Anderson E, McFarlane J, and Helton A: Community as client: a model for practice, *Nurs Outlook* 3(5):220, 1986.

Cassel J: The contribution of the social environment to host resistance, *Am J Epidemiol* 104(2):107, 1976.

Clayton R and Ritter C: The epidemiology of alcohol and drug abuse among adolescents, *Advances in alcohol and substance abuse,* 4(3/4):69-97, New York, 1985.

Dean PG: Expanding our sights to include social networks, *Nurs Health Care* 7(10):544, 1986.

Goeppinger J and Baglioni AJ Jr: Community competence: a positive approach to needs assessment, *Am J Community Psychol* 13:507, 1986.

Goeppinger J, Lassiter PG, and Wilcox B: Community health is community competence, *Nurs Outlook* 30(8):464, 1982.

Goeppinger J and Schuster G: Community as client: using the nursing process to promote health. In Stanhope M and Lancaster J, editors: *Community health nursing: process and practice for promoting health,* St Louis, 1988, Mosby–Year Book.

Hanchett E: *Community health assessment,* New York, 1979, John Wiley & Sons.

Hazzard M: An overview of systems theory, *Nurs Clin North Am* 6:383, 1975.

Higgs ZR and Gustafson DD: *Community as client: assessment and diagnosis,* Philadelphia, 1985, FA Davis.

Klein DC: Community and mental health: an attempt at a conceptual framework, *Community Mental Health J* 1:301, 1965.

Kopf EW: Florence Nightingale as statistician. In Spradley BW, editor: *Readings in community health nursing,* Boston, 1986, Little, Brown.

Lalonde M: *A new perspective on the health of Canadians—a working document,* Ottawa, 1974, Government of Canada.

Lassiter PG: A community development perspective for rural nursing, *Family and Community Health* 14(4):29, 1992.

McKay R and Segall M: Methods and models for the aggregate, *Nurs Outlook* 31(6):328, 1983.

McKinley JB: Social networks, lay consultation, and help-seeking behavior, *Soc Forces* 53(1):275, 1973.

Montero LA: Florence Nightingale on public health nursing, *Am J Public Health* 75(2):181, 1985.

Neuman B: *The Neuman Systems Model,* Norfolk, Conn, 1982, Appleton-Century-Crofts.

Reinhart UW: Rationing the health-care surplus: an American tragedy, *Nurs Econ* 1(4):210, 1984.

Robertson I: *Sociology,* ed 2, New York, 1981, Worth.

Rodgers S: Community as client—a multivariate model for analysis of community and aggregate health risk, *Public Health Nurs* 1(4):210, 1984.

Ruth J, Eliason K, and Schultz PR: Community assessment: a process of learning, *J Nurs Educ* 31(4):181, 1992.

Smith MC and Barton JA: Technologic enrichment of a community needs assessment, *Nurs Outlook* 40(1):33, 1992.

Shamansky SL and Pesznecker B: A community is . . ., *Nurs Outlook* 29(3):182, 1981.

Shumway SM and Wisehart D: How to know a community, *Nurs Outlook* 17:63, 1969.

Von Bertalanffy L: *General systems theory,* New York, 1968, George Braziller.

Williams CA and Highriter ME: Community health nursing: population focus and evaluation, *Public Health Rev* VII (3–4):197, 1978.

CHAPTER 7

NURSING DIAGNOSIS
Diagnostic Process

Wealtha Yoder Helland*

General Considerations

After client data have been collected, they must be interpreted and given meaning. The data alone are simply a number of cues or pieces of information obtained from the five senses. These data, or cues, may include client statements, observable signs and symptoms, laboratory values, census data, and reports from professional colleagues.

The terms *data* and *cues* are used interchangeably although they differ subtly. A cue is a signal or hint for action. In nursing diagnosis, a client behavior becomes a signal for nurse action, including cognitive action, when the nurse perceives and interprets the behavior (Gordon, 1994). These cues, or behaviors of the client, are the data used in nursing diagnosis.

Analysis and synthesis are the thought processes used to interpret client data and identify nursing diagnoses. In this chapter, analysis and synthesis are divided into phases. The phases are presented as guidelines to help the novice understand the elements of analysis and synthesis. The guidelines for analysis and synthesis are:

1. Data are categorized.
2. Data gaps and incongruencies are identified.
3. Cues are clustered into patterns.
4. Appropriate theories, models, concepts, norms, and standards are applied and compared with patterns.

5. Health concerns and strengths are identified.
6. Etiological relationships are proposed.

Definitions

The definition of *nursing diagnosis* arises from the definition of *nursing*. According to the American Nurses Association, "Nursing is the diagnosis and treatment of human responses to actual or potential health problems" (ANA, 1980, p. 9). The North American Nursing Diagnosis Association (NANDA) approved the following definition of nursing diagnosis at the Ninth General Assembly in March 1990. "A nursing diagnosis is a clinical judgment about individual, family, or community responses to actual or potential health problems/life processes. Nursing diagnosis provides the basis for selection of nursing interventions to achieve outcomes for which the nurse is accountable" (Carroll-Johnson, 1993, p. 306). The key phrases in both definitions will be explained below.

The word *judgment* has several meanings in the dictionary. Judgment is (1) "the process of forming an opinion or evaluation by discerning and comparing" and (2) "an opinion or evaluation so formed" (Woolf, 1979:620). Nursing diagnosis involves judgment of both types; it is a *process* (diagnostic process) and a *product* (diagnostic statement). *Clinical judgment*, then, is the application of judgment to nursing practice. This chapter describes the diagnostic process or *how* clinical judgments are made. The next chapter discusses the outcome of the diagnostic process, which is the diagnostic statement.

*Portions of this chapter were written by Phyllis Baker Risner in the third edition.

One purpose of nursing diagnosis is to identify the responses of the individual, family and community to health-related situations. According to the American Nurses Association, nurses are concerned with a wide range of health-related responses in both sick and well clients. Those responses can be reactions to an actual problem such as a chronic illness or they can indicate a potential health problem. Human responses to health problems are often multiple, episodic or continuous, fluid, and varying, and are less discrete or circumscribed than medical diagnostic categories tend to be (ANA, 1980). Examples of human responses are self-care limitations, pain and discomfort, self-image changes, and problems with significant relationships.

Actual or potential health problems/life processes activate human responses. The scope of nursing practice is broad and encompasses a wide range of responses. A nurse assists persons as they encounter life processes or maturational change throughout the life span. Nurses address client responses from pathophysiological states and treatment-related situations to personal situations, environmental factors, and maturation issues. Examples of actual or potential health problems include blindness, stroke, trauma, or surgery, while examples of life processes or events include pregnancy, relocation, financial problems, dying, or child rearing (Carpenito, 1991).

The term *health problem* can be confusing since it is used in several ways. A health problem may be a medical diagnosis or situation requiring medical intervention as described in the previous paragraph. *Health problem* or just *problem* may also refer to a problematic patient response requiring nursing diagnosis and intervention, such as inadequate self-care during pregnancy.

A *nursing intervention* is any type of direct care that a nurse performs with or for a client. These actions may include nurse-initiated care and strategies resulting from nursing diagnoses, physician-initiated treatments resulting from medical diagnoses, and performance of the daily essential functions for the client who cannot do these (Bulechek and McCloskey, 1989). The definition of what is and is not a nursing diagnosis relates to whether the health problem can be "definitively" treated by a nurse.

The *achievement of outcomes* beneficial to client health is the end point of nursing practice. Nursing diagnosis as a component of the nursing process provides direction for nursing practice. Nursing diagnosis is a professional responsibility for which the nurse is held accountable.

Historical Perspective

Nurses have reached conclusions about client health for many years. However, it has only been in the past two decades that nurses have formalized nursing diagnosis. In 1973 several nurse leaders convened the First National Conference on the Classification of Nursing Diagnoses at the St. Louis University School of Nursing. Attendees at the conference generated a list of health problems diagnosed and treated by nurses. These health problems were called *nursing diagnoses.*

The St. Louis conference was the beginning of what eventually became known as the North American Nursing Diagnosis Association (NANDA). NANDA conferences have been held biannually since 1973 and the Association is now international in scope and influence. For example, the current list of nursing diagnoses was revised into International Classification of Disease (ICD) code and submitted to the World Health Organization.

Importance of Nursing Diagnosis

The most frequently identified purposes for using nursing diagnoses are to improve delivery of care, to facilitate intraprofessional communication, to validate nursing functions, to measure nursing work loads, and to increase autonomy. Each of these purposes will be discussed as it relates to nursing practice and the profession.

Nursing diagnoses *improve client care delivery* by fostering research and individualizing care. Nursing diagnostic labels based on supporting theory and research augment and/or facilitate research-based practice. Also, since the diagnostic process is a careful, deliberate method of evaluating client data, conclusions arising from the diagnostic process are individualized to the client.

Nursing diagnoses *facilitate intraprofessional communication* by providing a common language for client health problems. Nurse-to-nurse communication promotes collaboration and continuity of care. Nursing diagnoses communicate professional judgment and provide a common frame of reference for nurse peers. Knowing the nursing diagnosis and the interventions commonly associated with the diagnosis helps nurses anticipate nursing care requirements.

Nursing diagnoses *validate nursing functions* by linking the problematic human response to treatment of the response. The rationale for nursing and client action becomes clearer when the client problem is stated. It is also easier to credit problem resolution to nursing intervention when client problems are specified as nursing diagnoses.

Adequate staffing is critical for effective care delivery. Nursing diagnoses are useful predictors of *nursing work load*. Nursing diagnoses have been used in patient classification systems to define staffing needs, as well as in patient acuity systems.

Finally, nursing diagnoses *increase professional autonomy* by providing a language to differentiate nursing from the practice of other health care providers. This differentiation increases the visibility of nursing and promotes the assumption of greater responsibility and accountability for practice. Nursing diagnoses also help nurses articulate their contributions to client care.

Diagnostic Process

The diagnostic process is the analysis and synthesis of data collected during assessment. *Analysis* is the separation of a whole into its component parts. It is examination of these parts and their relationships. In the nursing diagnostic process, analysis is organizing the client data base (the whole) by categorizing pieces of data according to the concepts of a model. Analysis also involves identifying information missing from the database (data gaps) that is needed to understand the client's health status. Data categorization and the identification of data gaps are the first two phases of the diagnostic process.

Synthesis is combining parts or elements into a whole. In nursing diagnosis, synthesis is the clustering or grouping of related data into patterns; the application of standards, norms, theories, frameworks, and models; the identification of human responses as strengths and health concerns; and the identification of factors contributing to the client's responses. These elements form the last four phases of the diagnostic process.

The diagnostic process requires several kinds of knowledge and complex thought. Diagnosis requires empirical or scientific knowledge, personal or self-knowledge, critical thinking, and decision-making. *Scientific knowledge* provides the information needed to analyze and synthesize client cues. *Personal or self-knowledge* and intuition can positively or negatively influence the accuracy of the diagnostic process. For example, the nurse may use empathy to heighten perception of a client's responses, or nurse bias may interfere with perception and result in a misdiagnosis.

The analysis and synthesis of client data involves critical thinking. *Critical thinking* is sifting through the data and generating ideas about what they mean. Processes such as imagining, conceiving, and inferring are used to interpret client data and formulate a nursing diagnosis. Factors influencing critical thinking include the knowledge base of the nurse, the experiences of the nurse, and the pressure of time.

Decision-making is discriminative thinking and includes the elements of deliberation, judgment, and choice. Decision-making is especially relevant to the analysis and synthesis of client data because it is used to test alternative explanations of client cues and to reach a conclusion about the client's health-related responses.

Guidelines for the Diagnostic Process

There are six phases in the analysis and synthesis of client data. These phases are not rigid, linear steps but guidelines for approaching this component of the nursing process. It is helpful to picture oneself working among the phases while the predominate movement is from the first to the last phase. More specifically, the meaning of client behavior is derived from interpreting single cues (first phase) as well as interpreting a pattern of client cues (third phase). Phases of the diagnostic process and decision questions for each phase are presented in Table 7-1. Contents of the table will be reviewed as each phase of the diagnostic process is discussed.

Phase 1

Data are categorized according to the concepts of the model selected for care. Nursing models such as Roy's (1991) adaptation model or Gordon's (1994) functional health patterns are examples of broad nursing models used with individuals. Other models for families and communities are described later in this chapter.

As shown in Table 7-1, decision-making questions that must be answered in this phase are: Is the model being used to categorize the data the most appropriate model for this client? Which cues, or pieces of data, belong in which category? Selecting an appropriate model means choosing a model with concepts useful for categorizing client data. The concepts and subconcepts of the model become the categories and subcategories used to organize client data. Categorization is then a matter of listing relevant client data under the concepts of the model. Organizing the data facilitates interpretation by revealing relationships among cues, thus making missing data more obvious.

Table 7-2 illustrates phases of the diagnostic process as columns using client data with the biopsychosociospiritual model. Columns are listed under either analysis or synthesis. In the first column, data about the client are categorized under the appropriate categories and subcategories of the model. For example, cues about the client's diet and body size are listed under the nutrition subcategory of biophysical health.

Data are categorized during or soon after assessment. Usually an assessment or admission form guides initial data collection. Such a form contains a prearranged method for organizing or categorizing client cues. The nurse needs to know the relationship between any assessment or admission form being used and the nursing model selected for client care. Forms have their limitations and assessment must always go beyond them, but the closer the relationship

Table 7-1	Phases in the Diagnostic Process and Decision Questions for Each Phase

Phase	Decisions
Categorize nursing assessment cues	Is the model appropriate to the client situation?
	Which cues belong in which category?
Identify data gaps and incongruencies	What additional data are needed to reach a conclusion? What data must be obtained before proceeding with analysis and synthesis? What data can be obtained later? What data are inconsistent and need clarification?
Cluster data into patterns	Which cues relate to each other?
	Which cues belong in which pattern?
	Which cues are relevant? nonrelevant?
Apply and compare theories, concepts, norms, and standards	Does the pattern match the defining characteristics of a nursing diagnosis?
	Which theories, and so on, are appropriate for interpreting patterns?
	What are the client's perceptions of "normal?"
Infer health concerns and strengths	What are all possible hypotheses, alternatives, and options?
	What is the probability that each option is present?
	Which alternatives are not valid? Which hypotheses are valid?
	Is there enough data to rule out an alternative?
	Is there enough data to confirm a conclusion?
	Which patterns are functional? Which patterns are strengths?
	Which patterns are actual, potential, or possible concerns?
	What is rationale for inferences?
Propose etiological relationships	Which cues or patterns may be the contributing factors?
	Which nursing diagnosis etiology is the "best fit" for data?

between the assessment/admission form and the model selected for care, the more useful the form will be in categorizing data according to the model.

Phase 2

Data gaps and incongruencies are identified. Data gaps are missing information needed to understand client health status. Table 7-2 identifies gaps in the example's categorized data. For example, the client's religious beliefs are unknown. Other examples of data gaps that may appear during the initial contact are sexual history, family history and genogram, past coping, and communication patterns.

The most complete assessment contains only a fraction of the information that might be collected. Identifying significant missing information involves clinical judgment and decision-making. As shown in Table 7-1, decision-making questions to ask are: What additional data are needed to reach a conclusion about the client's health-related responses? What data must be obtained before proceeding with analysis and synthesis? What data can be obtained later and what data are inconsistent, incongruent, and need clarification?

An incongruency occurs when data are conflicting or inconsistent. An example of an incongruency is a client denying a history of smoking while having an open pack of cigarettes and matches in a pocket and brown stains on two fingers. This incongruency needs

to be clarified or validated before defining specific client concerns. Data gaps and incongruencies indicate areas for further assessment.

Nursing diagnoses handbooks are available to assist with identifying data gaps. These books contain the defining characteristics or signs and symptoms of each nursing diagnosis (Carpenito, 1991, 1992; Gordon, 1993). The nurse can compare client data or cues with the defining characteristics of a possible nursing diagnosis and identify missing cues that would help form patterns. Reviewing the defining characteristics helps the nurse identify additional questions areas of data collection.

Phase 3

Cues are clustered into patterns. A pattern is a sequence of behavior over time. Repetitive behavior is more indicative of client health status than a single cue. For example, refusal to eat one meal is less significant than refusing to eat for a week. Client cues are observed and recorded over time to differentiate typical from atypical client behavior. Atypical client behavior is not carried forward in the analysis and synthesis of data. The term pattern also refers to a group of related cues constructed by the nurse. Repetitive client behaviors are incorporated into one or more patterns. Grouping or clustering data into patterns is the beginning of synthesis because it is combining elements into a whole.

Table 7-2 | **Analysis and Synthesis of Client Data: Phases in the Process Using the Biopsychosociospiritual Model***

Analysis			Synthesis		
1. Data categorization	2. Data gaps	3. Patterns	4. Application Comparison	5. Response	6. Etiology
Biophysical Health					
Nutrition		*Nutrition pattern*			
"I eat one meal a day, usually a hot dog, and drink three or four soft drinks." 5'2", 300 lbs. Skin folds on arms and ankles	Appetite Type and size of soft drink Availability of food Nutrition knowledge Client's perception of her weight	Eats one meal a day 5'2", 300 lbs. Skin folds Sits all day Lives alone 60 years old Female Wants no change Low income Black	Basic food groups Calorie intake Fluid intake Metropolitan Life height-weight chart	Actual concerns: Altered nutrition Obesity	Altered appetite Lacks nutrition knowledge Difficulty preparing food Inadequate income Loneliness
Exercise		*Exercise pattern*			
"I sit alone all day and watch TV with my cat." Walks with cane	Activities of daily living Range of motion Strength/energy	Sits all day Walks with cane 60 years old Wants no change Income is $200 a month	Physiology Developmental norms	Actual concerns: Sedentary lifestyle Impaired physical mobility Strength: mobile with cane	Lacks motivation Difficulty walking/ moving No money for diversional activities
Psychological health		*Interaction pattern*			
"I like my life as it is; I don't want any changes." Sits in chair staring out window; no eye contact. "I am 60 years old." Female	Self-concept Coping Developmental tasks	Sits alone all day watching TV with cat Sitting, staring, no eye contact Likes life as it is; wants no change Lives alone	Maslow's hierarchy of needs Communication Psychology	Actual concern: Limited social interaction Strength: Lives with cat	Self-concept disturbance No support system Limited physical mobility Depression
Sociocultural health		*Economic pattern*			
"I live alone. My income is $200 a month. Rent costs me $100 a month, and utilities are about $50." Black	Significant others Income source Insurance Transportation Values, traditions, and norms	Unemployed Income $200 a month, $50 left after paying rent and utilities 60 years old	Federal poverty guidelines	Actual concern: Income below poverty level Strength: Independent	Lacks knowledge of resources Inability to apply for resources Ineligibility for resources
Spiritual health					
	Religious beliefs and practices Values and valuing	No data available			Beliefs about asking for help

*Refer to pp. 122-127 for clarification of this table.

Grouping related cues facilitates interpretation of client data. A single cue may have multiple meanings depending its association with other cues. For example, in Table 7-2 a cue in the exercise subcategory of biophysical health states, "I sit alone all day and watch TV with my cat." The cue indicates a sedentary lifestyle. This cue also relates to the nutrition pattern in that the client burns few calories. This same cue relates to the client's psychological health and implies that the client has little contact with other people.

Patterns are constructed by examining the whole database and relating cues to each other based on ideas about the meaning of the client information. For example, in Table 7-2, the client's *exercise pattern* contains cues about activity and use of a cane (biophysical health), age and attitude toward change (psychological health), and income (sociocultural health). The aim is to construct patterns containing information about a client's response to an actual or potential health problem and the factors related to the response. Conclusions about the meaning of the pattern form the basis for the nursing diagnosis. To prevent diagnostic error, the nurse needs to accurately interpret cues, avoid overgeneralizing from too few observations, and cluster cues correctly.

Cues are incorporated into patterns depending on the significance of the cue and the priorities of the care. Cues collected from the client differ in level of importance. For example, a blood pressure of 210/115 is more significant than the sex of the client because the blood pressure is elevated. Single cues interpreted as abnormal or highly significant are incorporated into patterns because such cues are likely to signal care priorities.

Ideas for patterns come from many sources. Sources include the knowledge and experience of the nurse, the client's viewpoint, and contextual information, such as the medical diagnosis. The nursing model selected for care is an important source for clustering cues into patterns and naming the pattern. Another important source for identifying and naming patterns is a handbook of nursing diagnoses. The nurse can compare client cues in a pattern with the defining characteristics, or signs and symptoms, of likely nursing diagnoses. Such a comparison facilitates both the construction and naming of patterns. Sometimes there are no nursing diagnostic labels that match the client's pattern so the nurse must generate a pattern label.

In summary, Table 7-1 lists questions to ask in this phase: Which cues relate to each other? Which cues belong in which patterns? Does the pattern match the defining characteristics of a nursing diagnosis? These and other decisions must be made during this phase of the diagnostic process.

Phase 4

Appropriate theories, models, concepts, norms, and standards are applied and compared with patterns. The nurse compares the client's patterns to theories, models, concepts, norms and standards to identify the client's health-related responses. Nursing and nonnursing theories and models are used to interpret the client's data patterns. Some examples of nursing models that may be used to compare with the client's patterns are Roy's adaptive or ineffective behaviors, Orem's self-care deficits, and Friedman's family functioning. Other models and theories that may be useful include family systems, human needs, perception, communication, crisis, role, and stress theories. Decision-making questions in this phase (see Table 7-1) are the following: Does the pattern match the defining characteristics of a nursing diagnosis? Which theories, concepts, norms, and standards are most appropriate for interpreting the patterns? What does the client consider "normal"?

Knowledge of developmental and physiological norms in addition to psychological parameters is important when comparing and interpreting client patterns. Standards used for individuals may include the Metropolitan Life Insurance Company height and weight chart, the four basic food groups, normal ranges of vital signs and laboratory values, and developmental norms (such as Erikson's or the Denver Developmental Screening Test). Client data are compared with normal ranges, values, expectations, and client baseline information.

An important aspect of comparing the client's patterns to models or theories is the client's perception of "normal," because the nurse's assumptions and perceptions of normal may differ from the client's. One way to learn the client's perception of normal is to ask the client. When the nurse and client share an understanding of the client's view of his or her own health status, mutuality and cooperation are more likely.

Examples of comparing and applying data are given in Table 7-2. In this example, the client's nutritional pattern is compared with the basic four food groups, recommendations for daily caloric and fluid intake, and the Metropolitan Life chart for height and weight. The client's exercise pattern is compared to physiological and developmental norms. Her interaction pattern is compared with Maslow's hierarchy of needs, communication theory, and psychology. Although data gaps exist, the client's income and expenses may be analyzed mathematically and compared with federal poverty guidelines.

Phase 5

Health concerns and strengths are identified. In this phase the nurse identifies client responses as strengths and concerns by drawing conclusions about client patterns after comparison with theories, models, norms, and standards. The nurse hypothesizes about the results of the comparison and considers alternative possibilities. Reaching a conclusion is done by inferring the meaning of client cues, ruling out improbable explanations, and deciding the client's response to a situation or condition. Inferences are made about the client's health status, condition, or situation in each of the assessment categories.

As shown in Table 7-1, decision-making questions to ask in this phase are: What are all possible hypotheses or alternative explanations for the client's cue pattern? What is the probability that each hypothesis is accurate? Which alternative hypotheses are not valid? Are there enough data to rule out alternatives? Are there enough data to confirm a conclusion about the client's response? Which patterns are functional? Which patterns or cues are strengths? Which patterns are dysfunctional—that is, which are actual or potential responses of concern? What is the rationale for all the inferences and conclusions?

After interpreting the data, the nurse makes one or more of the following judgments regarding the client's health-related responses:

- No responses of concern. The client appears to be functioning/coping at an optimum level.
- Responses of actual concern. The client data indicate excesses, deficits, or stressors in one or more areas.
- Responses of potential concern. The client is at risk.
- Responses of possible concern. The nurse has reason to suspect a concern but needs more data or verification of existing data.

Examples of conclusions or inferences about the client's health responses derived from the application of theories, norms, and standards are shown in Table 7-2. An actual concern exists in this client's nutrition pattern because she is deficient in the basic food groups. Another actual concern is obesity, as the client is approximately 75% overweight, depending on the standard used. Insufficient information is available to reach a conclusion about her caloric and fluid intake.

There is also a concern about her exercise pattern because of her weight, impaired mobility, and sedentary lifestyle. Her interaction pattern is a concern because the data indicate that the client has limited social interaction. According to federal guidelines the client's income is below the poverty level, so her economic situation needs further exploration. Other possible concerns may need further exploration, such as self-care, elimination, and other biophysical patterns.

Client strengths are the client's mobility with a cane, having a cat, and independence. These strengths are integrated in the plans for nursing care. Examples of strengths and concerns for the individual, family, and community are shown in Table 7-3.

In reality, the next phase in data processing would also occur while hypotheses about client responses are being tested, that is, proposing an etiology or considering contributing factors to the identified response. However, in this text the two phases are described separately.

Phase 6

Etiological relationships are proposed. In this phase the nurse explores and identifies factors influencing or contributing to the client's responses. The nurse makes inferences and hypotheses about possible contributing factors relating to the client's responses based on cues in the pattern. These judgments are pivotal in data processing because the statement of etiological relationships helps direct nursing intervention.

Table 7-3	Examples of Strengths and Concerns Applied to the Individual, Family, and Community	
Client	**Strengths**	**Concerns**
Individual	Ability for self-care	Decreased self-care
	Feelings of independence	Dependence
	High morale	Lack of self-esteem
	Family support	No family
	Many friends	Social isolation
	Adequate housing	Inadequate housing
	Education	Lack of job skills
Family	Past coping experience	Crisis
	Open communication	Dysfunctional communication
	Adequate financial resources	Inadequate resources
	Extended family presence	No support system
	Flexible rules	Rigid rules
	Defined roles	Confused roles
Community	Adequate funding to meet health needs	Inadequate funding
	Enthusiastic leadership and interest in health concerns	Disinterest
	Health services available, accessible, acceptable	Health services unavailable, inaccessible, unacceptable

Application of Models

The choice of a model suitable to the client situation is made during the data collection component of the nursing process. The model then provides a structure for collecting, categorizing, and interpreting the data. It may also influence the wording of the diagnostic statement. Partial examples of how models are applied to the individual, family, and community client in the diagnostic process are described below.

Individual Client

Many different nursing models are useful in analyzing and synthesizing data about the individual client. Two models that are frequently chosen for the individual are Orem's (1991) self-care model and Roy's (1991) adaptation model. Model selection is influenced by variables relating to the nurse, the client, and the setting. Refer to Chapter 2 for more information about model selection.

When Roy's (1991) adaptation model is used, data are collected and categorized according to four modes: physiological, self-concept, role function, and interdependence. The patterns are interpreted as adaptive or ineffective. The following is a discussion of an individual case study using Roy's model. An application of the diagnostic process is given in Table 7-4.

Individual Case Study
Assessment: Subjective Data (from Record and Client)

Mrs. B is a 75-year-old widow of Appalachian origin who lives alone with her dog in the house she and her husband built in their urban neighborhood 50

As shown in Table 7-1, questions to ask in this phase are: Which cues or patterns may be the contributing factors to the response? Which etiology is the "best fit" for the identified response?

Examples of possible etiologies are shown in Table 7-2, where an actual nutritional concern is indicated by inadequate intake of the four basic food groups and the client's excess weight. Therefore the nurse would explore probable contributing factors. From the limited data available, factors could be altered appetite, lack of knowledge about nutrition, difficulty preparing food, inadequate income, loneliness, or some combination. These factors need to be explored further and validated with the client. The concern about exercise could be related to lack of motivation, difficulty in walking/moving, and/or inadequate income for diversional activities. The client's limited social interactions could be influenced by her self-concept, lack of social support, limited mobility, and depression. The client's inadequate income could be related to her lack of knowledge of resources, her inability to apply for resources, ineligibility, or her beliefs about asking for help.

A client response in one category may be the etiology of another response in a different category. For example, the client's inadequate income limits resources for nutrition and exercise. It is also possible that one etiological factor may be related to several concerns. For example, lack of motivation may be a contributing factor for both nutrition and exercise concerns. Guidelines for differentiating concerns and etiological relationship(s) are discussed in Chapter 8.

Table 7-4	Analysis and Synthesis of the Individual Client: Roy's Adaptation Model*

| | **Analysis** | | | **Synthesis** | |
1. Data categorization	2. Data gaps	3. Patterns	4. Application/ Comparisons	5. Response	6. Etiology
Physiological					
Activity/rest		*Activity/rest*		Ineffective:	
"I can't wear shoes." Walker beside bed	Range of motion, sleep, safety	All activity/rest cues *plus:* 5'3", 160 lbs. Edema of legs Wears glasses 75 years old	Physiology, nursing, aging theories	Mobility High risk for safety concerns	Discomfort from edematous feet Shortness of breath Advanced age
Nutrition		*Nutrition*		Ineffective:	
"Can't stay on low-salt diet." 5'3", 160 lbs. Edentulous	Nutritional assessment, knowledge of diet, effect on intake	All nutrition cues *plus:* Edema of legs 75 years old Lives alone	Metropolitan chart, aging theories	Excessive weight Noncompliance Possible chewing concern	Intake exceeds metabolic need Edema Unknown Edentulous

*Refer to pp. 129-130 for clarification of table.

Continued

Table 7-4 **Analysis and Synthesis of the Individual Client: Roy's Adaptation Model—cont'd**

Analysis			Synthesis		
1. Data categorization	2. Data gaps	3. Patterns	4. Application/ Comparisons	5. Response	6. Etiology
Elimination	Elimination				
Fluid & electrolytes		*Fluid & electrolyte*	Physiology, nursing	Ineffective: Excess fluid concern	Lack of medicine Inappropriate diet
Edema (4+) Right ankle 10″ Left 10.5″	Intake, salt, elimination	All fluid & electrolyte cues *plus:* Can't wear shoes Has not taken medicine			
Oxygenation		*Oxygenation*	Physiology, pathophysiology, nursing, aging	Ineffective: Oxygenation leading to altered tissue perfusion to extremities	Altered circulation
Color pink, lungs clear P 72, R 20, BP 200/ 100 Extremities cool to touch; unable to palpate pedal pulses Shortness of breath	Knowledge of hypertension Past medical history Skin and foot assessment	All oxygenation cues *plus:* Edema of legs States name, location Forgets medicine 75 years old			
Endocrine function		*Endocrine function*	Physiology, pharmacology, nursing, aging	Ineffective: Noncompliant with medication Adaptive: Temperature	Forgetfulness, unresolved grief
"I haven't taken my medicine in 2 weeks. I just forget to take it." T 98.6 degrees	Knowledge of medication, motivation, daily schedule	All endocrine cues *plus:* Can't stay on diet Edema of legs			
Protection function	Skin and foot assessment				
Senses			Physiology, aging	Adaptive: Glasses Vision Potential safety concern as visual acuity unknown	
Wears glasses	Hearing, smell, touch, date of last eye exam, acuity				
Neurological function	Neurological				
Self-concept					
Physical self		*Physical self*	Psychology, nursing, aging theories, Appalachian culture	Adaptive: Oriented; assess further as forgets medicine	
"My name is Sarah. I'm in the hospital for high blood pressure." Age 75 years Appalachian origin Sitting up in bed, smiling	Health maintenance practices, values and beliefs	All physical self cues *plus:* Can't wear shoes Edentulous 5'3″, 160 lbs. Has not taken medicine Wears glasses			

Table 7-4	Analysis and Synthesis of the Individual Client: Roy's Adaptation Model—cont'd					
Analysis			**Synthesis**			
1. Data categorization	**2. Data gaps**	**3. Patterns**	**4. Application/ Comparisons**	**5. Response**	**6. Etiology**	
Role function		*Role function*		Adaptive:		
Retired clerk	Developmental tasks	All role function	Role, family,	Several roles	Recent loss of	
Knits for	Past coping, grieving	cues *plus:*	Erikson, aging	Possibly maladaptive:	husband	
grandchildren	process	Age 75 years	theories; grief/	Widowhood		
Husband died 2		Lives alone with dog,	loss			
months ago		belongs to				
Four children		Methodist church				
Five grandchildren						
Interdependence		*Interdependence*		Potentially		
Lives alone with dog	Significant other, pet	All self-concept, role	Family, Maslow,	ineffective:	Lives alone, mobility	
Receives Social	care, diversional	function, and	aging, nursing	Socialization	Mobility	
Security, pension,	activities,	interdependence	theories,	Home maintenance		
Medicare	communication,	cues	economics	management		
Belongs to Methodist	transportation,			concern		
Church	home maintenance					
Children write or call	management					
once a month						

years ago. Her husband died 2 months ago. She has four children and five grandchildren, all of whom live out of town. The children write or call her at least once a month. Mrs. B knits items for her grandchildren. She is a retired clerk, and belongs to the Methodist church. Her income includes Social Security, a pension, and Medicare. She states, "My name is Sarah. I'm in the hospital for high blood pressure. I haven't taken my medicine for 2 weeks. I just forget to take it. My feet are so swollen that I can't wear my shoes. And another thing, I just can't keep to that low-salt diet."

Assessment: Objective Data

Client is sitting up in hospital bed, smiling; no teeth in mouth. She wears glasses. Walker is next to bed. Height 5'3", weight 160 lbs, temperature 98.6 F, pulse 72 beats per minute and regular, respirations 20 per minute; blood pressure 200/100 (right arm, sitting). Lungs clear but client exhibits shortness of breath. Color pink. Extremities cool to touch. Unable to palpate pedal pulses. Pitting edema 4+ of both ankles and feet. Circumference of right ankle 10 in, left ankle 10½ in.

Individual Analysis and Synthesis: Roy's Adaptation Model

This client's data are categorized according to Roy's four modes. An explanation of the analysis/ synthesis process for the activity/rest pattern within the physiological mode follows.

The *physiological mode* includes activity and rest, nutrition, elimination, fluid and electrolyte balance, oxygenation, endocrine function, protection, the senses, and neurological functions. The client's statement, "I can't wear shoes," and the presence of a walker beside the bed are cues categorized in the activity/rest category. These cues and related cues from other categories are used to construct the *activity/rest pattern*. Reviewing other categories for related cues reveals that the client is overweight (nutrition), has edematous legs (fluid and electrolytes), wears glasses (senses), and is 75 years old (self-concept). These additional cues provide more information about the client's pattern of activity/rest. For example, her edematous feet probably explain why she cannot wear shoes. Safety is a concern because she apparently uses a walker, is elderly, and her visual acuity is uncertain. Knowledge from physiology, nursing, and aging theories were used to interpret the client's cues. It can be concluded from the first-level assessment that her mobility response is ineffective and she is a safety risk for a fall. The activity/rest pattern also contains cues about etiology or factors related to her ineffective mobility and safety. Identifying the stimuli or stressors contributing to the ineffective human response is second-level assessment in Roy's model. The focal stimulus for her mobility problem is the discomfort of her edematous feet. Contextual and residual stimuli are her inability to wear shoes and noncompliance with medication and diet. Other stimuli that may contribute to her ineffective mobility response are her shortness of breath and advanced age. Data gaps for the activity/rest category pertain to her range of motion, sleep, and safety. Eliminating these data gaps would provide more information about her activity/rest health status and any factors contributing to difficulties with this aspect of health.

Table 7-4 shows how other data from the case study were analyzed and synthesized using Roy's model. The table provides additional opportunity to examine the diagnostic process in action.

Based on this analysis/synthesis of the individual, Mrs. B's strengths include adaptive temperature regulation, physical self-concept, and effective implementation of several roles.

Examples of this client's health concerns are:

1. Ineffective mobility related to foot discomfort, edema, inability to wear shoes, and altered circulation
2. High risk for safety concerns related to impaired mobility and possible decreased vision
3. Ineffective nutrition related to being edentulous, excessive caloric intake, decreased mobility, and unresolved grief
4. Potential social isolation related to living alone and impaired mobility
5. Incomplete database: elimination; nutritional and fluid assessment; knowledge of diet, medication, and hypertension; communication; effect of no teeth; visual acuity and range of motion; sleep; environmental safety; home maintenance management, including pet care; motivation; developmental tasks, including grieving and past coping; significant others; values and beliefs; health maintenance practices; diversional activities; transportation; daily schedule; sexual history; and past medical history.

Family as Client

Family models and frameworks are used to analyze family data. Four well-established family frameworks are systems theory, structural-functional framework, interactional models, and developmental framework. Conclusions from family data indicate whether family responses are functional or dysfunctional, adequate or inadequate, or altered or potentially altered. Functional or adequate family responses are strengths, whereas nonfunctional responses are identified as concerns. If a systems approach is used, the family is evaluated as an open or closed system

with rigid, diffuse, or permeable boundaries; functional or dysfunctional self-regulatory mechanisms (throughput); and system overload or deprivation (input or output). When Friedman's (1986) structural-functional framework is used, data about the structure and function of the family are categorized separately. Data about family structure is grouped and analyzed according to:

1. Role structure (position, behavior, conflict, strain, sharing, and modification)
2. Value systems (overt or covert rules, priorities, conflicts, and restrictiveness or flexibility)
3. Communication patterns (functional or dysfunctional)
4. Power structure (coalitions and decision-making, classified as dominated, autonomic, or leaderless).

Friedman's categories of family function are affection (personality maintenance), socialization and social placement, reproduction, family coping, economy, and health care. Family response patterns are diagnosed as either adequate or inadequate and functional or dysfunctional. An example of this approach is shown later.

The interactional approach focuses on ways family members relate to each other. Internal family dynamics are analyzed in this approach as functional, potentially alterable, or altered. Family interaction processes or dynamics are role, status, communication patterns, decision-making, coping patterns, and socialization. Satir (1972) uses the interactional process to identify four categories: rules, self-worth, communication, and links to society. The interactional model is limited and needs to be used in conjunction with another model. Duvall (1977) uses the developmental approach with family tasks and stages of progression through the life cycle. The collected data are analyzed for clues that identify the stage and tasks; then a descriptive statement is made, noting the developmental needs. An example of how to use the guidelines of the analysis/synthesis process with a family client is provided in Table 7-5, according to Friedman's (1986) structural-functional model.

Family Case Study
Assessment: Subjective Data (from Family Interview)

Mr. and Mrs. P. are expecting their second child in 2 months; they have a 3-year-old son, Brad. Both parents are college graduates and attend church regularly. They are buying their three-bedroom brick home in a suburban neighborhood. Mr. P. is 35 years old and owns a small business. Mrs. P., age 34, works in an architectual firm and co-supports the family.

Table 7-5	**Analysis and Synthesis of the Family Client: Structural-Functional Model***				
Analysis			**Synthesis**		
1. Data categorization	**2. Data gaps**	**3. Patterns**	**4. Applications/ Comparisons**	**5. Response**	**6. Etiology**
Structure					
Role		*Role*			
Mrs. P.: Age 34 yr, female, co-support, college graduate	Anticipatory plans, feelings	All role cues Share chores Attend church Holds child Council representative Works Gets prenatal care	Psychology, role, family theory, developmental	Potential concern: Stress	Multiple roles and role change
Mr. P.: Age 34 yr, male, co-support, college	Anticipatory plans, feelings	All role cues Share chores Attend church In Big Brothers Owns business		Potential concern: Stress	Multiple roles and added responsibilities
Brad: Age 3 yr, male	Feelings Preparation	All role cues Child care by grandparents		Potential concern: Sibling rivalry	Arrival of sibling
Values		*Values*			
"We share chores." Alone time Together time Attend church Child care by grandparents	Cultural assessment, spiritual assessment	College graduate Works Owns business Buying home Gets prenatal care	Philosophy, religion, culture	Strength: No apparent conflict	
Communication		*Communication*			
Couple takes turns speaking and listening, includes child Child speaks in sentences, calls parents Mommy and Daddy	Patterns with grandparents	All communication cues	Satir, communication, growth and development	Strengths: Functional communication pattern Child's pattern within normal limits	
Power structure		*Power structure*			
Couple makes decisions jointly	Past decisions: Outcome and process	Share chores Take turns speaking and listening, include child	Satir, decision-making	Strength: Shared power	

Refer to pp. 133, 135 for clarification of table.

Continued

Table 7-5	**Analysis and Synthesis of the Family Client: Structural-Functional Model—cont'd**

Analysis			Synthesis		
1. Data categorization	2. Data gaps	3. Patterns	4. Applications/ Comparisons	5. Response	6. Etiology
Function					
Affective function		*Affective*			
Child sitting on mother's lap	Need-response, recreation	All affective function cues	Psychology, developmental family, Maslow	Strength: Mutual nurturance	
Couple sitting close, occasionally touching		Share chores Together time Take turns speaking, include child			
Socialization		*Socialization*			
Husband in Big Brothers Wife representative on neighborhood council	Family history, child-rearing practices Developmental status of child	Working parents Parents college graduates Child care by grandparents Attend church	Psychology, developmental norms, communication	Strength: Community participation	
Reproduction		*Reproduction*			
Pregnancy in seventh month	Sexual history, family planning, maternal reproductive history	Wife 7 months pregnant	Psychology Family theory	Assess further	
Family coping		*Family coping*			
	Past crises, coping mechanisms, resources, anticipatory plans, feelings	All role cues Share chores, child care, attend church Take turns Joint decisions Sitting close Husband owns business Wife works	Satir, crises theory, developmental stress	Potential stressor: birth of child and sibling	Maturational crises
Economics		*Economics*			
Husband owns small business Wife plans to stop work in architectural firm when baby is born	Anticipatory plans	All economic cues Buying home Prenatal care Future child care Joint decision-making Future loss of income	Economics, family	Potential concern: Loss of income	Unemployment of wife after delivery
Health care		*Health care*			
Buying three-bedroom home Regular prenatal care	Health maintenance practices Individual health histories	All economic and health care cues	Economics, primary and secondary prevention	Strength: Adequate housing and regular prenatal care	

"We share chores and decision-making. We also have time alone at least once a week in addition to a night out together at least once a month." Mrs. P. is a representative on their neighborhood council. She visits her private physician regularly for prenatal care. Mr. P. is a member of Big Brothers and attends their functions. Child care is provided for Brad by his maternal grandparents. Mrs. P. plans to stay at home for 1 year after the birth.

Assessment: Objective Data

Brad walks across the room, climbs up on the couch with his parents, and sits on his mother's lap. Couple sitting close together on couch, occasionally touching. Couple takes turns speaking and listening, includes Brad in conversation. Brad calls parents Mommy and Daddy, speaks in complete sentences. His height is approximately 3 feet, weight approximately 30 lb.

Family Analysis and Synthesis: Structural-Functional Model

According to Friedman's structural-functional model (1986), family structural dimensions include role, values, communication patterns, and power structure. Family functions are affective patterns, socialization, reproduction, family coping, economy, and health care. In the structural component, *role* implies ascribed or achieved position in a family. Data from this family indicate that Mrs. P. is a 34-year-old woman with the roles of wife, pregnant mother, daughter, employee, volunteer, alumna, church member, client, and co-supporter. Mr. P. is a 34-year-old man who is a husband, father, businessman, church member, volunteer, alumnus, and co-supporter. Brad is a 3-year-old boy who is a son, grandchild, and potential brother. With the arrival of the new baby, there are three potential responses of concern. First, the change in Mrs. P.'s role from employed to unemployed, as well as her multiple roles, may cause increased stress. Data gaps include her anticipatory plans and feelings. Second is a potential for sibling rivalry to develop in the 3-year-old. Data gaps include preparation and feelings of the father and son. Third is a potential for stress in the husband due to his multiple roles and added responsibilities. Other data about the family's structure (values, communication patterns, and power structure) are entered and processed in Table 7-5.

The *economic* function involves the provision and allocation of finances, space, and materials. Data reflecting the economic function of this family include the husband owning a small business and the wife working in an architectural firm. Other cues with economic implications are purchasing their home, the costs of prenatal care, child care (if any), and joint de-

cision-making. The loss of Mrs. P.'s income after the baby is born is a potential concern. The data gap includes anticipatory plans.

The *health care* function includes the provision of physical necessities and health care. Data indicate that Mr. and Mrs. P. are purchasing a three-bedroom home and Mrs. P. gets regular prenatal care. These are strengths. Data gaps include eating habits, 3-day recall; immunizations; dates of last dental, vision, and breast examinations and Pap smear; use of alcohol and other substances, including over-the-counter drugs; exercise, family and individual health history; and knowledge of labor and delivery. Data about other family functions (affective pattern, socialization, reproduction, and family coping) are entered and processed in Table 7-5. The overall family strengths identified are nonconflicting values, functional communication patterns, shared power, mutual nurturance, links to society, adequate housing, and regular prenatal care.

The family concerns are:

1. Potential stress related to role change
2. Potential for sibling rivalry related to new baby
3. Potential concern about the loss of income related to Mrs. P's future unemployment
4. Maintenance of family health
5. Incomplete database: anticipatory plans, feelings, cultural and spiritual assessments, relationship with extended family, past decision outcomes and process, family need-response, family recreation, child-rearing practices, developmental level, reproduction history, sexual history, past coping and resources, and health care practices.

Community as Client

A community may be defined in several ways. Depending on the definition, a community can be the total population or an aggregate within a geographical area. Epidemiological, interactional, systems, and nursing models can be used for analysis/synthesis of community data at either level.

If systems theory is used, data are interpreted according to inputs (what the community obtains and feedback); throughput (decision-making and communication); output (what the community disposes of); boundary maintenance (what the community contains and retains, permeability, and system linkages with the subsystems and suprasystems); and system states of entropy, negentropy, and homeostasis.

Several nursing models are useful for providing nursing care at the community level. Gordon's (1994) functional health patterns have been adapted to communities. The Omaha Classification Scheme (Martin and Scheet, 1992) also may be used for categorizing community data and identifying patterns. The Omaha system has four major domains: environmental, psychosocial, physiological, and health behaviors. Neuman's (1989) health care systems model is frequently used with the community client. Its theoretical perspective focuses on stressors and stress reduction as a means of improving health. The two fundamental components of the model are the client and the environment. The client consists of a basic structure surrounded by protective layers. The basic structure of the client is described as having five variables: physiological, psychological, sociocultural, developmental, and spiritual. The innermost protective layer is the lines of resistance, the middle layer is the normal line of defense, and the outer layer is the flexible line of defense.

Regardless of the model used, analysis indicates patterns, resources, and influencing factors that identify strengths, concerns, and high-risk populations. Conclusions and judgments are made about community responses in each category of the models.

Community data are interpreted from histograms, frequency graphs, pie charts, statistical maps, tables, and narrative statements. The use of energy flow charts can graphically show interrelationships among systems. Concepts, theories, and standards that may be used for synthesis include the concepts of communication, group, leadership, and motivation; developmental, systems, and nursing theories; standards of public health, epidemiology; primary, secondary, and tertiary prevention; federal poverty guidelines; Environmental Protection Agency and Occupational Health and Safety Agency standards; and cultural, organizational, and political norms.

A community case study followed by an example of how to use the guidelines of the analysis/synthesis process with a community client is presented according to Neuman's Health Care Systems Model (1989).

Community Case Study
Assessment: Subjective Data

The following quotes are from clients in a session of an ongoing support group for battered women housed in a shelter. The group is led by a psychiatric nurse. Client #1: "My husband and I yelled at each other but he never hit me until I got pregnant. It hurt but he had been drinking so I thought he didn't mean it. After he sobered up he apologized and promised that he would never hit me again." Client #2: "Since he lost his job, it's (the abuse) worse than ever." Client #3: "I'm worried about the money too but I didn't get pregnant by myself! When he gave me a black eye my mother asked me what happened. When I told her she said I'd just have to live with it (being hit). I suppose she said that because my dad used to give her the back of his hand once in awhile when she aggravated him." Client #4: "I'm in this support group because the public health nurse said wife beating just gets worse unless people

get help." Client #5: "I'm living at the shelter now . . . I've had my last beating. Where do I go from here?"

Assessment: Objective Data

Data are based on participant observation and secondary analysis of shelter intake summary. A dozen women are in the support group. The majority of the women are white and said they had been abused by their husbands. One woman had a large bruise on her arm and three were pregnant. Most of the women looked younger than 30 years of age and came to the shelter with small children. Not all group members spoke but they listened attentively to each other, offering supportive comments. Several women cried when describing their life situation.

The intake summary revealed that the women suffered a variety of types of abuse ranging from being pushed and grabbed to being beaten unconscious. About half of the women reported that they had been injured in the last abusive incident and that the abuse occurred at least once a week. The duration of abuse was a matter of months to more than 10 years. The women varied in educational level, social class, income, and employment history.

Community Analysis/Synthesis:
Neuman's Health Care Systems Model

The community client is analyzed using Neuman's Model (1989). See Table 7-6 for analysis and synthesis of data obtained so far. According to Neuman the basic structure of the client consists of physiological, psychological, sociocultural, developmental, and spiritual variables. The physiological data showed that the group is all women, some are pregnant, and one woman had a bruise on her arm. The physical health status and resources of the women is a data gap. Data and data gaps about the psychological, sociocultural, and developmental variables are included in Table 7-6. More information needs to be obtained about the spiritual variable.

Neuman (1989) states that lines of resistance are activated when the stressor has penetrated the normal line of defense and the flexible line of defense. Data about the lines of resistance of the women include the statements, "I'm in the shelter"; "I've had my last beating"; and, "Wife beating just gets worse without help." Data gaps are the precipitating factors for shelter admission and any past treatment for abuse. The usual lifestyle and coping strategies of the women are a data gap. Such information relates to the normal line of defense. The women's usual attempts to avoid abuse is also a data gap. Behavior to avoid abuse relates to the flexible line of defense.

The environment in Neuman's model is located within the client (internal) and outside the client

Table 7-6 Analysis and Synthesis of the Community Client: Neuman's Care System Model*

	Analysis			Synthesis	
1. Data categorization	2. Data gaps	3. Patterns	4. Applications/ Comparisons	5. Response	6. Etiology
Client Basic structure: *Physiological* All women, some pregnant, large bruise on arm	Physical health status and resources	*Stressor: women abuse* "My dad used to . . ." Shelter admission ". . . last beating." "Wife beating. . ." "My husband . . . hit me . . ." Large bruise on arm Shelter intake survey results	Health assessment	Concern: validated woman abuse; Potential concern: future abuse, injury, and death	Progressive, escalating cycle of abuse
Psychological Women cried Group participation— shared and listened	Mental health status, e.g. self-concept, guilt, shame		Psychology Group theory Epidemiology	Assess further Strength: Group participation	Low self-esteem, high dependency needs Learned gender role behavior of abused women
Sociocultural "My dad used the back of his hand . . ." Most women were white; married; and varied by education, social class, income, and employment	Extent of personal resources, e.g. employment skills	*Etiology of abuse* "He grew up with it (abuse) too." "He had been drinking." "He lost his job . . ."	Psychology Sociology	Assess further	
Developmental Most women were less than 30 years old and had small children	Achievement of developmental tasks		Developmental theory	Concern: Generational cycle of abuse	Learned gender role behavior of children of abusers
Spiritual	Beliefs and values			Assess further	
Lines of resistance "I'm in the shelter now." "I've had my last beating." "Wife beating just gets worse without help."	Precepitating factors for shelter admission Past treatment for abuse	*Reaction to stressors* Admission to shelter Women cried Content of group sessions "I've had my last beating."	Psychology Epidemiology	Assess further	

*Refer to pp. 134, 136-137 for clarification of table.

Continued

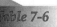

Table 7-6	Analysis and Synthesis of the Community Client: Neuman's Care System Model—cont'd				
Analysis			**Synthesis**		
1. Data categorization	**2. Data gaps**	**3. Patterns**	**4. Applications/ Comparisons**	**5. Response**	**6. Etiology**
Normal line of defense	Usual lifestyle and coping strategies	*Potential for reconstitution* Shelter admission Participation in support group Personal resources	Crises intervention Epidemiology	Strength: Readiness for treatment	
Flexible line of defense	Usual attempts to avoid abuse				
Environment					
Internal environment		*Fear*			
Intrapersonal stressors: Majority of women abused by husband "Where do I go from here?"	Personal goals	Powerlessness Future abuse Inciting attack Future for self and children	Psychology	Concern: Anxiety for future	
External environment					
Interpersonal stressors: "My husband . . . hit me . . ." "He grew up with it (abuse) too." "He had been drinking." Survey results of abuse Extrapersonal stressors:	Characteristics of abuser e.g. willingness to engage in treatment	Escalating forms of abuse	Epidemiology Crises intervention	Potential concern: treatment of abuser	History of exposure to violence as a child
"He lost his job."	Community stressors and resources e.g. employment and child care		Sociology	Concern: Adequacy of stress-relieving resources	Community acceptance of violence

stressors are forces from the far environment. In this example the family of each woman in the shelter is the near environment and the community surrounding the shelter is the far environment. Each part of the environment produces stressors. The abuse experience and the uncertainties of change are intrapersonal stressors of the women in the support group. The abuser(s) of each woman and the abusive encounters are interpersonal stressors. Unemployment, with all of its ramifications, is an extrapersonal stressor. Data gaps related to the environment include the personal goals of each woman, characteristics of the abusers,

and other community stressors and resources. Willingness of the abuser to engage in treatment is a priority data gap. Opportunities for such treatment must be available in the community.

Neuman's model requires identification of client stressors, determination of the client's reaction to stressors, and evaluation of the potential for reconstitution of the client system following invasion by stressors. The major stressor of this community client is abuse of women. Cues from the case study supporting the pattern of abuse include verbal statements by group members, physical injury, and data from the intake survey. The client group reacted to their abuse by coming to the shelter. Some women cried and one declared that she was not going to take any more beatings. Data about reconstitution is limited but admission to the shelter and participation in the support group are positive steps toward recovery. Another cluster present in the data is the client's ideas about the reasons for the abuse. Reasons stated were having grown up with abuse and the drinking patterns and loss of employment of the abusers.

Epidemiological information about abuse of women provides a description of the phenomena of abuse, abusers, women victims, child victims, and the quality and benefits of services for abuse (Illinois Coalition Against Domestic Violence, 1988). Determining the areas of similarity and difference between the client group and the epidemiological picture of abuse from a larger population is useful for decision-making about diagnosis and treatment. Health assessment, psychology, group theory, sociology, developmental theory, and crisis intervention were also used to interpret client data.

The major strengths of the women in the support group are their group participation and readiness for treatment. Responses of concern identified include validated abuse, the generational cycle of abuse, anxiety about the future, and the adequacy of stress-re-

lieving resources. Potential concerns are the likelihood of future abuse, injury, and death, and treatment for the abuser. More data are needed about sociocultural and spiritual variables of the client, as well as their defenses against abuse.

Factors known to be related to abuse of women are the progressive, escalating cycle of abuse; low self-esteem, high dependency needs, learned gender role behavior of abused women, and learned gender role behavior of children of abusers; history of exposure to violence as a child; and community acceptance of violence. Data from the women in this aggregate provided support for some of these contributing factors. Further assessment is needed to confirm or rule out other possible causes.

Summary

In this chapter the definition, importance, and history of nursing diagnosis was presented. Nursing diagnosis was discussed as a *process* of analysis and synthesis. Critical thinking and decision-making were integrated with the phases in the diagnostic process. Guidelines were given for interpreting the data and making inferences. Examples were included for the individual, the family, and the community in the application section.

Critical Thinking Exercises BY ELIZABETH S. FAYRAM

1. Justin is a 20-year-old college student who is being seen in the student health service for follow-up for mononucleosis diagnosed 4 days ago. Justin is single and lives with three other college students in an apartment near campus. His vital signs are: T 101; P 110; R 30; BP 110/84. He complains of a constant sore throat, frequent headaches, and weakness when he stands or walks. Before this illness he was in good health and biked 5 to 10 miles three times per week. He states he is worried about missing school and "giving the mono" to his roommates and girlfriend. He describes his urine output as dark; he has been eating "little" and has been drinking juice and pop. He takes two Tylenol tablets every 4 hours. He takes

naps during the day and is sleeping for short periods of time at night.
   a. Select a model for use in this situation. Categorize the data, using the model.
   b. Identify the most pertinent data gaps and additional information useful in this situation.
   c. List the client's strengths and health concerns.
   d. Identify factors (etiology) influencing the concerns.
2. Explain the relationship between the nursing diagnosis process and a nursing diagnosis statement.
3. Identify the advantages and disadvantages of using a nursing diagnosis classification system.

REFERENCES AND READINGS

American Nurses Association: *Nursing: a social policy statement,* Kansas City, 1980, The Association.

American Nurses Association: *Standards of clinical nursing practice,* Kansas City, 1991, The Association.

Bates B: *A guide to physical examination,* ed 5, Philadelphia, 1991, JB Lippincott.

Bulechek GM and McCloskey JC: Nursing interventions: treatments for potential nursing diagnoses. In Carroll-Johnson RM, ed: *Classification of nursing diagnoses: proceedings of the eighth conference,* Philadelphia, 1989, JB Lippincott.

Carpenito LJ: The NANDA definition of nursing diagnosis. In Carroll-Johnson RM, ed: *Classification of nursing diagnoses: proceedings of the ninth conference,* Philadelphia, 1991, JB Lippincott.

Carpenito LJ: *Handbook of nursing diagnosis,* ed 4, Philadelphia, 1991, JB Lippincott.

Carpenito LJ: *Nursing diagnosis: application to clinical practice,* ed 4, Philadelphia, 1992, JB Lippincott.

Carroll-Johnson RM: *Classification of nursing diagnoses: proceedings of the eighth conference,* Philadelphia, 1989, JB Lippincott.

Carroll-Johnson RM: *Classification of nursing diagnoses: proceedings of the ninth conference*, Philadelphia, 1991, JB Lippincott.

Carroll-Johnson RM: *Classification of nursing diagnoses: proceedings of the tenth conference*, Philadelphia, 1993, JB Lippincott.

Duvall EM: *Marriage and family development*, ed 5, Philadelphia, 1977, JB Lippincott.

Fagin CM: Collaboration between nurses and physicians: no longer a choice, *Acad Med* 67(5):295–302, 1992.

Friedman MM: *Family nursing: theories and assessment*, New York, 1986, Appleton-Century-Crofts.

Fitzpatrick JJ: Taxonomy II. Definitions and development. In Carroll-Johnson RM, ed: *Classification of nursing diagnoses: proceedings of the ninth conference*, Philadelphia, 1991, JB Lippincott.

Gordon M: *Manual of nursing diagnosis*, ed 6, St. Louis, 1993, Mosby.

Gordon M: *Nursing diagnosis: process and application*, ed 3, St. Louis, 1994, Mosby.

Illinois Coalition Against Domestic Violence: *Woman abuse* (brochure), Springfield, IL, 1988, The Coalition.

Kim MJ, McFarland GK, and McLane AM: *Pocket guide to nursing diagnoses*, ed 5, St Louis, 1993, Mosby.

Maslow AH: *Motivation and personality*, ed 2, New York, 1970, Harper & Row.

Martin KS and Scheet NJ: *The Omaha system: applications for community health nursing*, Philadelphia, 1992, WB Saunders.

National Commission on Community Health Services: *Health is a community affair*, Cambridge, Mass. 1967, Harvard University Press.

Neuman B: *The Neuman systems model: application to nursing education and practice*, Norwalk, 1989, Appleton-Century-Crofts.

Orem DE: *Nursing: concepts of practice*, ed 4, St. Louis, 1991, Mosby.

Roy Sr C and Andrews HA: *The Roy adaptation model: the definitive statement*, Norwalk, 1991, Appleton & Lange.

Sanford S: Administrative application of nursing diagnosis, *Heart Lung* 16(6):600, 1987.

Satir V: *Peoplemaking*, Palo Alto, Calif., 1972, Science and Behavior Books.

Turkoski BB: Nursing diagnosis in print, 1950–1985, *Nurs Outlook* 36(3):142, 1988.

U.S. Department of Health and Human Services: *Healthy people 2000: national health promotion and disease prevention objectives*, Washington, D.C., 1990, U.S. Government Printing Office.

Woolf HB: *Webster's new collegiate dictionary*, Springfield, Mass., 1979, Merriam.

CHAPTER 8

NURSING DIAGNOSIS
Diagnostic Statements

Wealtha Yoder Helland*

General Considerations

The *product* of the diagnostic *process* is the nursing diagnosis statement. The nursing diagnosis is an essential component of the nursing process for the purpose of planning client care. It flows from the analysis and synthesis, and is not identified in isolation. Writing nursing diagnoses is the responsibility of the professional nurse and is within the scope of professional nursing practice. The nursing diagnosis is a statement of nursing judgment.

This chapter discusses how to write, validate, and document nursing diagnostic statements. Examples of nursing diagnoses for individual, family, and community clients will be presented using several models. Guidelines for writing nursing diagnoses are explained in detail in the chapter and are cited here:

1. The nursing diagnosis is a statement of an actual, high-risk, or wellness health concern.
2. The nursing diagnosis is written as a descriptive and etiological statement.
3. The nursing diagnosis is concise and clear.
4. The nursing diagnosis is client centered, specific, and accurate.
5. The nursing diagnosis provides direction for nursing intervention.
6. The nursing diagnosis is the basis for independent and collaborative nursing actions/interventions.

*Portions of this chapter were written by Phyllis Baker Risner in the third edition.

7. The nursing diagnoses are validated with the client.

The NANDA System

In 1988 the American Nurses Association endorsed the North American Nursing Diagnosis Association as the official system of nursing diagnoses in the United States. The previous chapter described the history, work, and influence of NANDA. This chapter describes NANDA nursing diagnoses and the taxonomy or classification system for organizing the diagnoses.

Nursing Diagnoses and Human Responses

There are currently 108 nursing diagnoses approved by NANDA as shown in the box on page 138, which lists them according to the Classification of Nursing Diagnoses by Human Response Patterns. The human response patterns are exchanging, communicating, relating, valuing, choosing, moving, perceiving, knowing and feeling. Human responses refer back to individual, family, and community responses in the definition of a nursing diagnosis. The nine human response patterns are ways people can respond when confronted with a health problem, a life process, or both.

Each response pattern is defined, and nursing diagnoses within the scope of the definition are categorized under that response pattern. For example, the "relating" category includes diagnoses describing

Classification of Nursing Diagnoses by Human Response Patterns (NANDA Taxonomy I—revised)

Exchanging

Altered nutrition: more than body requirements

Altered nutrition: less than body requirements

Altered nutrition: high risk for more than body requirements

High risk for infection

High risk for altered body temperature

Hypothermia

Hyperthermia

Ineffective thermoregulation

Dysreflexia

Constipation

Perceived constipation

Colonic constipation

Diarrhea

Bowel incontinence

Altered urinary elimination

Stress incontinence

Reflex incontinence

Urge incontinence

Functional incontinence

Total incontinence

Urinary retention

Altered tissue perfusion (specify type) (renal, cerebral, cardiopulmonary, gastrointestinal, peripheral)

Fluid volume excess

Fluid volume deficit

High risk for fluid volume deficit

Decreased cardiac output

Impaired gas exchange

Ineffective airway clearance

Ineffective breathing pattern

Inability to sustain spontaneous ventilation

Dysfunctional ventilatory weaning response

High risk for injury

High risk for suffocation

High risk for poisoning

High risk for trauma

High risk for aspiration

High risk for disuse syndrome

Altered protection

Impaired tissue integrity

Altered oral mucous membrane

Impaired skin integrity

High risk for impaired skin integrity

Communicating

Impaired verbal communication

Relating

Impaired social interaction

Social isolation

Altered role performance

Altered parenting

High risk for altered parenting

Sexual dysfunction

Altered family processes

Caregiver role strain

High risk for caregiver role strain

Parental role conflict

Altered sexuality patterns

Valuing

Spiritual distress (distress of the human spirit)

Choosing

Ineffective individual coping

Impaired adjustment

Defensive coping

Ineffective denial

Ineffective family coping: disabling

Ineffective family coping: compromised

Family coping: potential for growth

Ineffective management of therapeutic regimen (individuals)

Noncompliance (specify)

Decisional conflict (specify)

Health-seeking behaviors (specify)

Moving

Impaired physical mobility

High risk for peripheral neurovascular dysfunction

Activity intolerance

Fatigue

High risk for activity intolerance

Sleep pattern disturbance

Diversional activity deficit

Impaired home maintenance management

Altered health maintenance

Feeding self-care deficit

Impaired swallowing

Ineffective breastfeeding

Interrupted breastfeeding

Effective breastfeeding

Ineffective infant feeding pattern

Bathing/hygiene self-care deficit

Dressing/grooming self-care deficit

Toileting self-care deficit

Altered growth and development

Relocation stress syndrome

Perceiving

Body image disturbance

Self-esteem disturbance

Chronic low self-esteem

Situational low self-esteem

Personal identity disturbance

Classification of Nursing Diagnoses by Human Response Patterns (NANDA Taxonomy I—revised)—cont'd

Perceiving—cont'd

Sensory/perceptual alterations (specify) (visual, auditory, kinesthetic, gustatory, tactile, olfactory)

Unilateral neglect

Hopelessness

Powerlessness

Knowing

Knowledge deficit (specify)

Altered thought processes

Feeling

Pain

Chronic pain

Dysfunctional grieving

Anticipatory grieving

High risk for violence: self-directed or directed at others

High risk for self-mutilation

Post-trauma response

Rape-trauma syndrome

Rape-trauma syndrome: compound reaction

Rape-trauma syndrome: silent reaction

Anxiety

Fear

Sample Human Response Pattern from NANDA Taxonomy I—Revised (1992)

Human Response Pattern: Relating

Y70 Family Processes, Altered

Y71 Role Performance, Altered

Y71.0 Parental Role Conflict

Y71.1 Parenting, Altered

Y71.2 Parenting, Altered: Risk

Y71.3 Sexual Dysfunction

Y72 Sexuality Patterns, Altered

Y73 [Socialization, Altered]*

Y73 0 Social Interaction, Impaired

Y73.1 Social Isolation

Excerpted from Carroll-Johnson, 1991:383–4.
*Items in brackets are not NANDA-accepted diagnoses.

connections, linkages, and associations between and among persons, places, or things. One nursing diagnosis of the human response pattern "relating" is *Altered Parenting.*

Taxonomy

The North American Nursing Diagnosis Association developed a taxonomy using the human response patterns. A taxonomy is a system of organization based on logic and the relationships among items to be classified. A taxonomy helps users find a diagnosis by arranging diagnoses in small groups under defined headings. The box above presents the hierarchical arrangement of the 11 nursing diagnoses in the human response pattern "relating." Nursing di-

agnoses can also be organized alphabetically or according to other systems such as Gordon's (1994) functional health patterns, Saba's Classification of Home Health Care Nursing Diagnoses (Gordon, 1994:387–9), and the Omaha Classification System (Martin and Scheet, 1992).

Types of Diagnoses

There are three types of diagnoses in the NANDA system: actual, high risk, and wellness. An actual diagnosis is selected when the client has an existing health concern related to excesses, deficits, or stressors in one or more areas. An example of an actual diagnosis is *Chronic Pain.* A high-risk nursing diagnosis is "a clinical judgment that an individual, family, or community is more vulnerable to develop the problem than others in the same or similar situation" (Gordon, 1994:385). An example of a high-risk diagnosis is *High Risk for Injury.* A wellness nursing diagnosis is a "clinical judgment about an individual, family, or community in transition from a specific level of wellness to a higher level of wellness" (Gordon, 1994:386). An example of a wellness diagnosis is *Family Coping: Potential for Growth.*

Components of a Nursing Diagnosis

Diagnoses in the NANDA system may have four components: a label or name, a definition, related or risk factors, and a list of defining characteristics.

Label

The label "provides a name for the diagnosis, a concise phrase or term that represents a pattern of related cues. [The] label may include a qualifier" (Gordon, 1994:384). A *qualifier* is a term added to the nursing diagnosis to describe the client situation more fully. The box at right presents NANDA's list of qualifiers and their definitions. Other qualifiers may be used. The term "potential for enhanced" is the designated qualifier for wellness diagnoses.

Definition

All nursing diagnoses have definitions. The definition "provides a clear, precise description which clarifies the meaning of the diagnosis and helps differentiate it from other similar diagnoses" (Gordon, 1994:384).

Defining Characteristics

Defining characteristics are "clinical cues that cluster as manifestations of a nursing diagnosis" (Gordon, 1994:384). Cues may be subjective or objective. All *actual* diagnoses have defining characteristics which can be considered the signs and symptoms of the diagnosis. The cues of some diagnoses are designated as major or minor. A cue is major if it occurs 80% to 100% of the time and minor if it occurs 50% to 79% of the time (Gordon, 1994:385). These designations are helpful in guiding the search for cues most likely to signal a particular diagnosis. Most *wellness* diagnoses have defining characteristics. These cues are behavioral indicators of a wellness state. *High-risk* diagnoses do not have defining characteristics because the problem or concern does not exist.

Related Factors

Related factors are "conditions or circumstances that may cause or contribute to a diagnosis" (Gordon, 1994:384). Actual and wellness diagnoses both have

---

◆ NANDA Descriptors for Constructing Nursing Diagnoses

Diagnostic labels may include but *are not limited to* the following qualifiers:

Altered A change from baseline.

Impaired Made worse, weakened; damaged, reduced; deteriorated.

Depleted Emptied wholly or partially; exhausted of.

Deficient Inadequate in amount, quality, or degree; defective; not sufficient; incomplete.

Excessive Characterized by an amount or quantity that is greater than is necessary, desirable, or useful.

Dysfunctional Abnormal; incomplete functioning.

Disturbed Agitated; interrupted, interfered with.

Ineffective Does not produce the desired effect.

Decreased Lessened, lesser in size, amount, or degree.

Increased Greater in size, amount, or degree.

Acute Severe but of short duration.

Chronic Lasting a long time; recurring; habitual; constant.

Intermittent Stopping and starting again at intervals; periodic; cyclic.

Potential for Enhanced (wellness diagnosis) Enhanced is defined as made greater; to increase in quality or more desired.

Excerpted from Gordon (1994:241).

	Table 8-1	**Descriptive Summary of Components of Nursing Diagnoses**

Component	Actual Diagnosis	High-Risk Diagnosis	Wellness Diagnosis
Label	Provides a name for the diagnosis, a concise phrase or term that represents a pattern of related cues. Label may include a qualifier.	Same as actual diagnosis label.	Same. The term *Potential for Enhanced* is the designated qualifier. Labels are one-part statements.
Definition	Provides a clear, precise description. Delineates its meaning and helps differentiate this diagnosis from similar diagnoses.	None	Same as actual diagnosis definition.
Defining Characteristics	Clinical cues that cluster as manifestations of a nursing diagnosis. May be major or minor.	None	Same as actual diagnosis defining characteristics.
Related or Risk Factors	*Related factors* are conditions or circumstances that may cause or contribute to a diagnosis.	*Risk factors* are behaviors, conditions, or circumstances that render a client more vulnerable to a problem.	*Related factors* are same as actual diagnosis-related factors.

Excerpted from Gordon (1994:384–6).

related factors, but the concept is different for the two types of diagnoses. For actual diagnoses, related factors may be the etiology of the problem or concern. Related factors for wellness diagnoses list conditions or circumstances that promote wellness. High-risk diagnoses have risk factors instead of related factors. Risk factors are behaviors, conditions, or circumstances that render a client more vulnerable to a problem (Gordon, 1994:385). The identification of client risk factors guides nursing interventions to prevent the health problem. Table 8-1 provides a descriptive summary of the components of nursing diagnoses.

The diagnosis *Ineffective Breastfeeding* will be used to illustrate the different components of an actual nursing diagnosis. The name of the diagnosis is *Breastfeeding;* the word *Ineffective* is a qualifier. The definition of *Ineffective Breastfeeding* is "the state in which a mother, infant, and/or family experiences dissatisfaction or difficulty with the breastfeeding process" (Kim, McFarland, and McLane, 1993:7). Examples of factors related to difficulty breastfeeding are prematurity of the infant and a poor infant sucking reflex. Defining characteristics of *Ineffective Breastfeeding* include nonsustained suckling at breast and nursing less than seven times in 24 hours (Kim, McFarland, and McLane, 1993:7). See the box at right for other related factors and defining characteristics of *Ineffective Breastfeeding.*

Differentiation Among Components

Differentiating among diagnostic labels, etiologies, and signs and symptoms is not always easy. A diagnostic label can be the etiology for another diagnostic label when it describes a condition or circumstance that causes or contributes to a problematic human response (e.g., *Impaired Physical Mobility related to Activity Intolerance*).

Another area of difficulty is differentiating between signs and symptoms and the etiology. For example, is "dysfunctional eating pattern" a defining characteristic or a related factor of *Altered Nutrition: More than Body Requirements?* According to NANDA (1993), it is a defining characteristic. A dysfunctional eating pattern can be a manifestation of obesity; however, it could also be a condition that contributes to obesity.

Differentiating among components of nursing diagnoses is not easy because nursing is committed to holism. "The process of diagnostic labeling takes apart that which we understand to be an inseparable whole" (Randell, 1991:75). Careful attention to the nursing diagnosis definition and the descriptions of the four components of diagnoses in the NANDA system will assist in writing useful nursing diagnoses.

Nursing diagnoses reference manuals and pocket guides contain diagnostic labels, definitions, related factors, and defining characteristics for each diagnosis. Some references separate subjective and objective

---

◆

Sample of NANDA-Approved Nursing Diagnosis

Breastfeeding, ineffective The state in which a mother, infant, and/or family experiences dissatisfaction or difficulty with the breastfeeding process.

Related factors
    Prematurity
    Infant anomaly
    Maternal breast anomaly
    Previous breast surgery
    Previous history of breastfeeding failure
    Infant receiving supplemental feedings with artificial nipple
    Poor infant sucking reflex
    Nonsupportive partner/family
    Knowledge deficit
    Interruption in breastfeeding

Defining characteristics
    Unsatisfactory breastfeeding process
    Actual or perceived inadequate milk supply
    Infant's inability to attach on to maternal nipple correctly
    No observable signs of oxytocin release
    Observable signs of inadequate infant intake
    Nonsustained suckling at breast
    Suckling at only one breast per feeding
    Nursing less than 7 times in 24 hours
    Persistence of sore nipples beyond first week of infant's life
    Maternal reluctance to put infant to breast as necessary
    Infant exhibiting fussiness and crying within first hour after breastfeeding; unresponsive to other comfort measures
    Infant arching and crying at breast; resisting latching on

Excerpted from Kim, McFarland, and McLane, (993:7).

---

defining characteristics. Other references contain prototype care plans, as in Kim, McFarland, and McLane (1993). Use of a current nursing diagnoses reference is essential.

Writing Diagnostic Statements

Diagnostic statements are written to communicate client concerns and direct planning and nursing intervention. The basic format for writing a nursing diagnosis is a two-part statement. The statement consists of a descriptive component naming the human response and an etiological component stating factors related to the response. The descriptive part of the statement is used to construct client expected outcomes. Outcomes communicate the desired state of the client upon resolution of the health concern, including client behaviors indicative of problem resolution. Human responses of concern to nurses are resolved by eliminating the factors that cause or contribute to the concern. Therefore, both parts of the diagnostic statement are important in directing the planning for nursing intervention.

Basic Format: Two-part Statement
First Part: Descriptive

There are several ways to name human responses of concern. The name or label can be selected from a taxonomy or classification system of nursing diagnoses, such as the NANDA-approved list. Concerns may also be worded according to the specific nursing model used in the diagnostic process—for example, *Ineffective Interdependence related to stress from relationship with mother* (Roy's model). Individual nurses can name client concerns in their own words when no published diagnoses adequately describe the client's response.

Several NANDA diagnoses include the word "specify" after the label, e.g. *Knowledge Deficit (specify)*. Tailoring the diagnoses to the client increases the precision of the diagnosis and contributes to individualized care. Wilkinson (1992:135) suggests adding a "specific descriptor" to other nursing diagnoses as needed for greater specificity. For example, *Impaired Physical Mobility related to decreased strength and endurance* becomes *Impaired Physical Mobility: inability to walk related to decreased strength and endurance*.

The NANDA-approved list of nursing diagnoses contains individual and family diagnostic labels. Examples of individual diagnoses are *Altered Urinary Elimination* and *Impaired Physical Mobility*. Examples of family diagnoses are *Altered Family Processes* and *Parental Role Conflict*. Currently there are no community level diagnoses on the list, but two community diagnoses were included on a "to be developed" handout circulated at the tenth NANDA conference (Kim, McFarland, and McLane, 1993). Also, some current NANDA labels may be adapted for the community client.

All three types of diagnoses—actual, high risk, and wellness—are named with a descriptive statement. When writing an actual diagnosis, do *not* state the word "actual" in the diagnosis. It is understood that the diagnosis is actual unless the label indicates otherwise.

The NANDA list includes high-risk diagnoses, but any diagnosis can be used to describe a client at risk. Add the words "high risk for" to the nursing diagnosis when modifing a NANDA label. An example of such a diagnostic statement is *High risk for Hopelessness related to long-term stress*.

There are several possible ways of writing wellness diagnoses. Some possibilities use the NANDA system and others do not. Presently there are four wellness diagnoses in the NANDA system: *Health-Seeking Behaviors; Family Coping: Potential for Growth; Effective Breastfeeding;* and *Anticipatory Grieving*. These diagnoses may be used when the client situation matches the diagnosis. Another option within NANDA is to express NANDA problem labels in positive terms using the designated qualifier "potential for enhanced." An example of a wellness diagnosis using this alternative is *Potential for Enhanced Individual Coping*. Lastly, other words can be used with NANDA diagnoses to describe client wellness. For example, community health nurses adapted the NANDA taxonomy for wellness by adding special modifiers to the diagnoses, such as *Adequate* Diversional Activity and *Healthy* Sleep Pattern (Wilkinson, 1992).

Other sources of descriptive statements for wellness diagnoses are available. Duespohl (1986) and Houldin, Salstein, and Ganley (1987) identify wellness nursing diagnoses in their manuals. An example for an individual client is *Adequate Self Care related to use of personal and family resources*.

An alternative to writing wellness diagnoses is to list client strengths at the conclusion of the diagnostic process. Client strengths are identified and documented for care planning. Strengths are the resources of the client for health promotion, maintenance, and restoration. The identification and use of strengths is especially important for client self care. Examples of individual strengths are "effective coping" and "knowledge of condition." Examples of family strengths are "effective parenting" and "open communication." Community strengths could be "enthusiastic leadership" or "adequate health resources."

Identification of client strengths and wellness diagnoses is receiving increased attention as health care delivery focuses on illness prevention and health promotion. At the same time, cost containment and other factors constrain health care services. Few third-party payors reimburse for health promotion services, and wellness is not a priority in many nursing care situations. Nevertheless, nurses need to develop and market their expertise in health promotion with sick and well clients. It seems wise to limit the identification of wellness diagnoses to situations in which specific nursing intervention is intended and valued by nurse and client.

Second Part: Etiology or Related Factors

The etiology part of the diagnostic statement gives the nurse's perception of conditions or circumstances that contribute to the health concern. There are various kinds of related factors such as:

Environmental: odors, lighting, noises
Sociological: language, finances, support system
Spiritual: rituals, practices, beliefs
Physiological: fluid deficit/excess, hypothermia
Psychological: fear, anxiety, low self-esteem

Etiologies or related factors are identified in most nursing diagnosis manuals, which may be consulted when writing the nursing diagnosis statement. An example of a two-part diagnosis for an individual client is *Self-feeding Deficit related to pain*. A sample family diagnosis is *Altered Family Processes related to hospitalization of income provider*. An example for the community level is *Social Isolation related to cultural beliefs*.

An error to avoid when writing a diagnosis is reversing the parts of the diagnostic statement. This means mistaking the etiology as the problem and the problem as the etiology. Check for this error by reading the diagnosis backwards using the sentence "Etiology leads to Problem." For example, the parts of the diagnostic statement are reversed in the diagnosis *Support System Deficit related to altered parenting*. It does not make sense to read it backwards. When the two parts of the above diagnosis are exchanged to read *Altered Parenting related to support system deficit*, it does make sense. Another method to avoid this error is to use a nursing diagnosis reference book to facilitate wording.

There are several variations used in writing the etiological part of the diagnostic statement. The variations increase the clarity, specificity, and conciseness of diagnoses. Other variations attempt to avoid redundancy and deal with the realities of clinical practice. The variations are described below.

No Etiology

Some diagnostic labels are acceptable as one-part diagnostic statements. Such labels are narrow in scope and describe specific client responses (e.g., *Post-trauma Response*). Also, the treatment of the response varies little according to the etiology. For example, *Stress Incontinence* is a specific diagnosis, and nursing intervention would be similar whether the incontinence was related to weak pelvic muscles or an incompetent bladder outlet.

Another reason to use one-part diagnostic statements for some diagnoses is to avoid redundancy. For example, the only etiology listed for *Reflex Incontinence* is neurological impairment. Adding the etiology is not necessary to specify the response or direct nursing care. Thus the specificity of the label and the predictive value of the etiology for nursing action are

key considerations when deciding whether to omit an etiology.

Unknown Etiology

Sometimes the nurse identifies a client response but does not know the etiology or related factor(s). In this situation write the first part of the diagnostic statement, and state the etiology as "unknown etiology." For example, write *Spiritual Distress related to unknown etiology*. This is a temporary label until a specific cue search can be undertaken to find the etiology or related factor(s). In the meantime, knowing the descriptive label may provide some direction for care planning.

Multiple Etiology

Many client concerns have several contributing factors. Stating more than one etiology in the diagnostic statement saves time and decreases the total number of client diagnoses. In addition, identifying more than one etiology is necessary when nursing interventions differ because of their related factors. For example, *Sleep Pattern Disturbance related to fear of impending surgery, noisy environment, and pain*, would be treated by strategies to reduce fear, noise, and pain. Intervening to reduce environmental noise but taking no action to reduce the client's fear and pain would probably not be effective.

Complex Etiology

Human beings are complex and sometimes the etiology of a human response is difficult to determine. Wilkinson (1992:134) suggests using the phrase "complex factors" when the etiology or related factor(s) can not be reliably identified. Indeed, some complex NANDA diagnoses do not have related factors listed. For example, the related factors of the three diagnoses about self-esteem are yet to be developed. When self-esteem is a client concern, it might be appropriate to write *Situational Low Self-esteem related to complex factors*. Obviously, it is more helpful to identify the etiology whenever possible to focus intervention strategies.

Secondary Etiology

At times the diagnostic statement would more clearly describe the client if the etiology included the name of a pathophysiological or disease process. In such cases the phrase "secondary to" as part of the etiology enhances the diagnostic statement. For example, adding "radical mastectomy" to the diagnosis, *Ineffective Individual Coping related to body image disturbance secondary to radical mastectomy* provides more specific direction for planning care. Use of this etiological variation may not be necessary since medical diagnoses are highly visible.

Descriptive and Etiological Parts of the Nursing Diagnosis Statement: Joined by the Words "Related To"

The words "related to" indicate a relationship between the health concern and related factor(s). These words are not as legally or causally defining as "due to." The symbol "r/t" can be used to represent "related to" and will be used in the rest of this chapter.

The PES Format

A three-part PES format was identified by Gordon (1976) to write nursing diagnoses. The letters stand for a health problem (P), etiology (E), and the defining cluster of signs and symptoms (S). This format may help students write nursing diagnoses because "S" is the rationale for naming the concern. Including the cluster of signs and symptoms as part of the statement encourages accountability and verifies the diagnostic process. The following is an example of a nursing diagnosis written in PES format: *Anxiety* (problem) *related to hospitalization* (etiology) *as evidenced by restlessness, insomnia, facial tension, and statement of increased helplessness* (signs and symptom). The words "as evidenced by" may be abbreviated as A.E.B.

Misconceptions: What Nursing Diagnoses Are Not

In defining what nursing diagnoses are and understanding their development, it is also helpful to clarify possible areas of confusion. The list of misconceptions begins with one of the most common problems in accepting the term *nursing diagnosis*—the misunderstanding brought about by its confusion with the term *medical diagnosis*.

1. *The nursing diagnosis is not the medical diagnosis.* Nursing diagnoses must be within the legal and educational parameters of nursing. One attempt to clarify the legal scope of nursing is to divide nursing practice into independent and interdependent functions. Independent nursing interventions include activities of health promotion and education, disease prevention, nursing treatment (restoration or maintenance), and referral. Nursing diagnoses are limited to independent nursing practice where nurses are directly accountable for client outcomes.

Interdependent nursing functions are shared with others. Nursing participation in medical diagnosis and treatment is an important aspect of interdependent practice. Nurses are accountable for responsibilities within interdependent nursing practice, but they are not accountable for the outcomes of medical care. This means that (1) aspects of medical care performed by nurses must be integrated into the nursing care plan, and (2) medical diagnoses are excluded from nursing diagnoses.

There is no consensus within the nursing profession about how to incorporate medical care into the client's care plan. Medical terminology is sometimes used in nursing diagnoses, especially in the etiology; for example, *Self-esteem Disturbance r/t disfiguring surgery.* Stating the etiology using medical terminology provides little direction for nursing intervention and violates the definition of a nursing diagnoses. Weber (1991) suggests checking to see whether the first part of the diagnostic statement (the problem) could be the etiology of another diagnostic label, such as *Ineffective Individual Coping r/t self-esteem disturbance.* Nursing intervention would then be directed to both parts of the diagnostic statement.

Carpenito (1992) presents another option for incorporating medical care aspects (collaborative problems) into the nursing care plan. She defines collaborative problems as complications of a disease, test, or treatment that nurses treat interdependently. She suggests using the term *potential complication* to describe collaborative problems. The diagnostic statement for a collaborative problem would include both the possible complication and the disease, treatment, or other factors producing it. Nurse-initiated interventions in relation to the medical diagnosis could then be recorded under the collaborative problem; for example, *Potential Complication of Congestive Heart Failure: Pulmonary Edema.* The interdependence and collaboration between nursing and medicine will continue to be an important part of care delivery. At present there is no consensus about how to incorporate the medical-related activities of the nurse into nursing care planning. However, there is consensus that collaborative practice benefits client care. Shared documentation contributes to mutual communication and understanding.

2. *The nursing diagnosis is not a diagnostic test.* The nursing diagnosis reflects the client's response to the diagnostic test, such as a gallbladder x-ray, a computed tomography (CT) scan, magnetic resonance imaging (MRI), a biopsy, or a glucose tolerance test. The nursing diagnosis states the client's reaction to the test as shown in the following:

Incorrect: Liver biopsy
Correct: *Anxiety r/t unknown outcome of liver biopsy*

3. *The nursing diagnosis is not a medical or surgical treatment.* The nursing diagnosis reflects the client's response to the treatment. Examples of treatments to which clients may have specific responses are cast immobilization and chemotherapy. Possible client responses are fear, anxiety (anticipatory), depression (reactive), and hopelessness. The nursing diagnosis states the client's individual response to the treatment as shown in the following:

Incorrect: Radiation therapy
Correct: *Fear r/t anticipation of radiation therapy*

4. *The nursing diagnosis is not the equipment.* The nursing diagnosis may reflect the client's reaction to specific equipment such as a pacemaker, insulin pump, urinary catheter, and mechanical ventilator. Possible client responses to the equipment may be one or more of the following, depending on the type of equipment: impaired verbal communication, high risk for infection, powerlessness, anxiety, and self-care deficit. The nursing diagnosis states the client's reaction to the equipment as shown in the following:

Incorrect: Nasogastric tube
Correct: *Skin irritation of nares r/t nasogastric tube*

5. *The nursing diagnosis is not a single conceptual label.* Labels such as "immobilization" and "constipation" are too general and do not define the specific concern or show necessary relationships that are needed to develop meaningful individualized nursing orders. Examples of more definitive nursing diagnoses are shown in the following:

Incorrect: Immobilization
Correct: *Immobile in bed r/t neuromuscular impairment secondary to quadraplegia*

6. *The nursing diagnosis is not a single cue, sign, or symptom.* A nursing diagnosis describes a pattern of client behavior, not an isolated behavior or cue. Also, a nursing diagnosis is not a sign or symptom of illness such as elevated blood pressure, increased pulse rate, edema, thirst, or weakness. Nurses may use a nursing diagnosis reference to identify additional defining characteristics when concerned about a single client behavior. A sign/symptom of illness could be incorporated into a nursing diagnosis in two ways as shown in the following examples. The first example includes dysuria as a symptom, whereas the second example specifies dysuria as the disturbance in urine elimination. The last example illustrates an incorrect nursing diagnosis.

Correct: *Altered Urinary Elimination r/t mechanical trauma A.E.B. dysuria*
Correct: *Altered Urinary Elimination: dysuria r/t mechanical trauma*
Incorrect: Dysuria r/t mechanical trauma

Nurses need to be aware of misconceptions about nursing diagnoses, so they can avoid errors and understand how to write appropriate nursing diagnoses.

Guidelines for the Diagnostic Statement

The content of a nursing diagnosis is evaluated during its construction and after its completion. Nursing diagnoses should be accurate, concise, clear, client centered, and specific, and should provide direction for planning care. The following guidelines amplify and summarize the desired characteristics of a nursing diagnostic statement.

1. *The nursing diagnosis is a statement of an actual, high-risk, or wellness health concern.* The three types of diagnoses—actual, high risk, and wellness—were developed to describe different client health states. Information has been presented about how to write each type of diagnosis. Nurses are well prepared to assist both sick and well clients with health promotion, maintenance and restoration.

2. *The nursing diagnosis is written as a descriptive and etiological statement.* The basic format for writing a nursing diagnosis is to label the client's response to an actual or potential health problem with a descriptive statement followed by an etiological statement identifying factors contributing to the response. Suggestions have been given for writing useful diagnoses and avoiding errors, such as writing legally inadvisable statements and stating value judgments. For example, it would not be correct to write *High risk for fall r/t inconsistent use of side rails.* This diagnosis is incorrect because nursing diagnoses are to be client centered; the etiology should relate to the client's response, not the nurse's behavior. While it may be true that side rails are used inconsistently, there are better ways to correct the situation that pose less legal risk. It is also best to avoid value judgments about clients when writing diagnoses. For example, it is unwise to write *Fluid Volume Deficit r/t uncooperative patient.* Try to elicit the client's explanation for his or her behavior as one means of identifying a more helpful etiological statement.

3. *The nursing diagnosis is concise and clear.* Conciseness and clarity facilitate communication among peers and health team members. A concise, clearly stated diagnosis will be read and understood as opposed to a lengthy paragraph that takes time to read and unravel. The PES format is not concise so it is used more in nursing education than nursing service. Clarity is achieved by avoiding jargon or esoteric abbreviations. Using NANDA terminology when it describes the client response is another means to achieve clarity. Indeed, the whole purpose for NANDA and other systems of diagnoses is to give practitioners terminology for clinical communication.

4. *The nursing diagnosis is client centered, specific, and accurate.* Client-centered diagnoses are stated in terms of the client's response to intrapersonal, interpersonal, and environmental stressors. The nursing diagnosis

focuses on the client rather than the stressor. An incorrect statement would be "cluttered home r/t impaired home maintenance management." A client-centered nursing diagnosis would be *Impaired home maintenance management r/t insufficient family organization or planning.*

The diagnosis must specifically identify the client's response to an actual or potential health problem/life process. Precision is necessary for accurate communication and appropriate nursing interventions to be planned and implemented. The need for specificity and ways to achieve it have been addressed earlier in the chapter.

An accurate diagnosis is essential if nursing intervention is to be appropriate and effective. Several nurse activities contribute to diagnostic accuracy. First, check that NANDA terminology matches the client response/situation. Review the components of the diagnosis, such as the definition, and validate it with the client. If the label does not match the client's concerns, name the response in your own words. Do not redefine NANDA terminology. Second, remember that clinical cues are probabilistic and not absolute indicators of a client's health. Collecting multiple, reliable cues increases the chances of making an accurate diagnosis. It is also necessary to remember that a nursing diagnosis is an inference, not reality itself. Be open to other possible diagnoses if the client or others reject a diagnosis you identified. The diagnostic process is not an exact science.

5. *The nursing diagnosis provides direction for nursing intervention.* Nursing diagnoses are the basis for planning nursing intervention. Both the descriptive and etiological parts of the diagnostic statement provide direction for individualized nursing intervention. It is helpful to think about what you are inclined to treat when selecting the diagnosis. For example, rather than writing the diagnosis *Impaired mobility r/t blindness,* consider how the nurse would intervene. The nurse would safeguard the client during ambulation. Therefore a more useful diagnosis might be *High Risk for Injury: impaired mobility r/t newly diagnosed blindness.*

6. *The nursing diagnosis is the basis for independent and collaborative nursing actions/interventions.* The nurse identifies all areas of health concerns, including those for which others' expertise is needed. Nursing diagnosis within the independent sphere of practice has been discussed. Client concerns needing referral to other providers are within the interdependent or collaborative sphere of nursing practice. These concerns must be addressed by referring the client to an appropriate resource. For example, if a nursing diagnosis is *Anxiety r/t inadequate finances,* the nursing action is referral of the client to a social worker, the welfare department, or the Social Security office. Because anxiety can affect the client's ability to respond to nursing interventions for other nursing diagnoses, it must also be considered.

Collaborative nursing diagnoses and interventions are frequently related to the biomedical domain of nursing. The physician is responsible and accountable for diagnosing, prescribing, and treating the client's pathological condition. Nurses are responsible and accountable for assessing and reporting the client's response to the medical diagnoses and the treatment regimen. The nurse's knowledge and expertise regarding signs and symptoms of progress or potential complications of the client's pathological condition contribute to the biomedical aspect of the client's care. Equally important is the nurse's holistic approach to the client's concerns and the identification of concerns appropriate for nursing interventions to promote, maintain, or restore health.

Nurses differ about the scope of nursing diagnoses related to collaborative practice. Some nurses believe that nursing diagnostic labels, such as *Decreased Cardiac Output,* do not belong in NANDA's taxonomy because treatment of the diagnosis requires physician intervention. Other nurses believe that such labels do describe nursing diagnoses because, although physician intervention is needed, the majority of interventions are independent nursing actions. This will be an ongoing area of controversy and development.

7. *The nursing diagnoses are validated with the client.* There are two elements in validating nursing diagnoses. The first relates to the cluster or pattern of signs and symptoms that defines the diagnosis. This validation involves reviewing the data that led to the judgment, and verifying their sufficiency and accuracy. The nurse also evaluates the rationale on which the diagnosis is based to reinforce the reasonable degree of probability.

The second validation is an important aspect of nursing diagnosis and the one most frequently omitted: collaborating with the client to confirm the nursing diagnosis. Collaboration is an essential component of successful change for three reasons. First, working together is the basis of a trusting relationship and is more likely to provide accurate and valid data. Second, the trusting relationship provides the client with the support needed for risking and changing behaviors. Third, the collaborative relationship indicates mutual influence. According to Orlando (1961), if there is no mutual validation, the nurse is engaging in a nontherapeutic activity. In presenting the perceptions and interpretations to the client, one approach is to state: "After reviewing the information you gave me, it seems to me that there are a few areas we may be able to help you with. You told me that _____ was bothering you. I was wondering if you also saw _____ as something we could work on. Here are some other areas I would like you to tell me about. _____ What do you think about this one?"

The client's acceptance of the diagnostic statements usually indicates mutuality. If the client does not perceive the nursing diagnosis as accurately indicating a health concern, there is no mutuality and even the most comprehensive and sensitive nursing plans will be meaningless. Nursing care cannot exist in a vacuum, striving for written perfection without client participation. When the client does not acknowledge a health concern, the nurse may record the diagnosis as inactive, indicating it is still a concern but unacknowledged by the client.

Client involvement from the beginning establishes a participatory relationship and encourages the self-care concept. The only exceptions to this second phase of validation would be an emergency or an unconscious client.

After the list of diagnoses is validated, priorities must be determined. When the client and nurse are in agreement with the list of health concerns, they must rank the diagnoses according to client need for nursing intervention. Setting priorities provides a logical approach to a multiplicity of concerns and is discussed in the next chapter.

Documenting Nursing Diagnoses

Nursing diagnoses are compiled into a list and recorded on the client's chart. Since the client's plan of care requires knowledge of all client health concerns, an interdisciplinary problem list is best. The problem list should provide a system for dating entries and a method of noting the status of the health concern—active, inactive, or resolved. The problem list provides a capsule view of the client's health status.

Because assessment is ongoing, it is important to provide a strategy for obtaining the client information identified as data gaps. One option is to simply write "incomplete database" followed by a list of data gaps at the end of the nursing admission/assessment form. As the information is obtained it can be crossed off and integrated into the record.

The list of nursing diagnoses is reflective of the client's changing condition and responses. The initial list is not a fixed entity; it is flexible with the expectation of being updated. Nursing diagnoses made after initial data collection are usually tentative and require further assessment and validation.

As long as the client has a health concern, there will be continued adaptation and change in response to it. The nurse needs to assess these changes and adapt the nursing diagnoses and interventions to them. For example, after additional assessment, the nursing diagnosis may be changed from *Anxiety r/t impending surgery* to *Fear r/t body image disturbance.* Professional nurses continually use the diagnostic process to update and individualize client care.

Application of Models to Nursing Diagnosis

Nursing diagnoses are written for all three types of clients: individual, family, and community. The following discussion and tables describe how to apply the content of this chapter for each. In Tables 8-2 through 8-5, the first column identifies the model or model category. The second column contains the client response to the situation, state, or condition, which forms the descriptive part of the nursing diagnosis statement. The third column lists the etiology (related factors or risk factors), which forms the second part of the diagnostic statement.

Individuals

Nursing models that may be used for the individual include Roy (1991) and Orem (1991). Orem's model has three categories of self-care requisites: universal self-care, developmental self-care, and health deviation self-care. Health deviation requisites are associated with illness care. The two nursing diagnoses using Orem's model in Table 8-2 communicate the difficulty a client is experiencing during illness.

Roy's model consists of four modes: physiological, self-concept, role, and interdependence. Data categorized and processed within these modes could yield nursing diagnoses such as *Ineffective blood pressure control r/t inappropriate application of medication patch.* This diagnosis describes ineffective adaptation of a client in the physiologic mode. The vast majority of NANDA labels are for individuals. Three examples are presented in Table 8-2. The diagnoses represent the human response patterns of exchanging, feeling, and choosing, respectively.

Table 8-2	**Nursing Diagnoses for the Individual Based on Selected Models**

Model	Response	Etiology
Orem	Self-care deficit: Medications	Denial of illness and absence of plans to obtain medication
	Inadequate activity: Bedrest	Exacerbation of disease process
Roy	Ineffective blood pressure control	Inappropriate application of medication patch
	Ineffective role transition	Lack of maternal role model
NANDA	High risk for poisoning	Medication accessible to toddler
	Chronic pain	Occupational back injury
	Decisional conflict (termination of pregnancy)	Conflicting personal values/beliefs

Family

Nursing diagnoses of the family may be stated as functional, structural, or developmental depending on the model used. The diagnoses may be from one model exclusively or from the NANDA-approved list of nursing diagnoses. As with nursing diagnoses of individuals, family diagnoses may be related to actual or high-risk concerns, or with promoting and maintaining optimum family health.

Table 8-3 offers examples of family nursing diagnoses using several family models. Satir's (1972) Interactional Family Model contains four major concepts: communication, rules, self-worth, and social linkages. The nursing diagnosis, *Inflexible Rules r/t authoritarian values* demonstrates how Satir's concepts are used to formulate a family diagnosis. Major concepts of Friedman's (1986) model include structural components such as values, communication, and roles, along with functional components such as affect, socialization, economics, and family coping. Examples of nursing diagnoses using Friedman's concepts are *Ineffective Bonding (affective function) r/t prematurity of infant* and *Reversal of Roles r/t chronic illness*. Duvall (1977) and Stevenson (1977) are developmental theorists who list tasks and stages that

can be used as diagnostic categories. Hart and Herriott's (1977) systems theory categories are processes of adaptation to the environment, integration of the parts, and decisions regarding the first two processes. These categories may also be used to structure family nursing diagnoses. The purpose in writing family nursing diagnoses is to help the family achieve or maintain optimum health as it is defined within the model(s) chosen for nursing practice with families.

Community

Three models for the community client have been presented earlier in the text: General Systems (von Bertalanffy, 1968), Community-as-Client (Anderson, McFarlane, and Helton, 1986), and Community Competence (Goeppinger, Lassiter, and Wilcox, 1982). The Community-as-Client Model is an adaptation of Neuman's Health Care Systems Model. Each model can be applied at the geopolitical community level or with a smaller aggregate community. All three models include the concepts of community structure and process, although the concepts are emphasized differently.

Community nursing diagnoses may be stated according to structure or process. Structural diagnoses

Table 8-3	**Nursing Diagnoses for Families Based on Selected Models**	
Model	**Response**	**Etiology**
Satir	Inflexible *rules***	Misunderstanding or authoritarian values
	Decreased *self-worth*	Inability to share feelings, altered body image, or confusion from medication
Friedman	Inadequate recreation	Closed *societal links*
	Bonding	Prematurity of infant, cesarean section, or absence of role model
	Impaired *parenting*	Inconsistent discipline or lack of knowledge
	Reversal of *roles*	Chronic illness or absence of extended family
	Reduced income	Discontinued employment
Developmental	Inability to accomplish stage-specific *developmental tasks*	Dysfunctional communication or lack of knowledge
Systems	Deprivation of system *input*	Institutionalization
	Impaired *decision-making*	Confusion from medication or crisis
	Decreased safety in *environment*	Physical abuse or alcoholic mate
	Maintaining *equilibrium*	Adequate coping or open communications
NANDA approved (1992)	Ineffective family *coping:* compromised	Incorrect information or temporary role change
	Ineffective family *coping:* disabling	Highly ambivalent family relationship or unexpressed hostility in one member
	Potential for growth: family *coping*	Adaptation and progress toward self-actualization
	Altered family *process*	Situational or developmental transition or crisis
	Altered *parenting*	Lack of available role model, physical abuse, or lack of support from significant other, lack of knowledge

*Italicized words indicate major concepts within models, as mentioned in text on p. 148

Table 8-4	Nursing Diagnoses for Community Health Concerns Based on Structure and Process	
Model	**Response**	**Etiology**
Structure		
Demographic characteristics	Increased respiratory diseases	Air pollution, overcrowded conditions, or inadequate ventilation
	Increased dog bites	Packs of roaming dogs, inadequate code enforcement, or inadequate personnel and facilities
	Increased infant mortality rate	Cause unknown, inadequate nutrition, or increased teenage pregnancies
Aggregates	Inadequate prenatal facilities	Lack of funds or planning
	Increased lead poisoning in toddlers	Substandard housing or lack of prevention or knowledge
	Increased dental caries in school-age children	Poor hygiene or lack of knowledge
	Increased child abuse	Cause unknown
	Inadequate programs for substance abuse	Lack of funds or priority
	Lack of genetic counseling	Lack of personnel or knowledge of need
	Lack of gerontological services	Lack of planning or funds
Systems	Substandard housing	Economic recession, lack of funds for improvement, or high unemployment
	Inadequate transportation	Lack of state or federal funds or interest
	Decreased maintenance of sewers	Lack of information, personnel, or leadership
Process		
	Decreased communication	Political associations, sectionalism, or anger
	Lack of neighborhood participation	Apathy, lack of information, or cultural beliefs

Table 8-5	Nursing Diagnoses for Community Health Concerns Based on Adaptation of NANDA Categories of Choosing, Knowing, and Moving	
Model category	**Response**	**Etiology**
Choosing	Ineffective community coping	Lack of leadership, lack of finances
	Noncompliance: reporting communicable diseases	Lack of knowledge, insufficient staffing
Knowing	Inadequate school health program	Lack of knowledge, lack of finances, apathy
Moving	Social isolation	Lack of public transportation cultural beliefs

include those related to demographic characteristics, aggregates (groups with similar characteristics), or systems. Systems include sociocultural, political, recreational, housing, transportation, educational, religious, environmental, economic, and health care systems. Process diagnoses include communication, decision-making, participation, and leadership. Examples are given for structure and process diagnoses in Table 8-4.

Nurses can identify health concerns and affect change in many areas, with intervention pertaining to health maintenance, health promotion, health education, consultation, and disease prevention. Many community health nurses are also using the concepts of partnership, participation, and community development. It is the nurse's responsibility to work with the community in identifying the concerns and resources.

The nine human response patterns of NANDA can also be adapted for use at the community level. The category *exchanging* could relate to the community's inputs and outputs, including resources, products, services, and waste, among others. *Communicating* could include formal and informal networks and methods of communication such as printed or electronic media. *Relating* may refer to cultural, societal, and neighborhood patterns including recreational and social service availability and accessibility. *Valuing* includes the community's values such as the work ethic, nondiscrimination, health, and environmental safety. Examples of nursing diagnoses for some of the other NANDA categories are given in Table 8-5.

Summary

Nursing diagnostic statements are the basis for planning and nursing intervention. It is important that they are clear, concise, definitive statements of the client's actual, high-risk, or wellness health status and concerns. The nursing diagnoses must be amenable to nursing action and be validated with the client. They are written as descriptive and etiological statements. The diagnoses may be derived from the approved list of nursing diagnoses or from the professional nurse's experience and use of selected models for practice.

Critical Thinking Exercises BY ELIZABETH S. FAYRAM

1. Identify whether the following are correctly written nursing diagnosis statements. If a statement is incorrect, rewrite it in the appropriate format.
   a. Hyperthermia r/t increased temperature
   b. Impaired skin integrity r/t incontinence when asleep
   c. Ineffective coping r/t chemotherapy
   d. Obesity r/t altered nutrition: more than body requirements
   e. Pain r/t surgery
   f. Self-care deficit r/t inability to dress and feed self
2. Analysis and synthesis of the client's data identified a problem not listed in the NANDA taxonomy. Describe how to formulate a nursing diagnosis statement when the problem identified is not in a classification system.
3. Explain the advantages and disadvantages of using a classification system for nursing diagnoses.

4. Discuss how the client's positive aspects and strengths can be addressed in nursing diagnoses.
5. Mrs. Swenson is being discharged from the hospital following knee replacement surgery. She states, "I will be glad to go home. I'm ready. You've prepared me well for what to expect and do. But there is one thing I'm concerned about. My husband is not able to drive because of his poor eyesight. And I'm laid up with this knee So many of our friends don't drive in the winter. And our farm is way out in the country. I guess I'm worried that we'll be all alone."
   a. From the data, formulate a nursing diagnosis statement.
   b. Identify additional data that would be beneficial to obtain.
   c. Discuss how the above nursing diagnosis would be validated.

REFERENCES AND READING

American Nurses Association: *Standards of clinical nursing practice,* Kansas City, 1991, The Association.

Anderson ET and McFarlane JM: *Community as client: application of the nursing process,* Philadelphia, 1987, JB Lippincott.

Carpenito LJ: *Nursing diagnosis: application to clinical practice,* ed 4, Philadelphia, 1992, JB Lippincott.

Carroll-Johnson RM: *Classification of nursing diagnoses: proceedings of the ninth conference,* Philadelphia, 1991, JB Lippincott.

Duespohl TA: *Nursing diagnosis manual for the well and ill client,* Philadelphia, 1986, WB Saunders.

Duvall EM: *Marriage and family development,* ed 5, Philadelphia, 1977, JB Lippincott.

Friedman MM: *Family nursing: theories and assessment,* New York, 1986, Appleton-Century-Crofts.

Goeppinger J, Lassiter PG, and Wilcox B: *Community health is community competence,* Nurs Outlook 30(8):464, 1982.

Gordon M: Nursing and the diagnostic process, *Am J Nurs* 76:1298, 1976.

Gordon M: *Nursing diagnosis: process and application,* ed 3, St. Louis, 1994, Mosby.

Hart SK and Herriott PR: Components of practice. In Hall J and Weaver B, editors: *A systems approach to community health: distributive nursing practice,* Philadelphia, 1977, JB Lippincott.

Kim MJ, McFarland GK, and McLane AM: *Pocket guide to nursing diagnosis,* St Louis, 1993, Mosby.

Little D and Carnevali D: The diagnostic statement: the problem defined. In Walter JB and others, editors: *Dynamics of problem-oriented approaches: patient care and documentation,* Philadelphia, 1976, JB Lippincott.

Martin KS and Scheet NJ: *The Omaha system: applications for community health nursing,* Philadelphia, 1992, WB Saunders.

Orem DE: *Nursing: concepts of practice,* ed 4, St. Louis, 1991, Mosby.

Orlando IJ: *The dynamic nurse-patient relationship,* New York, 1961, GP Putnam's Sons.

Randell BP: Signs and symptoms, etiologies, diagnostic labels: what do we mean and where do we want to go? In Carroll-Johnson RM, editor: *Classification of nursing diagnoses: proceedings of the ninth conference,* Philadelphia, 1991, JB Lippincott.

Roy Sr C and Andrews HA: *The Roy adaptation model: the definitive statement,* Norwalk, Conn, 1991, Appleton & Lange.

Satir V: *Peoplemaking,* Palo Alto, Calif, 1972, Science and Behavior Books.

Stevenson JS: *Issues and crises during middlescence,* New York, 1977, Appleton-Century-Crofts.

von Bertalanffy L: *General systems theory: foundation, development, and applications,* New York, 1968, George Braziller.

Weber G: *Making nursing diagnosis work for you and your client,* Nurs Health Care, 12(8):424–30, 1991.

Wilkinson JM: *Nursing process in action. A critical thinking approach,* Redwood City, Calif, 1992, Addison-Wesley Nursing.

CHAPTER 9

PLANNING
Priorities and Outcome Identification

Paula J. Christensen

General Considerations

Plans for implementation are based on assessment and diagnosis of the client's health status, strengths, and concerns. After nursing diagnoses are validated, they provide direction for determining how to assist the client in resolving concerns related to the restoration, maintenance, and promotion of health. The descriptive and etiological clauses of the diagnosis help guide the nurse's development of the plan of care. The planning component involves judging priorities, establishing long-term expected outcomes, developing short-term expected outcomes, identifying strategies, and specifying nursing orders for implementation.

Traditionally, planning for client care was done *by* the nurse *for* the client. Formerly, it was usually based on the medical diagnoses. The client was passive and followed without question what the nurse recommended. The client viewed the physician and the nurse as "knowing best," and accepted treatment accordingly. As clients' knowledge of health and illness increased and nurses assumed responsibility and accountability for care given, the traditional bases for care were no longer valid. Currently, nurses assess their clients' health status and formulate individual plans for care *with* their clients. Plans still reflect the client's *medical* problems but now equally address *nursing* concerns: the client's *responses* to actual or potential health problems.

Planning, or determining how to assist the client in resolving health-related concerns, is through deliber-ate critical thinking, decision-making, and problem-solving with each client. This mutual planning process holds nurses accountable and responsible to clients for the agreed-on actions and subsequent outcomes.

The nurse's level of proficiency affects the phases of the planning component. The novice or beginning nurse bases planning on empirical knowledge gained from basic education, other nurses' experiences, and his or her own limited experiences. Judgments about each phase are deliberate, conscious decisions. The new nurse may need to consult other nurses regarding which nursing diagnosis is the top priority or what is a realistic time frame for the client to achieve the expected outcomes. As the nurse's expertise develops, these judgments are based on empirical and personal knowledge. Thus the nurse's experience provides a foundation for clinical judgments. Decisions continue to be conscious ones, incorporating empirical knowledge, yet the nurse learns to trust clinical intuition, which is a part of personal knowledge.

Nursing care standards, guidelines, policies, procedures, laws, and regulations are used to influence planning. However, based on the nurse's assessment and diagnosis of the client's situation, an individualized approach to alleviate the client's health concerns is developed. Nurses may identify health concerns that call for interventions by other health professionals. Decisions regarding consultations, referrals, and collaborative approaches to care are included in the plan as well.

The nurse collaborates with others while developing the plan. Information and ideas are sought from the client, people directly involved with the client, other nurses, and health team members. A multidisciplinary approach to care is particularly important for clients with complex health concerns. Resource people for individual and family client plans include clinical nurse specialists, social workers, physicians, dietitians, activity therapists, nutritional support specialists, physical therapists, and chaplains. All these offer their own expertise to facilitate a comprehensive and effective plan. Resource people for a community client plan may include an organizational developer or trainer, a financial consultant and planner, a management educator, a long-range planning consultant, and a state representative. Goal-oriented group meetings of these and other experts often yield unique and varied ways to assist the client in attaining an optimal level of health and functioning. The ideas generated for the plan are then shared with the client to ensure mutuality of intent and accountability for action. The nurse must use professional judgment in choosing which plans to share in detail with the client. Some clients, because of their health status, limitations, and age, are not capable of being completely involved in the mutual planning process. However, decisions regarding which plans to use should involve the client as much as possible to increase the client's sense of personal control and commitment to the plan.

This chapter focuses on the first three phases of planning: judging priorities, establishing long-term expected outcomes, and developing short-term expected outcomes. Guidelines for these elements are as follows:

1. Prioritizing nursing diagnoses
   a. Actual or imminent life-threatening concerns are considered before actual or potential health-threatening concerns.
   b. Temporal, human, and material resources are examined deliberately.
   c. The client is involved in determining the priority of concerns.
   d. Scientific and practice principles provide rationale for decisions.
2. Establishing long-term expected outcomes
   a. Long-term outcomes are client-focused and reflect mutuality with the client.
   b. Long-term outcomes are appropriate to their respective diagnosis.
   c. Long-term outcomes are realistic, reflecting the capabilities and limitations of the client.
   d. Long-term outcomes include broad or abstract indicators of performance.
   e. Scientific and practice principles guide the establishment of long-term expected outcomes.

3. Developing short-term expected outcomes
   a. Short-term outcomes are client-focused and reflect mutuality with the client.
   b. Short-term outcomes are appropriate to their respective goal.
   c. Short-term outcomes are realistic, reflecting the capabilities and limitations of the client.
   d. Short-term outcomes include specific indicators of performance.
   e. Short-term outcomes are numbered in appropriate sequence to achieve the long-term outcome.
   f. Scientific and practice principles guide the development of short-term outcomes.

All phases of the planning component are necessary to give direction for quality nursing care. Identifying strategies and specifying nursing orders for implementation are discussed in Chapter 10. Individual, family, and community clients need effective planning to achieve desired outcomes.

Judging Priorities

The process of judging priorities begins with the list of nursing diagnoses. Arranging these diagnoses in priority involves thinking about and deciding on a preferential order of the client's concerns. Making this choice, however, does not mean that one concern must be totally resolved before another is considered. Usually several diagnoses are focused on concurrently.

The act of choosing one diagnosis as the most important is based on several factors. Threats to life and health; temporal, human, and material resources available; the client's involvement; and standards, guidelines, policies, procedures, laws, and regulations all play a part in judging priorities.

Guidelines for Judging Priorities

1. *Actual or imminent life-threatening concerns are considered before actual or potential health-threatening concerns.* Diagnoses that involve life-threatening concerns, such as severe depletion or loss of function, should be considered first. Examples of life-threatening concerns for the individual, family, and community are as follows:

Individual:	Loss of cardiac, respiratory, or mental function
Family:	Loss of parent(s), home, or job
Community:	Water pollution, hurricane, tornado, nuclear radiation accident

Actual or potential health-threatening concerns are those that may impair functioning, or growth and development if not corrected. Examples of health-threatening concerns for the individual, family, and community are as follows:

Individual: Increase in life stressors along with decreased ability to cope, acute illness
Family: Addition of family member, long-term illness of family member
Community: Loss of key health care facility, major industry, or tax base

2. *Temporal, human, and material resources are examined deliberately.* The amount of time that the nurse has to work with the client affects the actual and potential diagnoses chosen on which to focus. The client in particular benefits from a sense of accomplishment; therefore, diagnoses in which short-term gains can be achieved will be important at first. In regard to human resources, the nurse determines whether the number of people and their qualifications and skills are adequate to attend to the client's concern. Material resources such as money, equipment, and supplies also need to be sufficient for intervention to be successful. For example, the nurse working in a marginally funded inner-city clinic for indigent clients has different resources from those of a nurse working for a wealthy suburban home health care agency. The nurse in the clinic may see the client on an infrequent and irregular basis. Thus, time with the client is limited, and usually only high-priority actual health concerns are dealt with. Staffing, equipment, and supplies may also be inadequate because of lack of funds. Therefore the people and materials would be scarce and could negatively impact eventual attainment of outcomes.

3. *The client is involved in determining the priority of concerns.* The client's involvement is essential when arranging concerns in order of importance. Because nurses work mutually with clients, the nurse considers the client's (1) understanding of the health concerns and related situation; (2) values, thoughts, and feelings about resolving health concerns; (3) general state of health; and (4) ability to solve problems. The client must have an adequate knowledge of the health concerns and the situation. The nurse is responsible for assessing the client's knowledge level and teaching the client relevant information on which to make informed decisions. The client's values, thoughts, and feelings about resolving health concerns have an impact on the client's cooperation with certain interventions. For example, an individual client who smokes two packs of cigarettes per day and knows the health-related hazards may choose to continue to smoke. Plans to help the client quit smoking will be unsuccessful so long as the client does not *value* health promotion or does not *think* that facts will influence the decision to smoke. The client's general state of health influences the client's ability to be involved in judging health concerns. A client who is psychotic or uncon-

scious will have little involvement compared with the client who is awake and oriented. In the former situation, the client and the client's family should be informed of the priorities set by the nurse. If appropriate, the client's family is included in setting priorities for concerns. The client's ability to solve problems also influences how active the client will be in determining priorities. Severe anxiety, stress, and an altered level of consciousness often impair a client's thinking process, leading to disorganization and an inability to make decisions. If possible, the nurse facilitates improved problem solving by using the problem-solving strategy and clearly summarizing the specific problem so that the client can focus on it. Details of this strategy are given in Chapter 10. Individual, family, and community clients are involved in judging priorities.

4. *Scientific and practice principles provide rationale for decisions.* Judging priorities is facilitated by the use of theories, models, and principles. One model often used to evaluate the relative priority of diagnoses is Maslow's (1968) hierarchy of needs. Maslow identifies basic needs that all people share: air, food, safety, and love. Growth needs are not necessary for sustaining life but they promote self-growth, such as self-esteem and self-actualization. Basic needs are more important than growth needs; the individual must have basic needs met before focusing on growth needs. Using this model with a client who has unmet basic and growth needs, the nurse develops and implements plans for the unmet basic needs first.

Working with individual clients, physiological principles are also helpful in judging concerns. Consideration of these principles guides the nurse in giving immediate attention to life-threatening concerns. For example:

1. Knowledge that increased intracranial pressure can lead to changes in vital signs and to possible brain damage takes precedence over personal hygiene.
2. Knowledge that high blood pressure poses a threat to circulatory and cardiac status takes precedence over learning about borderline diabetes.

Isolated data and patterns of data give the nurse cues that aid in judging precedence. Examples of *isolated cues* that lead to immediate plans and interventions include vital sign readings significantly above or below general or client norms, and sudden changes in behavior. Examples of *patterns observed over time* that indicate a need for plans and interventions include gradual changes in vital signs and subtle changes in how the client relates to others. Table 9-1 provides an example of a client's prioritized health concerns using this rationale.

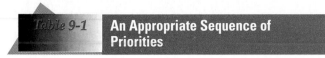

Table 9-1 **An Appropriate Sequence of Priorities**

Nursing diagnosis	Sequence of priorities	Rationale
Knowledge deficit related to nutrition in pregnancy	3	Latent health concern that can be dealt with concurrently with 2
Altered cardiopulmonary tissue perfusion: fluid volume excess	1	Most life-threatening concern at this time
Increased anxiety related to first pregnancy and fear of the unknown	2	Threatening mental health and potential threat to physical health

Standards, guidelines, policies, procedures, laws, and regulations influence the nurse's decision-making regarding priorities. They give direction—in varying capacity and degree—to nursing practice issues ranging from an authoritative principle or rule to suggested advice. Generally, though, nurses still use their own judgment along with these sources to individualize the client's priorities.

Outcome Identification

Client outcomes are labeled as long-term outcomes and short-term outcomes. Achievement of long-term outcomes results in the resolution of the health concerns indicated by the nursing diagnoses. Attainment of short-term outcomes leads to the achievement of their respective long-term outcome. The time frame of expected outcomes is related to the nature of the health concern, the availability of resources, the type of agency in which the care is being provided, and the characteristics of the clients.

For example, consider a male client who recently had a myocardial infarction and is still in an acute care setting. This person has a nursing diagnosis of "alteration in nutrition related to inadequate dietary intake." A long-term outcome for this client is to improve nutritional habits and adhere to recommended dietary guidelines (on his own volition). This outcome is beyond the time limits of his anticipated stay at this setting. Some short-term outcomes that are needed to achieve the long-term outcome are well within the time and resources available. The client is able to learn about food groups, dietary guidelines, and food preparation, and to adhere to the recommended diet as prepared by the institution. In this situation then, the long-term outcome reaches into the future, even past the client's discharge from the agency, and beyond the constraints of the immediate situation. The short-term outcomes focus on current means to alleviate the concern and to develop the client's knowledge, skills, and abilities in order to attain the long-term outcome. Continuity of care is facilitated through planning for both short-term and long-term resolutions to health concerns. Nurses work with clients to promote, maintain, and restore their optimal level of health through enhancing the achievement of expected outcomes.

Establishing Long-Term Expected Outcomes

After priorities have been determined, the nurse establishes long-term outcomes that flow directly from the nursing diagnosis, especially the descriptive clause. These are statements that lead to alleviation of the concern indicated by the diagnosis. A long-term outcome reflects a goal that states a broad or abstract intent, state, or condition (Mager, 1984).

Long-term outcomes often reach beyond the time a client is in direct care or service within an institution. These outcomes lead to the client altering physiological and psychological responses, attaining psychomotor skills, increasing knowledge, and developing abilities. Because these statements describe a *client's* outcome, they are used as one basis to evaluate progress. If the nursing diagnoses reflect specific client concerns, then only one long-term outcome is needed per diagnosis. However, diagnoses stated in broad terms usually require more than one long-term outcome statement.

Example

Nursing diagnosis (specific):	Inadequate exercise related to lack of frequency per week
Long-term outcome:	The client will increase frequency of exercise within 1 month.
Nursing diagnosis (general):	Alteration in metabolism related to inadequate insulin production
Long-term outcome:	The client will stabilize metabolism within 1 week.
Long-term outcome:	The client will decrease susceptibility to altered metabolism within 1 month.

Nature of Long-Term Outcomes

The nature of the long-term outcome depends on the diagnosis: long-term outcomes reflect health restoration, maintenance, or promotion. *Health restoration outcomes* are appropriate when a client's internal or external resources are inadequate or diminished.

Example

Nursing diagnosis:	Depleted nutritional state related to anorexia
Long-term outcome:	The client will develop an adequate nutritional status within 1 month.

Health maintenance outcomes are appropriate when the client wants to increase the existing internal or external resources or continue using those resources.

Example

Nursing diagnosis: Decreased use of open communication skills related to busy schedule
Long-term outcome: The client will increase use of open communication skills within 2 weeks.

Health promotion outcomes reflect a desire to function at a higher level of health, to grow beyond merely maintaining health.

Example

Nursing diagnosis : Increased concern regarding lack of knowledge of parenting skills for adolescence
Long-term outcome: The client will increase knowledge of parenting skills for adolescence within 3 weeks.

Long-term outcomes need to be realistic so that the client can achieve them. Therefore in determining the nature of the outcome, the nurse assesses the client's available internal and external resources. If resources are not readily available to achieve the outcome, it may need to reflect resource development first and include modification to realistically align the outcome to available resources.

Differences and similarities between client's and nurse-expected client outcomes must be considered. The nurse may have a greater knowledge base than the client, which could help the client understand the nature of the identified diagnoses; the client can help the nurse understand his or her own concerns and motivation. The nurse is responsible for establishing long-term outcomes for the client that are mutually acceptable to both the client and the nurse.

Relationship to Theories, Models, and Principles

The models used in the analysis and synthesis of data provide direction for establishing long-term outcomes. Theories and principles describe norms of behavior and functioning, and determine the rationale for the outcome.

Satir's (1967) model, for example, discusses healthy communication, describing in detail the concepts of functional and dysfunctional communication. This information assists the nurse in establishing a long-term outcome for a client with dysfunctional communication.

Example

Nursing diagnosis: Dysfunctional interpersonal communication related to the use of blaming and projection
Long-term outcome: The client will use functional (leveling) communication with the family within 3 months.

Immobility is an example of a physiological concept with principles that gives direction to long-term outcome development. Most nursing texts elaborate on the concept of immobility and its effects on body functions as well as on the psyche. That baseline knowledge about the concept and its related principles guides the client and nurse in planning to reduce the effects of immobility.

Example

Nursing diagnosis: Potential hazards of immobility related to prolonged bed rest
Long-term outcome: The client will decrease susceptibility to hazards of immobility within 6 days.

Any reliable source that describes norms of behavior can be used to assist the nurse in developing client long-term outcomes. Table 9-2 gives examples of long-term outcomes for different clients and shows how a variety of sources is used in establishing them.

Table 9-2 | Long-Term Expected Outcomes with Different Theoretical Bases

Client	Nursing diagnoses	Long-term outcomes	Theoretical bases
Individual	Altered health maintenance related to inadequate exercise	The client will exercise adequately within 1 month	Diekelmann (1977)
Family	Impaired affective functioning related to lack of separateness	The family will demonstrate affective functioning within 6 months	Friedman (1992)
Community	Inadequate decision making related to use of coercion	The client will develop a democratic form of decision making within 1 year	Hart and Herriott (1985)

Developing Short-Term Expected Outcomes

After long-term outcomes are established for the diagnoses, short-term expected outcomes are developed to specify client performances and behaviors related to the long-term outcome. Whereas long-term outcomes are derived from the descriptive clause of the nursing diagnosis, short-term outcomes flow from the etiological clause. Short-term outcomes are more immediate in nature and are usually achievable while the client is in the direct care of service of an institution. A short-term outcome describes an intended result of a particular action, not the process of the action itself (Mager, 1984). Usually three to six short-term outcomes are needed for each long-term outcome.

Three reasons exist for developing short-term outcomes (Mager, 1984). First, short-term outcomes *give direction* for selecting or designing nursing strategies and orders. Second, a properly stated short-term outcome *implies* the content of, potential materials needed for, and method of the strategy or order. Third, short-term outcomes provide a *means* for the nurse and client to *organize effort*. Short-term outcomes are therefore useful tools in the design, implementation, and evaluation of client care.

Characteristics of Short-Term Outcomes

Three characteristics of short-term outcomes that communicate their intent are performance, conditions, and criterion (Mager, 1984).

Performance

A performance is any activity engaged in by the client. It can be an activity that is directly observable or not directly observable but assessable. Overt client performances are those that can be directly seen or heard. Verbs that indicate overt performances, which are directly observable behaviors, include recite, list, sort, verbalize, demonstrate, name, select, and state.

Covert performances are mental—invisible or cognitive—but have a direct way of being assessed. Verbs that indicate covert performances include identify, solve, use, compare, and determine. Whenever the performance stated in a short-term outcome is covert (such as identify), an indicator behavior (such as state) needs to be added to the   statement.

Example

Overt verb:	The client will demonstrate proper insulin administration according to the American Diabetic Association within 1 week.
Covert verb (with indicator behavior):	The client will identify (state) three complications of bed rest within 2 days.

The short-term outcome creates a picture of what is expected of the client, communicating its intent to the client and those reading it. Each important outcome or performance is written in a separate statement. Therefore each short-term outcome contains only one performance verb.

Conditions

A short-term outcome may indicate the conditions under which the client is to complete the performance. Conditions may include the experiences that the client is expected to have had before completing the outcome, the resources available for use during the performance of the outcome, and the environmental conditions under which the client will carry out the performance. The conditions are included if they are essential to meeting the outcome. Conditions need not be included if the performance clearly states what is expected.

Example

Short-term outcome with clear expectations:	The client will state three barriers to effective communication within 1 week.

Below are examples of the three ways that conditions may be stated in a short-term outcome.

Condition	Example
The experiences before completing the short-term outcome	*After attending* two group sessions of diabetic classes, the client will name two major types of diabetes.
The resources available during the performance of the short-term outcome	*Given a menu* of a variety of foods, the client will circle the foods comprising a 2000-calorie intake for 1 day.
The environmental conditions during the performance	*When at home* the client will maintain a 2000-calorie diet according to the American

Criterion

The criterion is the standard by which a performance is evaluated (Mager, 1984). Criteria within the short-term outcome statement may be stated in one of four ways:

1. *Speed:* Set a time limit that is reasonable, given the client's health and the client's and nurse's capabilities and limitations.
2. *Accuracy:* Identify a specific degree of performance quantitatively.
3. *Quality:* Indicate the standard that is expected in terms of given acceptable procedures.

4. *Criterion referenced:* Use books, pamphlets, or other resources as a guide. Criteria give direction to nursing orders for meeting the short-term outcome. They also provide a measure to evaluate the achievement of the outcome.

Below are examples of the four ways of stating criteria in short-term outcomes.

Criterion

Speed	The client will name four complications of bed rest *within 3 days.*
Accuracy	The client will list *four or five* symptoms of high blood glucose concentrations.
Quality	The client will catheterize self using *aseptic technique.*
Criterion referenced	The client will describe (state) three components of the self-breast examination *according to* the American Cancer Society.

Domains of Short-term Outcomes

Short-term expected outcomes related to client learning situations can be classified into three domains, which provide direction for selecting and individualizing the strategies and orders. This is a classification of the *intended* behaviors, or the way people are expected to *think, feel,* or *act* as a result of participating in given learning experiences.

The three identified domains are cognitive, affective, and psychomotor (Bloom, 1956). *Cognitive outcomes* are associated with changes in knowledge or intellectual abilities and skills. A hierarchy of six major classes within this domain vary from simple recall of material to complex mental processes, such as analysis, synthesis, and evaluation of ideas. The six classes are as follows:

1. *Knowledge:* ability to remember and recall specific information as well as major schemes and patterns; the ability to organize, study, judge, and criticize
2. *Comprehension:* ability to make use of material or information without understanding its full implications
3. *Application:* ability to use abstractions in particular and concrete situations
4. *Analysis:* ability to clearly differentiate elements of a whole and their relationships
5. *Synthesis:* ability to constitute a pattern or structure not clearly there before; to create a whole out of its elements
6. *Evaluation:* ability to judge the value of material or methods for given purposes based on a standard of appraisal

Each class within this hierarchy requires achievement of behaviors within the preceding classes. As the behavior becomes more complex, the person is more aware of its existence. The nurse determines the level of understanding expected by the client in a learning situation and helps determine what is necessary to accomplish the outcome identified.

Affective outcomes emphasize changes in interests, beliefs, attitudes, values, or feelings, and may be expressed by adjustments or behavioral changes (Krathwohl and others, 1964). They include a degree of acceptance or rejection on the part of the participant. The hierarchy of five major affective categories reflects levels of internalization of an interest, belief, or attitude. The categories range from minimal awareness of a value to the commitment to that value that guides or controls the person's behavior. These categories are described as follows:

1. *Receiving* (attending): being aware of and willing to receive or attend to the existence of certain phenomena and stimuli (e.g., values, beliefs, attitudes, feelings)
2. *Responding:* having a low level of commitment or interest in the phenomena and stimuli to receiving a sense of pleasure or satisfaction accompanying the behavior
3. *Valuing:* being motivated by a value to display behavior consistently with held value; displaying loyalty and conviction to a value
4. *Organization:* determining interrelationships among values for self and establishing those that are most important
5. *Characterization by a value or value complex:* acting consistently in accordance with internalized values; integrating beliefs, ideas, and attitudes to one's own philosophy or world view

The person eventually makes adjustments or changes in behavior based on the interests, beliefs, attitudes, values, and feelings as they are increasingly internalized. Clients usually state their acceptance of a new value or attitude before acting on it. Working with clients in the affective domain is subjective and personal. The nurse exercises discretion, showing respect for the client's choices while providing necessary information and care to promote the client's optimal level of health. Affective outcomes, in particular, include the performance (verb), condition, *and* criterion—or evaluation criteria—to evaluate the client's achievement.

Psychomotor outcomes focus on developing the ability to perform a manipulative or motor skill. These skills are usually achieved in a complex combination with cognitive and affective abilities (Singer, 1972). The seven major levels vary from a basic awareness of senses involved to creating new motor acts. Simpson

(1966) and Urbach (1970) classified the psychomotor skills as follows:

1. *Perception:* awareness of objects, qualities, or relations through the use of the senses; knowing what is essential to the act being performed
2. *Set:* mental, physical, and emotional readiness for an experience or action
3. *Guided response:* experience or action is attempted on the part of an individual under the guidance of an instructor or self using imitation or trial and error; performance is judged using a model or example
4. *Mechanism:* some confidence and proficiency is gained by performing the action; the learned response has become habitual
5. *Complex overt response:* smooth, efficient, and automatic performance, with minimal expenditure of time and energy
6. *Adaptation:* ability to master the challenge of a problem situation requiring adjustment of learned response
7. *Origination:* ability to create new motor acts based on previously acquired awareness, performance, and psychomotor skills

Psychomotor outcomes are appropriate when the client needs to learn a particular technique or skill. The level of proficiency expected is determined by the client's health status, functional ability of the senses, previously learned (related) skills, dexterity, motivation and interest, cognitive abilities, biophysical strengths and limitations, sociocultural influences, environment, nurse-client relationship, and the nurse's knowledge and expertise as a teacher.

Cognitive, affective, and psychomotor domains are separated for purposes of categorizing behaviors, yet they are not mutually exclusive. People usually do not think without feeling, act without thinking, or feel without acting. When developing educational outcomes related to a learning situation, the nurse identifies the domain of each outcome to facilitate selecting strategies and orders. However, the nurse must be aware of the interplay among the cognitive, affective, and psychomotor aspects of the client. Therefore more than one domain may be involved in the achievement of expected outcomes.

The following are examples of short-term outcomes in three domains that each meet one long-term outcome:

Example

Nursing diagnosis: Alteration in nutrition (more than body requirements) related to imbalance of intake and excess eating

Long-term outcome: The client will consume an adequate nutritional diet following the rec-

ommended guide to daily food choices within 3 weeks.

Short-term outcomes: 1. The client will recall the food-guide pyramid and recommended servings within 3 days (cognitive).
2. The client will identify (state) the importance of a balanced diet within 1 week (affective and cognitive).
3. The client will incorporate the recommended American Diabetic Association diet into eating patterns within 2 weeks (psychomotor and cognitive).

Different verbs indicate client behaviors within each of the domains. These action verbs help differentiate the expected outcomes of the client. Below are lists of verbs that represent the three domains:

Cognitive	Affective	Psychomotor
Recall	Accept	Show
Inform	Appreciate	Imitate
List	Enjoy	Demonstrate
Discuss	Desire	Practice
Interpret	Listen	Assist
Distinguish	Relate	Perform
Apply	Regard	Master
Compare	Participate	Adapt
Evaluate	Judge	Create

Relationship to Theories, Models, and Principles

The specific performances included in short-term expected outcomes are based on the same theories, models, and principles used in establishing long-term expected outcomes. When short-term outcomes are developed, an in-depth understanding of the approach is necessary. The following example shows how the nurse's knowledge of the concept of immobility, related principles, hazards, and ways to prevent complications influences the development of short-term outcomes.

Example

Nursing diagnosis: Increased susceptibility to hazards of immobility related to decreased mobility

Long-term outcome: The client will decrease susceptibility to hazards of immobility while hospitalized.

Short-term outcomes: 1. The client will participate in four preventive measures four times a day within 1 day.
2. The client will verbalize four hazards of immobility within 2 days.
3. The client will identify (state) one way to decrease susceptibility to each hazard within 2 days.

4. The client will incorporate at least three preventive measures into daily routine four times a day within 4 days on client's own volition.

The specifics of range of motion, skin care, deep breathing, and turning could be included in the short-term outcomes themselves or referred to in the nursing orders.

Below is another example of long- and short-term outcomes, based on Satir's (1967) model. This example demonstrates the use of specific information about the importance of functional communication, barriers to it, and techniques of it. The examples of short-term outcomes show varying degrees of specificity.

Example

Nursing diagnosis: Dysfunctional communication related to the use of blaming and projecting.

Long-term outcome: The client will increase functional communication within 1 month.

Short-term outcomes: 1. The client will describe why functional communication is important, according to Satir, within 2 days.
2. The client will state three barriers to functional communication within 1 week.
3. The client will identify (state) two verbal and three nonverbal functional communication techniques within 1 week.
4. The client will use three functional communication techniques while talking to family within 3 weeks.

Guidelines for Outcome Identification

The following guidelines for outcome identification are derived from the ANA Clinical Standards of Practice (1991):

1. *Expected outcomes are client-focused and reflect mutuality with the client.* The long- and short-term outcomes are worded in *client* terms. Beginning each outcome with the terms "the client will" facilitates client focus. Mutuality is attained through communication with the client and involved persons about identified health concerns and strengths. The nurse discusses nursing diagnoses and related long-term outcomes with the client to determine whether the client also recognizes the strength or concern and is willing to direct energy toward supporting, diminishing, or alleviating the conditions identified in the diagnoses.

Situations can arise when individual clients are unable to participate in the development of long- and short-term outcomes because of an alteration in health status or age. The nurse is then responsible for including the client's family in decision-making. The expected outcomes still need to be worded in client terms.

Example

Nursing diagnosis: Altered sensory perception related to decreased level of consciousness

Long-term outcome: The client will maintain or improve present level of consciousness indefinitely.

Short-term outcomes: 1. The client will participate in the assessment of level of consciousness daily.
2. The client will accept auditory and tactile stimuli provided by the nurse at least every 2 hours.

2. *Long-term outcomes are appropriate to their respective diagnosis, and short-term outcomes are appropriate to their respective long-term outcome.* The nursing diagnosis is the basis for each respective long-term outcome. Therefore long-term outcomes should clearly relate to the nursing diagnosis. Attainment of the long-term outcome supports the strengths or diminishes or alleviates the concerns identified by the nursing diagnosis.

Example

Nursing diagnosis: Alteration in nutrition (less than body requirements) related to inadequate food intake

Long-term outcome: The client will consume an adequate nutritional diet within 1 month (clearly relates to diagnosis).

Long-term outcome: The client will learn about adequate nutrition within 1 month (limited relationship to diagnosis).

Learning about adequate nutrition does not necessarily lead to better nutrition. The first long-term outcome clearly states that the client will consume an adequate nutritional diet. The long-term outcome is the basis for its respective short-term outcomes and should be sufficient for the attainment of the long-term outcome.

3. *Expected outcomes are realistic, reflecting the capabilities and limitations of the client.* The client must perceive the expected outcomes as realistic to be motivated to achieve them. Being realistic involves developing long- and short-term outcomes that reflect the client's capabilities and limitations of internal and external resources. Examples of external resources to consider are time, money, family support, social agencies, personnel, and equipment. Examples of internal resources to consider are biophysical status, mental health, and coping patterns.

Inasmuch as health is a relative term, not all long-term outcomes can reflect maximum health status.

Each client has an optimum potential for health that is reflected in the long-term outcomes.

Example

Client:	40-year-old recently divorced man
Nursing diagnosis:	Lack of socialization related to recent divorce
Long-term outcome:	The client will develop a social support system within 6 months.

Example

Client:	20-year-old single, mentally retarded woman
Nursing diagnosis:	Lack of socialization related to overprotection of family
Long-term outcome:	The client will increase participation in activities involving people other than family within 3 months.

4. *Long-term expected outcomes include broad or abstract indicators of performance.* Because a long-term outcome is broad or abstract by nature, the use of verbs such as improve, decrease, increase, maintain, promote, develop, and restore is appropriate. General criteria can be included in a long-term outcome to give more direction to strategies and nursing orders.

Example

Nursing diagnosis:	Decrease in neighborhood safety related to poor lighting and limited patrols
Long-term outcome:	The client will increase neighborhood safety within 6 months (without general criterion).
Long-term outcome:	The client will improve neighborhood safety by increasing street lights and patrols within 6 months (with general criterion).

Either outcome statement is correct; both are client-focused and give a general direction for further plans.

Another aspect of stating long-term outcomes is their reference to a time element. The length of time is determined by considering the client's health status and available resources. The resources include both the client's and nurse's capabilities and limitations.

5. *Short-term outcomes include specific indicators of performance.* Short-term expected outcomes need to be more specific than long-term outcomes, referring to observable and measurable behaviors to meet the long-term outcome. Each short-term outcome statement includes the person, the performance, and a specific criterion. Conditions may be added to clarify the meaning. The performance needs to be assessable, and the criterion for assessment can be stated in terms of time, accuracy, quality, or reference. Time is usually included in all short-term outcomes because it gives the client and the nurse a guideline for pacing activities realistically. Refer to pp. 156-157 for examples of short-term outcomes with a variety of specific performances and criteria. These specific indicators of performance serve as a basis for evaluating the client's progress toward the long-term outcome.

6. *Short-term outcomes are numbered in the appropriate sequence to achieve the long-term outcome.* Proper sequencing or time ordering of short-term outcomes gives direction to and understanding of what is expected. Communicating this sequence helps the client recognize success in movement toward long-term outcome achievement.

7. *Scientific and practice principles guide the establishment of long-term outcomes and the development of short-term outcomes.* Expected outcomes are based on norms of behavior and functioning indicated in biophysical, psychological, sociocultural, and spiritual sciences. Theories, models, and principles from nursing and other practice disciplines provide the rationale for the outcomes. Standards of nursing care such as those developed by the American Nurses Association (1991) and specialty nursing organizations also give direction for client outcomes. In addition, state nurse practice acts define the scope of nursing practice, and health care institutions develop standards and mores of practice.

Summary

The planning component of the nursing process is based on a sound assessment and diagnosis of the client's health status, strengths, and concerns. Judging priorities, establishing long-term outcomes, and developing short-term outcomes constitute the first three phases of planning for implementation. Long-term outcomes are broad and abstract; short-term outcomes reflect specific behaviors and a shorter time for achievement. Identifying strategies and specifying nursing orders for implementation are the last two phases of planning. These elements are discussed in Chapter 10.

Each phase of planning is based on the nurse's knowledge of theories, models, and principles. Sources describing norms of behavior and functioning serve as the rationale for planning. To ensure client motivation and cooperation, the client must be involved in decision-making regarding priorities and expected outcomes.

Critical Thinking Exercises BY ELIZABETH S. FAYRAM

1. Prioritize the following nursing diagnoses and state the rationale for your decisions:
   a. A 6-month-old infant admitted to the pediatric unit with dehydration and vomiting.
      Fluid volume deficit
      High risk for altered body temperature
      High risk for altered nutrition: less than body requirements
      Interrupted breastfeeding
   b. A 78-year-old woman hospitalized for uncontrolled diabetes and leg ulcer.
      Altered thought processes
      Impaired skin integrity
      Pain
      Self-care deficit: hygiene and toileting
   c. A family, whose mother is dying, involved with a hospice agency.
      Altered role performance
      Anticipatory grieving
      Caregiver role strain
2. Kevin is 15 years old and has leukemia. He is undergoing chemotherapy. A priority nursing diagnosis is *High risk for infection r/t decreased immune function.* Write expected client outcomes for this specific nursing diagnosis.
3. Discuss how the nurse involves the client in the planning component. Explain why it is beneficial for clients to be involved in planning. Identify the consequences when clients are not as actively involved as possible.
4. You are working with a 32-year-old woman with rheumatoid arthritis. You have selected Orem's Self Care Theory of Nursing to guide the nursing process. One of the nursing diagnoses is *Impaired physical mobility r/t pain and joint inflammation.*
   a. Describe how Orem's model influences the planning component, including long-term and short-term expected outcomes.
   b. Write expected client outcomes for the above nursing diagnosis: include at least one outcome related to the teaching/learning process.
   c. For the outcome(s) related to client learning, identify the appropriate domain and its respective level (e.g., cognitive—application; psychomotor—guided response; affective—receiving).

REFERENCES AND READINGS

American Nurses Association: *Standards of clinical nursing practice,* Kansas City, 1991, The Association.

Atkinson L and Murray M: *Understanding the nursing process,* ed 4, New York, 1990, McGraw-Hill.

Bloom B, editor: *Taxonomy of educational objectives: the classification of educational goals. Handbook I: cognitive domain,* New York, 1956, David McKay.

Carpenito LJ: *Nursing diagnosis: application to clinical practice,* ed 5, Philadelphia, 1993, JB Lippincott.

Diekelmann N: *Primary health care of the well adult,* New York, 1977, McGraw-Hill.

Friedman MM: *Family nursing: theory and assessment,* ed 3, Norwalk, Conn, 1992, Appleton-Century-Crofts.

Hart SK and Herriott PR: Components of nursing practice: a systems approach. In Hall J and Weaver B, editors: *Distributive nursing practice: a systems approach to community health,* ed 2, Philadelphia, 1985, JB Lippincott.

Iyer PW and Camp NH: *Nursing documentation: a nursing process approach,* St Louis, 1991, Mosby–Year Book.

Iyer PW, Taptich BJ, and Bernocchi-Losey D: *Nursing process and nursing diagnosis,* ed 2, Philadelphia, 1991, WB Saunders.

Krathwohl D, Bloom B, and Masia B: *Taxonomy of educational objectives: the classification of educational goals. Handbook II: affective domain,* New York, 1964, David McKay.

Mager R: *Goal analysis,* ed 2, Belmont, Calif, 1984, Pitman Learning.

Maslow AH: *Toward a psychology of being,* New York, 1968, D Van Nostrand.

Maslow AH: *Motivation and personality,* ed 2, New York, 1970, Harper & Row.

Peplau HE: *Interpersonal relations in nursing,* New York, 1952, GP Putnam's Sons.

Pinnell NN and deMeneses M: *The nursing process: theory, application, and related processes,* Norwalk, Conn, 1986, Appleton-Century-Crofts.

Reilly D: *Behavioral objectives in nursing: evaluation in nursing,* ed 3, New York, 1990, National League for Nursing.

Satir V: *Conjoint family therapy,* rev ed, Palo Alto, Calif, 1967, Science and Behavior Books.

Simpson EJ: *The classification of educational objectives: psychomotor domain,* Urbana, Ill, 1966, University of Illinois Press.

Singer RN, editor: *The psychomotor domain: movement and behavior,* Philadelphia, 1972, Lea & Febiger.

Singer RN: *The learning of motor skills,* New York, 1982, Macmillan.

Urbach F, editor: *The psychomotor domain of learning,* Papers presented at Teaching Research, Salishan, Oreg, 1970, The Department of Higher Education, Monmouth, Oreg.

CHAPTER 10

PLANNING
Strategies and Nursing Orders

Elizabeth S. Fayram
Paula J. Christensen

General Considerations

The identification of strategies and specification of nursing orders are the last two phases of the planning component. These phases build on the priorities and expected outcomes, becoming even more specific in determining how to assist the client in resolving health-related concerns. The model incorporated with the nursing process influences the selection of strategies and nursing orders within the planning component.

Strategies and nursing orders are prescriptive in nature. That is, the *nurse* identifies which actions are most appropriate, based on the nurse's knowledge base, experience, and familiarity with the client situation. The nurse considers the autonomy and individuality of the client when choosing actions; yet the client now, more than ever, depends on the nurse to provide direction and support.

After expected outcomes are established, the nurse decides which strategies will facilitate their achievement. Similar to expected outcomes, strategies are directly related to the nursing diagnosis. A strategy is an overall method or approach that serves as a guide for individual nursing orders. Strategies are accepted methods and approaches that stem from many science and practice disciplines. Examples of strategies discussed in this chapter include teaching and learning, therapeutic use of self, contracting, and principles of nursing practice.

Nursing orders are individualized prescribed behaviors that flow from the strategies identified and lead to predictable client outcomes. The client as well as the nurse is included in the actions, along with others needed to achieve the desired outcomes.

This chapter focuses on the description of various strategies, how to choose strategies, and implications for their use. Nursing orders are discussed in terms of specific actions relating to the client's unique situation. Nursing care plans are addressed as tools that facilitate achievement of expected outcomes and implementation of strategies and nursing orders. The guidelines emphasized are as follows:

1. Strategies
   a. Major strategies for implementation are identified.
   b. Strategies are appropriate to their expected outcomes.
   c. Strategies are based on scientific rationale.
   d. Strategies are mutually determined with the client.
2. Nursing orders
   a. Nursing orders are appropriate to their respective outcomes and strategy.
   b. Scientific and practice principles provide rationale for orders.
   c. Nursing orders incorporate the autonomy and individuality of the client.
   d. Nursing orders indicate specific intended behaviors, giving direction to the nurse, client, and others.
   e. Nursing orders reflect consideration of human, temporal, and material resources.

f. Nursing orders are numbered in the appropriate sequence to achieve the short-term outcome.

g. Nursing orders are dated and include the signature of the responsible nurse.

h. Nursing orders are kept current and are revised as indicated.

i. Nursing orders include plans for termination of nursing services.

Strategies

An important part of the planning component is the selection of strategies. As discussed previously, a *strategy* is an overall method or approach that serves as a guide for individual nursing orders. Strategies arise from the science and practice disciplines, including psychology, sociology, education, and nursing.

Critical thinking skills are used when strategies are selected. The nurse begins by identifying possible strategies, then evaluates the merits of each strategy and makes a decision as to which strategy is likely to achieve the desired client outcome.

Strategies are selected based on the model incorporated into the nursing process, as well as on the nursing diagnosis and expected outcomes that have been formulated. The model and its concepts provide guidance to the nurse in the selection of strategies. When using Orem's Self-Care Theory of Nursing (1991), the nurse considers strategies fostering self-care such as teaching and learning, contracting, and problem solving. Neuman's Health-Care Systems model (1989), with its emphasis on stressors, reaction to stress, and levels of nursing interventions, guides the nurse in the selection of strategies such as stress management and teaching and learning.

More than one strategy may be appropriate to achieve the desired outcomes for a given client. The nurse suggests the strategy most appropriate at that particular time based on the client situation, age of the client, and the nurse's expertise with the various strategies. When selecting strategies, the nurse considers the client's strengths, such as the ability to problem solve and to communicate; the client's limitations, such as health problems; and the client's internal and external resources, such as coping patterns and support from family members. Several strategies could be considered for a client with the nursing diagnosis of "alteration in nutrition, more than body requirements," for example—teaching and learning, contracting, and behavior modification. Based on client variables such as the client's knowledge of the food pyramid and cognitive development, the nurse suggests the strategy (or strategies) best suited for the situation. Having a variety of strategies to choose from provides the nurse and client with additional choices if revision of the plan is necessary.

Many situations are appropriate for client participation in the selection of strategies. An example is the client who desires to try a behavior modification program in an attempt to lose weight. The nurse, however, has the expertise concerning the strategies and is best able to determine which strategy is likely to be successful based on the nursing diagnosis and expected outcomes. The nurse educates the client and explains the rationale for the choice of the strategy, especially if it differs from the one the client chose. Then, a mutual decision regarding which strategy to use is made.

Strategies discussed in the following section are (1) teaching and learning, (2) problem solving, (3) therapeutic use of self, (4) caring, (5) stress management, (6) behavior modification, (7) contracting, (8) group process, and (9) principles of nursing practice. Guidelines, principles, or steps are presented whenever possible to direct the nurse with specific nursing orders when using the selected strategy.

Teaching and Learning

The teaching and learning process is a strategy frequently used by professional nurses in a variety of settings and with various types of clients: individuals, families, and communities. The teaching and learning process is useful when dealing with health promotion and with health maintenance or restoration. Examples of when the teaching and learning process is appropriate are (1) a community group learning the benefits of, and foods included in, a high-fiber diet (health promotion); (2) an individual client with newly diagnosed diabetes mellitus learning the symptoms of hyperglycemia and the appropriate actions to take (health maintenance); and (3) a spouse learning to care for the client's ulcerated lesion (health restoration).

Bloom (1956) identified three domains of learning: cognitive, affective, and psychomotor. The cognitive domain deals with intellectual ability such as recall or recognition; the affective domain deals with changes in attitudes and values; the psychomotor domain involves skill or motor development. The teaching and learning process is an appropriate strategy for use with all three domains of learning.

The nurse, as teacher, becomes the facilitator of learning. The nurse involves the client in the teaching and learning process, including assessment of the need for learning, planning learning experiences, implementing the learning experiences, and evaluating learning outcomes.

The teaching and learning process is integrated into the nursing process based on the expected outcomes that have been formulated. Principles of teaching and learning are used to facilitate learning. These principles are presented according to the components of the nursing process (Pohl, 1981; Redman, 1993; Rordan, 1987; Whitman, 1992).

Assessment

The nurse may find it necessary to return to the assessment component when the strategy of teaching and learning has been selected.

Learning needs of the client must be determined. Before a teaching plan is developed and implemented, the client's learning needs must be assessed. The client's learning needs vary based on previous knowledge and experience, and the present situation.

Perception of the need to learn by the learner facilitates learning. Perceived needs for learning and priorities placed on learning by the client influence whether learning occurs. Perception of the need to learn is influenced by the person's beliefs, values, and previous experiences.

Physical and mental readiness are necessary for learning. A learner must have the physical and mental ability to learn. Physical readiness is related to developmental level and physical health status; mental readiness refers to the cognitive abilities to understand, assimilate, and apply. The nurse considers the effect of developmental levels and health status on the client's physical and mental readiness. The level of readiness is evaluated in relation to the level of learning to be accomplished. When the client is not physically or mentally ready to learn, the nurse includes significant others in the learning situation.

A client must be motivated in order to learn. For learning to occur, the client must have a willingness or desire to learn or change. A client may be motivated for numerous reasons, such as need, status, fear, and achievement. Motivation may be constant or temporary, strong or weak, and will be directed toward the most pressing concern at the time. Frequently the nurse is involved in stimulating the client's motivation to learn. This may be accomplished by helping the learner to know what is to be learned and the reason for the learning. Providing incentives to learn, such as benefits of learning, and dealing with other more pressing concerns first, such as anxiety or discomfort, also facilitate motivation.

The emotional climate affects learning. The client's emotions have a strong influence on ability to learn. The nurse examines the client's feelings about the topic and his or her current emotional state. When intense emotions are present in the learner, such as extreme anxiety or fear, very little learning can occur. Through effective communication techniques, the nurse helps the client deal with the emotions before attempting teaching and learning.

Knowledge of the client's cultural-ethnic patterns is essential. The health practices and beliefs of clients based on cultural diversity must be identified. To in-

dividualize the learning situation requires knowledge of the cultural pattern of the various groups that the nurse most frequently encounters.

Diagnosis

Following analysis and synthesis of the assessment data, a nursing diagnosis is formulated for which the teaching and learning process is the selected strategy. Examples of nursing diagnostic statements are as follows:

Knowledge deficit (parenting skills) related to lack of experience as a parent and lack of role models

Ineffective individual coping related to lack of knowledge of effective stress management (e.g., relaxation techniques)

Planning

The planning component for the teaching and learning process includes formulating expected outcomes related to learning and selecting learning activities with suitable materials and techniques.

Expected outcomes serve as guides in planning teaching-learning experiences. The client and nurse determine what learning needs are to be accomplished and establish long-term and short-term expected outcomes to be achieved. The desired outcomes serve as criteria for evaluating achievement of learning.

New learning must be based on previous knowledge and experience. Building on previous knowledge and experience increases the effectiveness and efficiency of the teaching and learning process. Determining the client's current level of knowledge and experience about a topic before providing new information reduces the chance of misunderstanding by the client who lacks specific information or is misinformed. The nurse can also avoid repeating information the client is already familiar with, a repetition that might hinder the client's interest in learning.

Learning is a sequential process that proceeds from simple to complex. The nurse determines nursing orders to achieve the desired outcomes, being aware of the sequencing of content and experiences. For example, a client learning new nutritional habits may read about foods included and excluded in the diet and the reasons for the nutritional change, discuss with the nurse how extensive a change would be required in the client's nutritional pattern, plan a 3-day food plan incorporating the guidelines, and prepare food at home for a week based on the new nutritional guidelines.

Teaching/learning techniques and materials are selected based on client needs. A variety of teaching/learning techniques are available, such as explanation, discussion, demonstration and practice, and experiences such as role playing. In addition, teaching/learning sessions may occur on a one-to-one basis or in group sessions. The short-term expected outcomes, the domain of learning (cognitive, affective, psychomotor), and the specific client's developmental level and learning style determine the techniques used. For example, a 4-year-old client learning about the surgical experience is provided with a role-playing situation using real equipment such as masks and intravenous (IV) equipment. Written and audiovisual materials are selected to facilitate and reinforce learning. They are used in combination with the interactive techniques. Written materials are reviewed for accuracy, content, the ability to meet the short-term outcomes, and the appropriateness of the material for the client. Learning is aided by involving as many of the learner's senses as possible.

Implementation

Implementation of the teaching and learning process occurs through active involvement of the client and significant others when appropriate. The nurse's ability to develop an effective nurse-client relationship is an important factor in the effectiveness of the teaching and learning.

An effective nurse-client relationship is important for learning. A positive interpersonal relationship enhances learning. Client learning is facilitated when the nurse and the client have a relationship that is trusting, cooperative, comfortable, and caring.

Effective learning requires active participation. Active involvement on the part of the learner through participation in the teaching and learning process facilitates learning. The client (and significant others as appropriate) is an active participant during identification of learning needs and the planning, implementation, and evaluation of learning experiences. During implementation, active participation may involve a variety of activities, such as using the senses (e.g., sight and hearing), performing a physical activity, and using cognitive processes. The nurse provides opportunities for participation and encourages the client to ask questions. The more actively the client participates, the more effective the learning.

Teaching and learning require effective communication. New information is learned through effective verbal and visual communication techniques. Effective communication is accomplished when the listener grasps the meaning conveyed by the speaker. The nurse uses feedback from the client to validate that the client understands the information correctly.

Effective teaching and learning require time. First, the nurse sets aside time to develop an effective teaching plan. Second, the nurse collaborates with the client to find the most appropriate time for implementing the teaching plan.

Control of the environment is an aspect of teaching. The nurse considers personal and environmental factors that influence client learning. The comfort of the client and the elimination of distracting interruptions are important factors that promote an effective learning environment.

Repetition strengthens learning. Continued practice enhances the learner's retention of new information and the formation of new behavior patterns. Different clients need varying numbers of repetitions for effective learning, depending on the complexity of the content to be learned and the client's abilities to learn.

Reinforcement influences learning. When a person receives satisfaction in learning new behaviors, these new behaviors will be retained longer. Personal pride in accomplishment is a strong incentive for learning and retaining new skills. The nurse considers both internal (personal) and external (reward or praise) factors that facilitate client satisfaction in learning.

Evaluation

Evaluation involves evaluating the expected outcomes, client responses to the learning, and the nurse's ability to use the teaching and learning process.

Long-term and short-term expected outcomes serve as the basis for evaluation of learning. Because the nurse "taught" the client does not mean the client has learned. The client exhibits achievement of the learning outcomes to validate having achieved the newly learned behaviors. Various evaluation methods are used, such as verbal statements and return demonstrations. Revision of the plan may be necessary to achieve the desired outcomes.

The nurse evaluates his or her own ability to use the teaching and learning process. The nurse identifies his or her own strengths and limitations in applying the principles of the teaching and learning process and ways to improve in that ability.

The basic principles presented describe methods of learning and factors that the nurse considers when facilitating client learning. Many of these principles provide the scientific rationale for nursing orders when implementing the teaching and learning process.

Problem Solving

The use of the problem-solving process as a strategy involves assisting clients in identifying a specific problem, generating alternative solutions, analyzing consequences, and making a thoughtful decision regarding an identified concern. The nurse, as in the teaching and learning process, is the facilitator. The nurse guides the client toward making a decision and supports the client in the process.

For the client to participate in the problem-solving process, several factors are necessary. The client must have the authority to participate in the problem-solving process and to make the decision. The client's ability and desire to generate and analyze alternatives, as well as the client's beliefs and preferences, are also factors. Last, the client must accept participation in the problem-solving process and in making the decision.

The problem-solving process consists of the following steps:

1. Identification of the problem and purpose/goal of the problem-solving process
2. Development of alternative solutions to the problem
3. Consideration of consequences for each of the alternatives
4. Selection of a specific alternative
5. Implementation of the decision
6. Evaluation of the effectiveness of the problem-solving process

When using problem solving as a strategy, the *first step* is to ensure that all involved have accurately identified the problem (e.g., nursing diagnosis) and factors influencing the problem. Those involved also need to understand the purpose of the problem-solving process and the outcome to be achieved by implementation of the decision.

The *second step* is to explore possible alternatives to resolve the problem. The client, from previous knowledge and experience, may be able to generate alternatives. Additional alternatives also may be generated from the nurse's knowledge and experiences, as well as from other health team members and resource material (e.g., community resources).

Factors identified by Bower (1982) as influencing the generation of alternatives are (1) the number of alternatives being considered at one time, (2) the number of people participating in the problem-solving process, and (3) the amount of time available in which to make the decision. Creativity, such as the use of brainstorming techniques, is another factor that influences the generation of alternatives (Gillies, 1989).

Usually two to four alternatives are generated. More than four becomes confusing and consumes more time when the consequences of each alternative are considered. If too much time is spent generating alternatives and making the decision, then action to deal with the problem is delayed. When generating alternatives, resources and constraints are considered, including finances, people, equipment, policies, and procedures.

The *third step* is to consider the consequences of the various alternatives. Each alternative is analyzed to determine whether it could achieve the goal and is also analyzed for cost and risk. Cost factors not only include financial support necessary but also time, en-

ergy, equipment, and people. Risk includes consideration of safety, comfort, and side effects. Feasibility is also deliberated, including policy considerations and the protection of the rights of others. Acceptance of the alternative by those affected must also be weighed. The nurse plays an important role in helping the client analyze the various options.

Selection by the client of a specific alternative is the *fourth step*. The chosen alternative is one that satisfies the stated long-term outcome and has many of the desirable consequences. The nurse facilitates the client in making the decision, but it is ultimately the client who decides.

The *fifth step* involves implementation of the decision as agreed on by the nurse and client. It should be clear to all involved as to who is to implement what and when.

Evaluation is the *final step* of the problem-solving process. Evaluation methods are considered and planned before the decision is implemented. Evaluation of the decision includes the determination of expected outcome attainment, the consequences that have occurred, and the need to reconsider the alternative that was selected.

Bailey and Claus (1975) have identified several *obstacles* to effective problem solving. One such obstacle is *failing to specify purposes and goals*. If the outcome is unclear, then appropriate alternatives may not be considered. *Plunging into action* occurs when a decision is made before considering relevant alternatives. *Jumping to conclusions* may occur when the cause of the concern is incorrectly identified, and the decision may or may not solve the concern. *Failing to look at probable consequences* means not considering the costs or risks adequately; thus undesirable consequences may occur. The nurse, who facilitates problem solving by the client, can minimize these obstacles to effective problem solving.

Problem solving is an appropriate strategy to use with clients in a variety of situations. For example, the problem-solving process could be used by the individual client who must make a decision regarding living arrangements following discharge from an acute care facility, or the community client in deciding about the distribution of health care services. The strategy requires active participation by the client. The greater the involvement by the client, the greater the client's commitment to the decision and the greater likelihood of follow-through. This promotes feelings of independence and esteem and provides problem-solving skills for future use.

Therapeutic Use of Self

In considering strategies to use with clients, nurses may consider using their own personalities. This strategy is known as therapeutic use of self and is the conscious effort by the nurse to use his or her personality for the purpose of benefitting the client. In a therapeutic nurse-client relationship, the client's identity is maintained and self-esteem is enhanced (Sundeen, 1993).

Therapeutic use of self is appropriate when clients need to express feelings, enhance their self-esteem, or clarify values. This strategy may be useful with a client who has recently undergone body changes, whether from trauma, illness, surgery, or growth, and needs to adjust to a change in body image. Using this strategy, the nurse assists the client to express feelings about body changes and what they mean to the client. This strategy may also be useful with family members, such as parents of a child with a chronic illness. Other examples include a new mother who lacks self-esteem regarding parenting abilities or a pregnant teenager clarifying her values.

Values clarification facilitates a person's identification of meaningful values and the priorities of these values (Stuart and Sundeen, 1991). Exploration of the relationship of a person's values with the decisions made and actions taken occurs through the values clarification process (Steele and Harmon, 1983). This process is facilitated by a therapeutic nurse-client relationship. The values clarification process identifies what is meaningful to the client, fosters the client's ability to make choices regarding significant values, and aids in understanding self. The nurse assists the client in realizing conflicting values and making decisions for the reestablishment of values and their priorities. An example involves a nurse, who through a therapeutic nurse-client relationship, facilitates a 21-year-old spinal cord–injured client's clarification of values in terms of sexuality and self-care.

The nurse, to be effective in therapeutic use of self, must commit to develop and grow in four areas: self-awareness, use of facilitative communication techniques, ability to develop a nurse-client relationship, and acceptance of others.

Self-awareness is the understanding of oneself. Nurses need to understand themselves before understanding others. This involves questioning one's own feelings and actions, maximizing one's strengths, minimizing limitations, and accepting self. Four aspects of the personality are considered in the process of self-awareness (Sundeen, 1993): body image (how one feels about one's body), self-ideal (who one wants to be), self-concept (who one is), and self-esteem (judgment of one's own worth). The more one's self-ideal and self-concept are similar, the greater will be one's self-esteem. These four aspects of personality influence the nurse's actions and interactions and are therefore an important aspect of self-awareness.

Using facilitative communication techniques includes congruent verbal and nonverbal communication,

which fosters the client's sharing of feelings or information. Facilitative techniques include sitting down with a client, using open-ended questions and encouragement for the client to express feelings, seeking clarification, respecting that the client may not want to interact at a particular point in time, actively listening, and using silence and touch appropriately.

In therapeutic use of self, the nurse develops a *collaborative relationship* with a client for the client's benefit. Characteristics of a nurse-client relationship include trust, empathy, caring, autonomy, and mutuality (Sundeen, 1993). *Trust* develops when the nurse is consistent and reliable. *Empathy* involves accurate perception of the client's feelings. *Caring* is demonstrated by showing respect and concern for the client. *Autonomy* involves recognition of the client's need for control. *Mutuality* is the active participation by the client to the extent possible.

Last, therapeutic use of self involves *acceptance of the client* and the client's values. Accepting the client's feelings, respecting differing values, and being responsive to individual differences are examples of nurse behaviors in accepting the client.

Nurses who use therapeutic use of self have certain characteristics and abilities. They have a stable self-concept and positive self-esteem, as well as the abilities to face the reality of situations. In addition, they are able to use verbal and nonverbal communication techniques effectively, relate to clients in a natural, congruent manner, and function as a role model. The nurse who uses therapeutic use of self assists clients to face reality and promotes their own self-acceptance.

Caring

Caring is a crucial element for health, human development, and human relationships (Leininger, 1988). Professional nursing care, with an emphasis on personalized caring, involves cognitive and culturally learned behaviors that enable an individual, family, or community to improve or maintain health status.

One dimension of caring is that it is an integral part of nurse-client relationships. A client's health status is influenced by the relationship that the nurse establishes and maintains. Clients themselves indicate that person-to-person communication is an important ingredient of the caring behavior (Leininger, 1988). Watson (1985) states that caring is effectively demonstrated interpersonally and that the quality of the nurse-client relationship is the most significant element. Characteristics of this relationship include congruence, empathy, and nonpossessive warmth.

Another dimension of caring builds and expands on the first. This second dimension is concerned with helping the client to grow and develop (Mayeroff, 1971). This aspect of caring develops over time and enhances the quality of the client's life. It is selected as a strategy for use with a particular client based on the client's concerns. An example involves a nurse and the caring relationship that forms with a pregnant teen-aged client who has few social supports. The teenager has been sexually abused by a relative but is not believed by other family members. The nurse forms a long-term relationship with the client, providing support and guidance as the client gives birth to a child and completes high school.

Second-dimension caring activities are intentional activities by the nurse to bring about a positive change in the client. Effective caring accepts who the person is and who that person may become. An important activity involves gaining knowledge. The nurse obtains knowledge of the client, including the client's needs, strengths, and limitations, and how to respond to those needs. Caring activities also include determining outcomes related to the identified need, planning, and implementing care to meet desired outcomes, which results in a positive change for the client. By using the nursing process effectively, the nurse demonstrates caring activities.

Leininger (1988:49-50), in studying caring behaviors in a variety of cultures, identified more than 30 components of care, including:

Comfort	Touch	Restoration
Support	Protection	Tenderness
Attention	Surveillance	Trust
Compassion	Personalized help	Instruction
Empathy	Presence	Direct assistance

These components of caring have been classified into four general areas (Ray, 1988:104-108):

1. *Psychological*
   Affective: empathy, compassion, patience
   Cognitive: teaching, observation, decision-making
2. *Practical*
   Social organization: time, coordination, safety
   Technical: skill, equipment
3. *Interactional*
   Physical: comfort, touch
   Social: communication, listening, reassurance, support
4. *Philosophical*
   Spiritual: spiritual concern, faith
   Ethical: attitude, trust, individualized care, respect
   Cultural: understanding of cultural care

This framework provides the nurse with a means of categorizing caring behaviors. Thus the nurse has several means of exhibiting caring toward clients.

Second-dimension caring makes a significant difference in the health of individuals, families, and communities. It involves deliberate, individualized actions by the nurse, with a sense of commitment to assist the client in resolving concerns and meeting expected outcomes.

Stress Management

Stress management is a strategy that facilitates the client's ability to deal effectively with the stress confronting people in contemporary society. As a strategy, it emphasizes active participation by the client to develop skills to manage stress. Stress management involves identifying the stressors present, evaluating the effectiveness of existing coping mechanisms, and developing more effective coping mechanisms.

An important aspect of stress management is the client's ability to cope. Coping is the effort to master a situation that is perceived as being harmful, threatening, conflicting, or challenging (Monat and Lazarus, 1977). The ability of a client to cope with a particular situation is influenced by (1) personal characteristics, (2) resources available, (3) the situation, and (4) coping patterns the client has developed.

Personal characteristics that influence coping include stage of development, personal values and goals, beliefs about self, roles, and responsibilities. The client's perception of the situation and past experiences in coping with similar situations are also individual characteristics that influence coping.

Resources available to the client include both internal and external resources, such as health status, time and energy available, financial status, and an interpersonal support system.

The *situation* may be short-term or long-term, and is classified as physical, psychological/intellectual, social, or environmental. A physical situation may be an illness, surgery, overwork, or physical danger. Psychological or intellectual situations include overstimulation, striving for success, lack of defined goals, and boredom. Social situations include multiple role demands, pressure to conform, change in employment, and isolation. Environmental situations involve the weather, crowded living conditions, and pollution.

Coping patterns are individualized and develop to assist the individual in dealing with harmful, threatening, conflicting, or challenging situations. Coping patterns are described as direct or indirect (Pines and Aronson, 1981). Indirect coping patterns are actions to reduce anxiety caused by a particular situation, with no alteration of the situation. Direct coping patterns are actions that deal with the specific situation. Both types of coping patterns are useful. However, indirect coping patterns are more temporary and do not change the situation in the long run. Examples of each type are shown in the boxes on p. 171.

Physical coping patterns include using relaxation

Examples of Indirect Coping Patterns

Physical	Psycho/intellectual	Social	Spiritual
Walking	Meditation	Social clubs	Prayer
Swimming	Woodworking, crafts, painting	Recreation with others	Attending religious services
Relaxation techniques	Fantasy	Attending social gatherings	Reading spiritual books
Biofeedback	Cognitive reappraisal	Talking with friends	Talking with clergy

Examples of Direct Coping Patterns

Use problem-solving skills to resolve the situation
Seek information and use it to act
Set limits on self or others
Use assertive techniques
Change or modify the situation

techniques, regular exercise, or biofeedback. Biofeedback is a process whereby the client learns voluntary control over an autonomically regulated physiological function, such as muscle tension, fostering relaxation (Betrus, 1991). Psychological/intellectual indirect actions include meditation, cognitive reappraisal, and creative activities such as painting or writing. Cognitive reappraisal, also known as cognitive therapy and attitude restructuring, involves changing one's perception of the situation (Scandrett-Hibdon, 1992). Social actions include talking with others. Through talking with friends, support and advice are often obtained. Spiritual activities also offer ways to cope for individuals who find prayer or meditation helpful. These indirect coping patterns help the client to reduce the anxiety associated with a stressful situation.

Direct coping patterns indicate that positive action is being undertaken to resolve the situation. Problem-solving skills can be used to identify various actions and outcomes and to choose the best action. A person may need additional information on direct actions to deal with a situation. For example, a mother who is returning to work obtains information about licensed day-care centers for her toddler. This information aids in the choice by providing direction and information. Setting limits on time and energy is another direct coping pattern. It may involve spending a specified time on an activity or interactions. Changing the situation is also a direct coping pattern. For example, a family living in crowded living conditions may look for a new apartment.

Some coping patterns are healthier and more effective than others. For example, the client who copes with a stressful job situation by consuming alcoholic beverages and withdrawing from others exhibits unhealthy coping, compared with the client who uses assertive communication techniques and exercise to cope with a similar situation. Coping patterns are considered to be *effective* when the uncomfortable feeling is reduced, the integrity of the individual is preserved, the client functions adequately in relationships and roles, and a positive self-concept is maintained (Miller, 1992).

Individuals usually have a variety of established coping patterns and do not frequently change patterns. They may adopt different coping patterns when they recognize that their present coping patterns do not alleviate their anxiety or that their patterns cost too much time, energy, or self-esteem.

The goals of stress management (Betrus, 1991) are as follows:

Developing an awareness of stress (e.g., stressors)
Recognizing own response to stress (e.g., coping patterns)
Developing and supporting effective coping behaviors
Using stress management techniques in everyday life

Consideration of the goals of stress management is part of the nurse's role in the restoration, maintenance, and promotion of client health. Nurses assist clients to assess their coping patterns and to identify which situations require additional coping efforts. When effective coping patterns are used, the nurse's role consists of providing support. If the client wishes to increase available coping patterns or to develop more effective coping patterns, the nurse's role is to provide knowledge and direction on how to use new coping behaviors. For example, if the nurse and client choose to use a more direct approach, such as problem solving, to deal with a situation, then the nurse assists the client in the problem-solving process. Or, the client may choose to learn assertive communication techniques, requiring the teaching/learning process and role playing. Relaxation techniques are indirect actions that help the client handle feelings that occur before, during, or after a stressful situation. For clients who have difficulty organizing their time, time management principles are appropriate interventions to include in a plan. Clients are also encouraged to use the resources available to them, such as support and self-help groups.

Another important aspect of stress management is clarification of values and goals. People need to sort out what is most important to them in a given situation. For example, a woman who is wife, mother, and career woman may find that she must reconsider her goal of a spotlessly clean house. Or, a man overwhelmed by a variety of roles may find that increasing organizational skills, such as planning tasks on a daily basis, are beneficial to stress management.

Nurses can use a variety of interventions to assist clients to develop or strengthen their coping patterns and to manage stress. The type of intervention depends on the client and the situation. Together, the nurse and client work to establish effective coping patterns.

Behavior Modification

Behavior modification is a strategy to assist clients to increase desirable behaviors or decrease undesirable behaviors. Behavior modification attempts to structure the effect of the environment on human behavior.

Behavior has been defined as any "observable, recordable, and measurable act, movement, or response of the individual" (Peddicord, 1991:797). Two theories of conditioning are used to explain the effect of controlling the environment on behavior: classical conditioning and operant conditioning (Reakes, 1993). *Classical conditioning* refers to the stimulus-response theory, in which an antecedent event (stimulus) influences behavior (response). For example, whenever a man has a cup of coffee (stimulus), he lights up a cigarette (response). *Operant conditioning* stresses that behavior is influenced by the consequence that follows the behavior. *Reinforcements* (positive or negative) are consequences that tend to increase behavior, and *punishments* are consequences that tend to decrease behavior. *Extinction* involves ignoring undesirable behavior while positively reinforcing the desired behavior. An example of operant conditioning involves a dieter who stops eating desserts and snacks (behavior) and loses weight (consequence). Assumptions of the operant conditioning theory are that people tend to repeat behaviors that lead to pleasant consequences and stop behaviors that lead to unpleasant consequences.

Behavior modification applies the principles of classical conditioning and operant conditioning to change behavior. The antecedent event *or* the consequence can be changed to increase or decrease behavior. *Increasing a desired behavior* may be accomplished by either (1) changing the antecedent event to one that will elicit the desired behavior or (2) following the desired behavior with a positive or negative reinforcer. An example of the use of a positive reinforcer involves a pregnant client who desires to practice breathing exercises daily. She enjoys watching the evening news and agrees to spend 10 minutes exercising (behavior) before watching the news (consequence).

Decreasing an undesirable behavior may be accomplished by (1) changing the antecedent event to one that will decrease the behavior, (2) using extinction, or (3) using a punishment, such as time out, loss of something valued, or adding an unpleasant consequence. In most nursing situations, the first two types of punishments should be used before considering an unpleasant consequence. An example of the loss of something valued involves a child on a pediatric unit who refuses to eat. The child likes time in the playroom; therefore, playroom time is suspended if the child does not eat half of the food at each meal.

Often situations call for decreasing an undesirable behavior while at the same time increasing a desirable behavior. Therefore, a combination of reinforcers and punishments are used.

The following steps are implemented in a behavior modification program:

1. *Assessment of the client's behavior pattern.* The behavior is defined accurately, is observable and measurable, and does not consist of inferences or personal interpretations. The phrase "fights all the time" needs further clarification. The antecedent events and the consequences of the behavior are identified. A record is kept of the baseline behavior patterns of the client, the antecedent events, the frequency of the behavior, and events that reinforce or punish the behavior after it has occurred.

2. *Formation of a nursing diagnosis regarding the behavior problem.* The nursing diagnosis must clearly state the specific behavior to be changed. Examples are inadequate weekly exercise, irregular contraceptive use, or excessive intake of between-meal snacks.

3. *Develop the behavior modification plan.* Whenever possible, the plan regarding the behavior to be changed is mutually agreed on by the nurse and client. The method used and the type and frequency of reinforcement or punishment are discussed by the client and the nurse.

When the plan is being developed, methods to increase desirable behavior or decrease undesirable behavior are identified. If antecedent events can be altered, alternative events preceding the behavior are identified. For example, if the person usually eats a snack while watching evening TV, the person might give up watching TV and try reading or another hobby at that time.

Reinforcers are determined with the client and are of importance to the client. Reinforcers are categorized as social, such as attention, praise; material, such as prizes, redeemable tokens; and activity, such as attending movies, playing games (Reakes, 1993). The reinforcer must be available and realistic. A reinforcer that is dependent on someone else, such as the nurse or family member, needs to be identified as such.

Punishment, to be effective, has to be valued by the client as well. For example, loss of watching TV may not be important to a client who does not like TV and enjoys reading. Punishment must not deprive persons of basic human needs, such as a meal or the attention of a parent or loved one. Punishments that impair the health of the client must be avoided.

The speed with which the reinforcer or punishment follows the behavior is considered and depends on the client's age, the behavior to be changed, and the situation. The schedule of the reinforcer or punishment is also determined. Reinforcement or punishment can occur each time the behavior occurs (continuous) or on an intermittent basis. In early stages of behavior change and with young children, reinforcers and punishments should follow soon after the behavior occurs and each time the behavior occurs.

The plan must be communicated to significant others and to other health team members. Family members can support the client, provide reinforcement or punishment, or alter the antecedent events.

4. *Implement the plan as specified.* Either by changing the antecedent event or providing reinforcement or punishment, implementing the plan *as written* is crucial to its success or failure. Consistency is necessary to determine whether the plan is working. Inconsistent application of the behavior modification plan undermines the situation, and the desired change in behavior will probably not occur.

5. *Evaluate the effectiveness of the plan in changing the client's behavior.* Compare the baseline behavior frequency with the frequency of the "new" behavior. If there is no change or only minimal change, the antecedent events, reinforcers, or punishments may not be effective. Modify the plan as needed by changing the antecedent events, reinforcers, or punishments, or by breaking the desired behavior change into smaller units to be accomplished.

Self-modification programs are an adaptation of behavior modification in which clients actually develop their own behavior modification programs. The client voluntarily selects a behavior to develop or change, such as a change in lifestyle (Pender, 1987). The behaviors are usually health promotion or health maintenance activities (e.g., cessation of smoking, weight loss).

The nurse's role is to facilitate the client's self-modification of behavior through use of the steps of the behavior modification program. The nurse assists the client to assess the behavior pattern, the reasons for the behavior change, the knowledge and skills to be used, the perceived benefits of the new behavior, and the support for the new behavior in the client's social and physical environment (Pender, 1987). The nurse also supports the client's use of the principles of classical and operant conditioning.

A behavior modification program is a useful strategy when a change in a client's behavior is desired. Clients can actually set up their own self-modification programs with encouragement and support by the nurse, or they can participate in programs set up by the nurse and other health professionals.

Contracting

Establishing contracts between a nurse and client may be beneficial when the client wants to change complex behaviors to adhere to the health care regimen. Contracts may also be considered for clients who want to maximize their health potential.

Contracting provides a systematic method of increasing desirable behavior. The nurse and client explicitly identify the desired behavior and the responsibilities of both client and nurse. The specific behaviors and responsibilities of each are outlined. The desired behavior must be measurable and specific. Contingency contracting adds the element of reinforcement. Some form of reinforcement is provided in return for the performance of the specified behavior (Boehm, 1992).

Contracts may be either written or verbal. An advantage of a written contract is that it signifies a more formal agreement between the nurse and the client. There is a greater chance for communication to be clearly understood (e.g., responsibilities) when the contract is written. The use of written contracts has been shown to be beneficial in a variety of situations, such as with clients desiring to modify diet (calories, cholesterol, fat, sodium, fluids), reduce smoking, establish an exercise regimen, cough and deep breathe, and ambulate after surgery (Boehm, 1992). It is particularly useful with clients experiencing long-term solutions to health problems or concerns that necessitate changes in lifestyle. Examples for individual, family, and community clients include the following:

Examples

Individual: Learn relaxation techniques
Establish a social support system
Adjust to a chronic illness

Family: Develop new communication styles
Improve parenting skills
Use seatbelts

Community: Develop a neighborhood "watch" program
Adhere to a new health regulation
Incorporate problem solving into meetings

As can be seen, contracting is useful with health promotion activities and with health restoration and maintenance. Contracting is a strategy that strongly encourages client adherence to a new health care practice.

Contracting uses many of the principles of behavior modification and problem solving. Elements of the contracting process are as follows:

1. The client is an active participant in the process.
2. The behavior must be clearly identified and measurable by the nurse and the client.
3. The behavior may need to be broken into smaller, more manageable steps.
4. Responsibilities of both the client and the nurse are identified.

5. Time for evaluation is specified.
6. A reinforcer is identified by the client if contingency contracting is used.
7. Signatures of both the client and the nurse are obtained.
8. Both the client and the nurse receive a copy of the written contract (if written).
9. The contract is evaluated and revised as necessary (Brykcznski, 1982; Steckel, 1982).

An example of this process (shown in the box below) involves a man who wants to control his blood pressure. This behavior needs to be broken down into more measurable and achievable steps. After discussing the variety of measures to control his blood pressure, the client chooses to establish a regular exercise regimen as a first step. It is important for the client to choose the behavior because this will increase the potential for success. A written contract is formulated to establish an exercise regimen including the behavior to be achieved, the responsibilities of the nurse and client, and the time frame in which the behavior should occur.

◆

Sample Contract

I, _____(client)_____, would like to achieve the following expected outcome:
Walk three times per week for 30 minutes.

To achieve this outcome, I,_____(client)_____, agree to the following responsibilities:
1. Arrange my weekly schedule to provide 30 minutes three times per week for walking.
2. Record dates and times spent walking.
3. Bring the record of the walking schedule to the next clinic appointment in 1 month.
4. Meet with the nurse monthly for counseling, support, and encouragement.
5. Reward myself for achieving the objective on a weekly basis by treating myself to a paperback book, movie, or long distance telephone call to a friend or relative.

Signature: _____(client)_____   Date: _____

I, _____(nurse)_____, agree to assist _____(client)_____ with the expected outcome of walking 30 minutes three times per week. My responsibilities include:
1. Meet with _____(client)_____ on a monthly basis for 1 hour.
2. Review the walking record monthly.
3. Monitor _____(client's)_____ blood pressure on a monthly basis.
4. Listen to the achievement and/or disappointment in the accomplishment of the outcome. Offer support and encouragement and assist in problem solving during monthly meetings.

Signature: _____(nurse)_____   Date: _____

Date of evaluation: _____
Results/Revisions:
Record brought to appointment. Thirty minutes of walking three or four times per week recorded. Walking time established as after work. Rewarded self with book or telephone call after achievement of weekly outcome. BP 152/90. Nurse and client agree to continue the contract and reevaluate in 1 month.

It is important to note that the results include whether the responsibilities of nurse and client were met. Reinforcement such as praise should be given on achievement of the desired outcome and responsibilities. Note that the nurse is unable to evaluate whether the client walked 30 minutes three times a week but is able to evaluate whether the client recorded the information.

There are many benefits in using contracting as a strategy. Contracting enables the client to actively plan and carry out changes in behavior. Through active participation, the client becomes more responsible for the behavior change, is given needed support and reinforcement, and is more likely to continue the desired behavior change. Through open communication between the nurse and client, expectations are clarified and feedback provided. Emphasis is placed on accountability of the nurse and the outcomes of the contracting process. The client is also provided with a strategy that can be used in future situations.

Group Process

Group process is a strategy that is useful when two or more people have a common goal or purpose. Types of groups frequently used within nursing are community, family, therapeutic, and psychotherapy groups (LaSalle and LaSalle, 1991). Examples of therapeutic groups are self-help groups such as Alcoholics Anonymous, and the educational group, "I Can Cope," for clients with cancer and their families.

Groups used in nursing practice are planned gatherings of persons designed to accomplish a common desired outcome. Examples are a group of older women from a community health center wanting to discuss mutual health concerns, or teenagers wanting support or information about parental divorce. Clients experiencing a stressful situation (e.g., heart problems, new parents, rehabilitation) may find it useful to be involved in a group with other members experiencing similar situations and concerns.

Examples of nursing diagnoses in which group process could be considered are as follows:

Altered family process
Altered parenting
Anxiety
Self-concept disturbance
Grieving
Knowledge deficit
Powerlessness
Rape-trauma syndrome
Social isolation

Factors to consider before setting up or referring a client to a group (Kinney, 1992) include the following:

• Type, purpose of the group in relation to the client's concern

• Client's perception of need
• Group leadership
• Location and cost
• Duration, frequency, and timing of meetings

The nurse, when effectively using and leading groups, considers the following factors of group process:

Stage of development of the group. Groups develop in stages: orientation, working, and termination phases. Being aware of behaviors of group members and tasks within each stage is beneficial to nurses working with groups.

Structure. Structure includes the size, membership, communication within the group, decision making, and roles. Effective groups consist of 5 to 15 members, have a cooperative rather than a competitive spirit, have a cohesive membership, and are meeting the purposes/goals of the group.

Leadership. A nurse who is in a leadership role within the group needs additional knowledge of leadership styles and strategies and their effect on the group. Functions of leaders within the group include obtaining and receiving information, helping to develop the group's goals, facilitating communication, helping to integrate various perspectives and possible alternatives, and evaluating proposals and decisions (Sampson and Marthas, 1990).

Effective interpersonal skills are essential to effective group leadership. The specific skills used, such as support, confrontation, summarizing, and clarification, are based on the goals of the group and the needs of its members.

Group process is an effective strategy to use with clients when two or more have the same concern and desired outcome.

Principles of Nursing Practice

A strategy frequently used by nurses involves the principles of nursing practice. A principle is considered to be an accepted rule of action or a basis of conduct or operation. Principles are found in the form of standards, guidelines, policies, and procedures. Many principles of nursing practice are unique to nursing; others have been adapted by nurses from other disciplines for application to the nursing process. Principles of nursing practice provide the scientific base of nursing by guiding many of the nursing orders included in the plan of care. Principles of nursing practice have evolved from a variety of sources, including nursing specialities, professional organizations, and agencies and institutions.

A large number of the principles have evolved from nursing specialities such as gerontological, maternal-child, mental health, family, community health, and oncology nursing. The principles, often in the form of guidelines, are developed by nurses with knowledge and expertise in the care of clients who have concerns related to that specialty. Guidelines are found in nursing textbooks, as well as in journal and research articles. An example involves the planning of nursing care with a client with recently diagnosed chronic obstructive pulmonary disease. The nurse selects nursing orders related to activity tolerance, breathing exercises, and precautions from guidelines developed by nurses experienced in the care of clients with respiratory concerns.

Principles of nursing practice have been developed by nurses in professional organizations such as the American Nurses Association and the American Association of Critical Care Nurses. For example, the ANA developed the Standards of Clinical Nursing Practice (1991) and Standards of Psychiatric Mental Health Nursing Practice (1982). ANA standards exist for all areas of specialty nursing practice.

Agencies and institutions have also developed principles of nursing practice, which are often in the form of policies and procedures. Policies are statements of institutional standards. An example is the standard an institution establishes in regard to frequency of changing the site for intravenous administration of drugs or fluids. A procedure is a particular course or method of action formulated by the agency or institution. An example is the procedure to be used when a client is being discharged. These written policies and procedures should be based on nursing research and provide rationale and consistency for nursing care within agencies and institutions.

Examples of *principles of nursing practice* for an *individual client*, a *family client*, and a *community client* are provided below.

For an *individual client*, guidelines for communicating with a hearing-impaired person are as follows:

1. Talk directly to the person.
2. Speak slowly and articulate clearly, but not in an artificial manner.
3. Talk in a normal tone of voice; do not shout.
4. Speak toward the ear that has the best hearing.
5. Restate with different words when not understood.
6. Provide visual cues to augment communication (Schuring, 1991:1979-1980).

For a *family client*, guidelines for family health practice are as follows:

1. Work with the family collectively.
2. Begin where the family is.
3. Plan nursing interventions based on the family's stage of development.
4. Recognize the validity of family structural variations.

5. Emphasize family strengths (Spradley, 1990:458-64).

For a *community client*, guidelines for occupational health nursing practice are as follows:

1. Assess health needs of employees and promote and maintain their health.
2. Analyze factors in the work environment that are hazardous to employee health and minimize their impact or prevent their occurrence.
3. Provide early diagnosis and prompt treatment for injury or illness on the job.
4. Provide programs for employees with disease or disability aimed at restoring and maintaining their maximum level of functioning.
5. Maintain accurate records of employee illness and injury for research and program planning (Spradley, 1990: 550-551).

Many principles of nursing practice are based on medical diagnoses, such as myocardial infarction and fractured hip. Principles of nursing practice are currently being developed in relation to specific nursing diagnoses, such as self-care deficit and spiritual distress. Nursing research is being conducted to substantiate and expand the principles of nursing practice, which will increase the scientific base of nursing, help direct nursing care, and add to the predictability within nursing practice. Opportunities are also available for nurses to communicate principles to other nurses. Nurses have the responsibility for being knowledgeable in regard to the principles of nursing practice that involve the concerns of clients with whom they interact. These principles are valuable when dealing with care plans for health maintenance, restoration, or promotion.

Guidelines for Strategies

1. *Major strategies for implementation are identified.* At least one strategy is identified for each long-term expected outcome and related short-term outcomes. One strategy or a combination of strategies provides direction to nursing orders. For example, the strategies of teaching/learning and problem solving help the client to learn about community resources and decide which services to use. The teaching/learning strategy gives suggestions for nursing orders through principles. Application of this strategy facilitates the client's increased knowledge regarding available and pertinent community resources. Identifying the exact problem or need for community resources, generating alternatives, and analyzing and choosing from alternatives are promoted through problem solving.

2. *Strategies are appropriate to their expected outcomes.* The strategy is directly related to the long- and short-term expected outcomes. Inasmuch as the outcomes

are mutually established with the client, the nurse has determined the client's willingness to achieve the outcomes. Different methods or approaches are used to achieve the outcomes. The nurse's knowledge of the client and the situation guides the choice of strategies that can truly facilitate the achievement of desired outcomes without the use of trial and error.

An example is that of a client who is experiencing a biophysical crisis of altered respiratory function related to a partially obstructed airway and who also has anxiety. The nurse prioritizes diagnoses, determines that the altered respiratory status is the more life-threatening diagnosis, and determines an expected outcome that the client will improve respiratory function by clearing the airway. The principles of respiratory nursing practice or guidelines from the American Heart Association (basic life support choking procedure) facilitate specific nursing orders and actions. Second, the nurse deals with the outcome of decreasing anxiety based on the strategy of principles of mental health nursing practice. In this situation one strategy cannot be interchanged for the other; each is specific to its respective outcome.

More subtle differences among diagnoses, expected outcomes, and client situations call for more discretion by the nurse. Two community neighborhood clients may have the same desired outcome relating to improvement of street conditions and sidewalks. One neighborhood group has already looked into the different kinds of materials that could be used and their costs. Therefore the decision-making step of the problem-solving strategy would probably be the place to start. The other neighborhood needs to explore the materials and options before making a decision about them. In this case, the nurse would start the problem-solving strategy at the second step of determining possible solutions.

3. *Strategies are based on scientific rationale.* Strategies stem from the science and practice disciplines. Theories, models, concepts, and principles provide rationale for some of the strategies. Others have their foundation in accepted methods or approaches determined by long-standing practice. Research findings and current literature may reveal new strategies, or substantiate the use of identified strategies. Nurses need to recognize the scientific bases of all strategies used in their practice. Knowledge of scientific rationale for strategies facilitates nurses' own self-confidence, increases their ability to justify methods or approaches to care, and establishes accountability for nursing practice.

4. *Strategies are mutually determined with the client.* The nurse, through knowledge and experience, provides the expertise on which strategies are appropriate given the client situation. The nurse also provides rationale for a strategy and the possible outcomes.

There are many situations where the client actively participates in the selection of the strategy, with the nurse facilitating the selection. Client involvement is likely to enhance client outcomes.

For example, a nurse working with a family who identifies ineffective coping as a concern assists the family in the selection of a strategy, such as stress management techniques. Often the nurse is helpful in offering strategies to try "first" or strategies clients may not have considered. Even when the client cannot actively participate in the selection process, the nurse communicates the strategy and its rationale to the client and/or significant others.

Nursing Orders

Nursing orders represent the independent function of the professional nurse: specifying the intended behaviors of the nurse, client, and others to achieve the desired outcomes. Nursing orders are directly related to their respective expected outcome and the related content area. The specific nursing orders are also determined by the selected strategy. Strategies provide steps, principles, concepts, guidelines, and rules that serve as a basis for choosing appropriate nursing actions. The nurse individualizes care to the client's unique situation: the personal human responses to actual or potential health problems and concerns. The nurse considers the client's strengths and limitations, and internal and external resources available. The unique way in which the client integrates psychological, developmental, biophysical, spiritual, and sociocultural aspects influences the nursing orders. In addition to specifying nursing orders for independent nursing actions, the nurse also develops nursing orders related to the client's biomedical health concerns. The nurse uses clinical judgment and critical thinking when planning nursing orders related to collaborative actions. For example, the nurse considers the physician's order for an intravenous diuretic when planning nursing orders for a client with chronic heart failure.

The nurse uses decision-making skills of deliberation, judgment, and choice (Schaefer, 1974) to determine which nursing orders are most likely to achieve the desired outcome. Either alone or with other nurses and health team members, the nurse considers the available options, using knowledge of nursing practice and other disciplines. Then the nurse forms an opinion and chooses among the options. During this process the nurse must consider the feasibility of the actions in relation to the client situation, the risks and costs involved, temporal, material, and human resources, and the skills and knowledge of the practitioners.

Guidelines for Nursing Orders

1. *Nursing orders are appropriate to their respective outcomes and strategy.* The nature of the long- and short-term expected outcomes leads to the nature of the orders. The orders reflect health maintenance, promotion, or restoration, depending on the focus of the desired outcomes.

Examples

Maintenance: Turn client every 2 hours during the day and night, maintaining proper body alignment of the client.

Promotion: Teach client basic nutrition patterns, explaining the food guide pyramid with the use of pamphlets and pictures; use the dietitian or nutritionist as a resource person.

Restoration: Assist client with range-of-motion exercises for the affected leg and hand every 2 hours during the day; maintain the limbs in a position of use and in good alignment during the night by using pillows and splints.

The content area of the expected outcomes also needs to be addressed in the nursing orders to reflect internal consistency. For example, if the outcome addresses use of open communication (content area), the orders need to include reference to achievement of open communication.

The strategy gives direction to the order specified through principles, concepts, guidelines, and rules. Therefore if the nurse uses principles of mental health nursing practice and teaching/learning as strategies to promote the use of open communication, nursing orders will reflect those principles. Examples of the use of strategies are provided on pp. 181-183.

An adequate number of nursing orders is needed to achieve the given short-term expected outcome. Usually two to six orders are sufficient. To determine "adequacy," question whether the actions named in the nursing orders will achieve the respective outcome.

2. *Scientific and practice principles provide rationale for orders.* Theories, concepts, models, and principles are the scientific bases for nursing orders. Current literature and research findings from nursing and other disciplines give direction to actions. The nurse needs to have a broad scientific knowledge base to justify a wide variety of nursing orders.

There are two major types of rationale for nursing orders: strategy oriented and content oriented. Strategies provide rationale for some nursing orders. Statements reflecting the strategy's principles, guidelines, steps, rules, and concepts are used as rationale for the *strategy-oriented nursing orders*. Rationale for the content area must also be included. *Content-oriented nursing orders* refer to the topic or focus of the expected outcomes. The content area is identified for each short-term outcome. The content area can be the same for all short-term outcomes, leading to some long-term outcomes that are more specific. The short-term outcomes for more general long-term outcomes probably have a varied content. Statements citing rationale from each content area provide a scientific basis for those nursing orders.

For example, if a client is to name the six categories in the food guide pyramid as the first short-term outcome in attaining the long-term outcome of improved nutritional status, nursing orders and rationale statements for teaching and learning (*strategy*) and nutrition (*content*) must be included. Therefore the scientific rationale statements for nursing orders include reference to the strategy identified and to the content of the order itself.

Using this scientific base deliberately leads to predictability in nursing practice. Through purposeful nursing actions, the nurse determines which orders are more successful in achieving projected client outcomes.

The scientific basis for orders is not usually documented in nursing practice settings. Documentation of the rationale along with the orders may be important if other health team members need to understand the rationale in order to follow through. For example, a psychiatric/mental health facility may place all teenagers in a behavior management program. In a client situation in which the therapeutic effect of this program is counterproductive, the nurse postpones and recommends not using the behavior management approach with a particular client. It would be helpful to communicate the scientific rationale for that decision in writing to other members of the health care team. Whether the rationale is written or not, the nurse should be prepared to state the rationale for nursing orders and defend decisions made regarding nursing practice.

3. *Nursing orders incorporate the autonomy and individuality of the client.* The uniqueness of the individual is reflected in the nursing orders. Based on a comprehensive and multifocal assessment, the nurse has identified the client's strengths, limitations, and internal and external resources. This information helps the nurse decide what is realistic to expect from the client. Nurses encourage clients' participation and responsibility to increase their sense of personal control and esteem. However, the client's strengths determine the level of participation and amount of responsibility that can be expected. For example, the client's cognitive level determines the extent of material and the manner in which the nurse presents information in a learning situation. Cultural and developmental aspects are also considered in specifying nursing orders. Historical in-

formation regarding patterns of behavior give direction for individualizing the approach to care.

Whenever nursing orders are based on the client's unique situation, a rationale statement supporting the nursing order is provided or readily available. These rationale statements indicating *individuality* may come from previously collected data or from literature and research citing differences among people based on culture or development.

4. *Nursing orders indicate specific intended behaviors, giving direction to the nurse, client, and others.* Nursing orders are detailed statements of *who* is to do *what* and *when* (within a given time frame). Each nursing order includes a subject, verb, and conditions or criterion for completion (see Chapter 9). Each order indicates the anticipated date of implementation.

Examples

Specific nursing orders: 1. The client will use walker to ambulate 50 feet four times a day, beginning 2/7/94.
2. The nurse will accompany the client during ambulation to provide verbal support and monitor safety and response to ambulation.

These examples state who is to perform what and under what conditions or purpose. The statements are concise and clear. Depending on the setting and expertise of the practitioners, one might explicitly define "verbal support" and "monitor safety and response to ambulation." Based on a professional nurse's education and the practice of the institution, agency, or practice, those phrases would have definable interpretations.

Nursing orders reflect behavior of all people involved in the client's care, that is, the nurse, client, family members, and other health team members. When appropriate, referrals, consultation, and collaborative approaches to care are given. For example, if the nurse writes an order for social service referral, the order should specify the intent of the referral. This clarity of intent gives direction to the social worker and facilitates accuracy and efficiency of service.

Example

Specific nursing order for referral: Social service referral to provide family support and evaluate home care needs in conjunction with primary nurse.

The use of audio and visual aids is specifically indicated. Pamphlets, tapes, brochures, and books are used to facilitate understanding and increase the client's participation in care. These aids are named to give direction to the appropriate health team members and to inform others of the intended content and level of material being addressed.

5. *Nursing orders reflect consideration of human, temporal, and material resources available.* The assessment of available resources is necessary before specifying nursing orders. As in judging priorities, many variables are considered to determine realistic means to the client's achievement of the expected outcomes. The nurse considers human resources, or people who can participate in the client's care. The number and type of services, employees, staff, and family members and their qualifications and expertise are analyzed. Also, abilities, motivation, and willingness to be involved influences follow-through.

Temporal resources, or time available for outcome achievement, influence nursing orders. In general, acute care settings for individual clients mandate shorter term achievements than do community settings. Some types of client outcomes and their related nursing orders take much more time than others. When outcomes and nursing orders involve many people or alteration of long-standing patterns of behavior, more time is needed, and the nurse can anticipate some resistance. People who seek out health care services or consultation are usually looking for guidance and direction to solve problems and concerns. Even with this motivation, if the guidance and direction involves a change in behavior (which it usually does), there will probably be resistance at some level. Anticipating this resistance helps the nurse set realistic expectations while writing nursing orders.

Material resources such as money, equipment, and supplies are also important to evaluate. The options from which the nurse chooses actions vary with the amount and types of material resources. The costs, risks, and benefits of using certain services, equipment, and supplies affect the choice. The source of funds may determine the actions chosen. For individual and family clients, local, state, federal and private payers and services are all involved. For community clients, funding sources and services include grants, special project funding, property tax income, and community programs.

After consideration of human, temporal, and material resources for nursing orders, the nurse may reassess the achievability of the client's expected outcomes. Modification of the outcomes is necessary if they are not aligned with resources available.

6. *Nursing orders are numbered in the appropriate sequence to achieve the short-term outcome.* Listing the nursing orders in recommended succession gives direction to the nurse, client, and others. Similar to the proper sequencing of short-term expected outcomes to reach a long-term expected outcome, the nursing orders should be in sequence to meet their respective short-term outcome. This sequence is used by the

nurse to review with the client progress toward achieving the expected outcome.

Some strategies guide the sequencing of nursing orders. For example, the strategies of behavior modification, problem solving, and contracting follow a recommended order of events. Principles of nursing practice based on procedures usually provide a step-by-step process to follow. Other strategies such as teaching/learning imply a sequence. Stating that the client must show readiness to learn implies that the nurse assesses readiness before actually teaching.

Sequencing of orders also promotes predictability in nursing practice. Through experience and knowledge, nurses learn prescriptions of events that lead to expected client outcomes. Studying and communicating these prescriptions adds to the scientific base of the discipline of nursing.

7. Nursing orders are dated and include the signature of the responsible nurse. Dating the nursing orders when written provides the nurse and others with a point of reference for the actions prescribed. The nurse uses the date while reviewing, modifying, updating, and evaluating the effectiveness and realistic nature of the nursing orders. Certain orders are discontinued and others initiated based on progress or lack of progress toward outcome achievement. By knowing when orders were initiated, the nurse determines whether the stated approach has had sufficient time to effect change.

The signature of the responsible nurse is necessary to determine accountability for the orders written. The nurse's signature is a personal and professional statement of responsibility. Other health team members will know who to contact with questions regarding the orders, recommended changes, and positive feedback. The client's responses to the actions prescribed are communicated accordingly. Individual nurses are increasingly determining their own case loads of clients in a variety of settings. The nurse's signature on orders indicates responsibility and accountability to clients and to others.

8. Nursing orders are kept current and are revised as indicated. Nursing orders reflect a client's concerns, strengths, and limitations at a given moment in a given situation. Inasmuch as health is a dynamic pattern of behavior and functioning, those patterns can and do change. The nurse is sensitive to those changes through ongoing assessment and evaluation of the client's situation and progress. The nurse recognizes when a given order is no longer appropriate and a revision is indicated. This may take place before the intended achievement of an expected outcome. The need for a revision in orders does not necessarily reflect on the validity of the original orders or competence of the practitioner. Many variables affect the client; some are anticipated and expected, others are not. Through evaluation and self-reflection, the nurse

determines whether the variables causing a change in the situation could have been (or were) predicted. An in-depth review of the previous components of the nursing process can explain the change and subsequent need to modify the orders.

Nursing orders are reviewed on a regular basis to determine the need for modification and updating. At a minimum the orders are reviewed on the expected dates of order implementation and short-term outcome achievement. In acute care settings, that probably indicates review at least every 24 hours. In long-term care settings, review is less frequent and determined by expected implementation and outcome dates. Family and community client orders involve many people and tend to be long-term. Therefore, a minimum review guideline includes the dates of implementation and projected outcomes.

9. Nursing orders include plans for termination of nursing services. Plans for termination of nursing services are included for clients with health promotion, maintenance, or restoration outcomes. From the inception of services, the nurse and client consider the time frame for expected outcome achievement in terms of continuation of care. Nursing orders reflect anticipation of the need for education, referrals, special instructions, follow-up, and community linkage. This anticipation facilitates the transition to the client's increased independence and self-reliance. Whether clients receive residential, overnight, clinic, day care, home care, or consultation services, expected outcomes and nursing orders reflecting the period after service are often necessary.

Guidelines for writing expected outcomes and nursing orders were used to develop the examples of plans for implementation for the individual, family, and community client given on pp. 181-183.

Nursing Care Plan

The nursing care plan is the tool for documenting and communicating the client's nursing diagnoses, expected outcomes, strategies, nursing orders, and evaluation (Fig. 10-1). The care plan serves as the key vehicle to promote an individualized and consistent approach to client care. Through documentation of the client's major concerns and plans to alleviate or modify the concerns, the nurse facilitates coordination of all the members of the health care team. If the plans are written according to recommended guidelines, long- and short-term expected outcomes provide the intended direction for care and an eventual basis for evaluation. Also, the strategies and nursing orders guide and coordinate the client, nurse, and others in their actions to promote outcome achievement. A completed care plan needs to be *used* to fulfill its purposes. A well-developed plan can prevent the use of time-consuming trial and error, avoid duplication of effort, and alleviate costly and timely omissions of care.

Example of Individual Client Plan

Situation: The client, a 58-year-old woman with diabetes, receives health care in a storefront clinic. Her diabetes was diagnosed 3 years ago, and she visits the clinic infrequently. She is able to give herself insulin, but the nurse, on assessment, has discovered that the client has been giving herself the injections in the thighs only. The client remembers being taught "something" about other "places" for injection, but has since forgotten them and does not realize the importance of rotating sites. She says that if it is important she will use other sites, if she knows what they are. The nurse recognizes the client's need to learn about and use other areas appropriate for insulin injection.

Nursing model: Orem's Self-Care Theory of Nursing (1991) is selected because the client is responsible for carrying out insulin injections. The client, being in the supportive-educative nursing system, influences the selection of strategy and development of goals, objectives, and nursing orders.

Nursing diagnosis: Knowledge deficit (insulin injection sites) related to lack of recognized need (12/6/94).

Long-term expected outcome : Client will increase knowledge of insulin injection sites by 12/13/94.

Short-term expected outcome 1: Client will list three appropriate sites for insulin administration and when to change sites by 12/6/94.

Nursing Orders

1. Nurse and client will discuss reasons for rotating sites on 12/6/94.

2. Nurse and client will discuss alternate injection sites and a rotation schedule, using pictures and pamphlets on 12/6/94.

Rationale

Strategy: Teaching and learning
Content: Insulin administration

Development of concepts is part of learning (strategy) (Pohl, 1981). Insulin, if given in the same site over time, causes scarring and decreased absorption (content) (Phipps, 1991).

Teaching requires effective communication; repetition strengthens learning (strategy) (Rorden, 1987). Audiovisual aids appropriate to client situation promote communication and repetition.

Short-term expected outcome 2: Client will demonstrate administration of insulin using three sites by 12/13/94.

Nursing Orders

1. Nurse will demonstrate how to give an injection in the abdomen, arms, and buttocks on 12/13/94.

2. Client will demonstrate injection into three areas without puncturing the skin on 12/13/94.

Rationale

Learning occurs through demonstration-practice (strategy) (Redman, 1993). Variety of sites decreases scarring and increases absorption (content) (Phipps)

Effective learning requires active participation of the learner; evaluation is an integral part of teaching (strategy) (Redman).

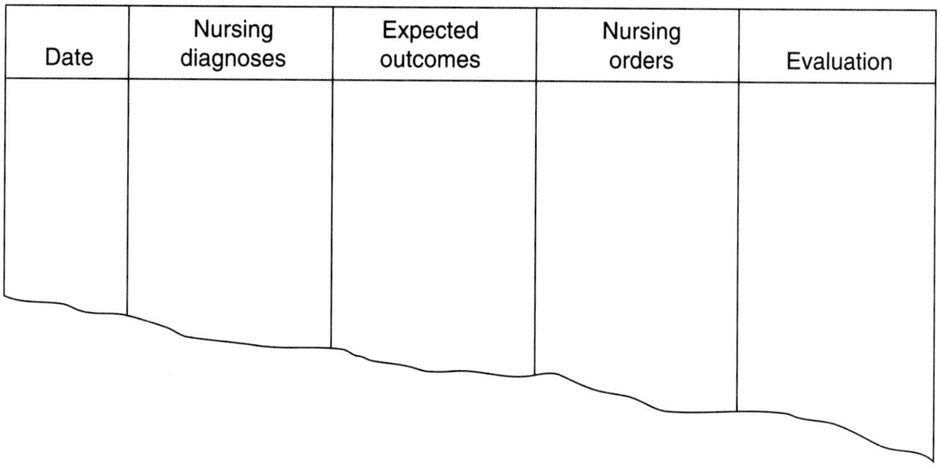

Date	Nursing diagnoses	Expected outcomes	Nursing orders	Evaluation

Figure 10-1 Components of nursing care plan.

Example of Family Client Plan

Situation: In June 1994, the home health care nurse began seeing a family with two children, a 3-year-old boy (John) and a 4-month-old boy (Adam). Both parents live at home, and both work outside the home during the day. The 3-year-old was toilet trained, but has been wetting his pants intermittently for the past few months and is starting to act out (fighting, arguing with others) at the day care center. The nurse was referred to the family by the day care center to assess the home situation and to recommend/implement actions as appropriate. After two home family visits, the nurse concludes that John's behavior is a symptom of the recent change in family dynamics with the addition of Adam in the home.

Nursing model:	Friedman's Structural/Functional Family model (1992) is selected for its focus on interaction among family members.
Nursing diagnosis:	Alteration in family processes related to John's reaction to a new family member (Adam) (6/23/94).
Long-term expected outcome:	Family will adjust to Adam's presence within 3 months, by 9/30/94.
Short-term expected outcome 1:	Family will name at least three ways that Adam has influenced their lifestyle by 7/1/94.

Nursing Orders	**Rationale**
1. Nurse will establish rapport with the family using facilitative communication techniques on 7/1/94.	*Strategy:* Therapeutic use of self *Content:* Sibling rivalry Effective use of communication techniques promotes development of the nurse-client relationship (strategy) (Sundeen, 1993).
2. Nurse and family will discuss the changes in family interactions that have occurred since Adam's birth and their feelings about the changes on 7/1/94.	Verbalization of the event and responses to it promotes understanding and decreases anxiety (strategy) (Stuart and Sundeen, 1991).
3. Parents will state how they relate to John and his behavior since Adam's birth on 7/1/94.	Changes in a child's behavior (daytime/nighttime wetting "accidents"; aggressive/quarrelsome) can be the result of decreased attention from parents and child's own fears (content) (individuality) (Whaley and Wong, 1991).

Short-term expected outcome 2: Parents and day care center will use a behavior modification approach to decrease John's acting out by 8/1/94.

Nursing Orders	**Rationale**
1. Parents, teacher, and nurse will record baseline of incidents and preceding situations that led to John's acting out behaviors by 7/8/94.	*Strategy:* Behavior modification and therapeutic use of self Identification of behavior pattern is necessary before determining approach: all key people need to be involved in developing the plan (strategy) (individuality) (Peddicord, 1991).
2. Nurse will assist the parents and teacher in naming potential reinforcements/punishments that are realistic and valued by John by 7/8/94.	Reinforcements/punishments need to be valued and appropriate to the client and situation (strategy) (content) (individuality) (Peddicord). Facilitative communication techniques promote expression of thoughts and feelings (strategy) (Sundeen).
3. Parents and teacher will develop a plan to decrease John's undesirable behaviors using identified reinforcers/punishers by 7/15/94.	People implementing the plan need to be a part of developing it (strategy) (Peddicord).
4. Parents, teacher and nurse will determine implementation and evaluation dates for plan on 7/15/94.	Consistent implementation and evaluation are essential to successful behavior modification (strategy) (Peakes, 1993).

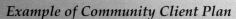

Example of Community Client Plan

Situation: A women's community organization became concerned about single mothers who could not afford health care services. Through various community contacts and an informal survey, the organization ascertained that services were provided to the poor and unemployed, as well as the middle- and upper-income people. However, a certain group of employed, low-income single mothers could not afford health care services. This assessed need was taken to the organization's board, which decided to investigate the potential of solving this problem. With board approval, a task force was formed, and a nurse consultant contracted to develop a plan to meet this community need. Based on the information presented, the nurse concluded that lack of services in the community was creating inadequate health care to low-income single mothers.

Nursing model:	Neuman's Health-Care Systems model (1989) is selected for its systems orientation and nursing focus on primary, secondary, and tertiary prevention.
Nursing diagnosis:	Insufficient health care to low-income single mothers related to lack of services in community (1/15/94).
Long-term expected outcome :	Community will develop health care services for low-income single mothers within 1 year (1/15/95).
Short-term expected outcome 1:	Organization board will accept a written plan for health care services to low-income single mothers within 6 months using recommendations from the task force and nurse consultant.

Nursing Orders	*Rationale*
1. Nurse and task force will review the community's health care situation, problem, organization's board commitment, and identified goal. These issues will be discussed and clarified on 2/1/94.	*Strategy:* Problem solving *Content:* Adequate health care services People involved need to understand the situation (strategy) (Sullivan and Decker, 1992).
2. Task force will determine four potential alternative solutions to the situation with nurse's guidance by 2/30/94.	Potential solutions need to be generated by the people concerned to provide anticipated resolution to the unique situation. Options are limited to focus group on goal attainment (strategy) (individuality) (Bower, 1982).
3. Task force and nurse will examine the risks and costs of each alternative by 3/30/94.	Consequences of alternatives are analyzed prior to selecting one (strategy) (Sullivan and Decker, 1992).
4. Task force will choose one alternative to recommend to the organization board for approval by 4/15/94.	Client (organization task force) needs to choose an alternative most likely to achieve intended goal (strategy) (Sullivan and Decker, 1992).

(Another short-term outcome is needed regarding implementation and evaluation of the alternative chosen.)

The professional nurse is responsible and accountable for developing the nursing care plan. Ideally the primary nurse, case manager, or nurse responsible for the ongoing care of the client completes the care plan. Many implications are made in developing a plan. An accurate and multifocal assessment is the necessary basis for the plan. Nursing diagnoses evolve from data analysis and synthesis, which require a comprehensive knowledge base and critical thinking abilities. The diagnoses are put into order of priority, long-term expected outcomes established, short-term expected outcomes developed, strategies identified, and nursing orders specified using scientific rationale. Other health team members may have input and feedback regarding the approach to the client, but the professional nurse is responsible for the care plan's development.

The care plan is initiated on the inception of nursing services. After an initial assessment of the client's situation is completed, the nurse consolidates that information for current and future use. Even if more data are needed to verify nursing diagnoses, the nurse records inferences of diagnoses and recommended approaches to those concerns. Subsequent data collection may lead to alteration or validation of the nurse's initial judgment. The expected outcomes, strategies, and nursing orders are modified accordingly.

Typically the nursing care plan includes the *individualized* plan for a client's situation. Yet some actual or potential health problems and concerns create *common patterns of human responses* among people. These similarities of altered patterns of behavior and functioning usually call for similar approaches to care by the nurse (e.g., general postoperative nursing care, elements of cardiac rehabilitation programs). Nursing care guidelines, policies, procedures, and standards are developed by various nursing organizations, institutions, agencies, and practices. These approaches are based on scientific and practice principles and are intended for use in predictable circumstances. Advantages of using routinized approaches in select situations are that they provide standards of care and criteria for evaluation of care, increase predictability in nursing practice, and save the nurse's time by decreasing repetitive documentation. Reference to these approaches on the care plan is appropriate *only* in terms of the *commonalities* with which clients are treated for *similar patterns* of human responses. *Individualized* nursing diagnoses and related plans that reflect the client's unique situation are still needed. All nursing care guidelines, policies, procedures, and standards should be kept current and readily available as a reference for nurses while writing nursing care plans.

The nursing care plan, the key vehicle for nursing care, needs to be a part of the client's permanent record. Therefore the care plan is completed in ink and follows the guidelines suggested in this and other chapters regarding the nursing process components.

Summary

Strategies and nursing orders are considered the *prescriptive* elements of the planning component. The nursing model, nursing diagnoses, and expected outcomes form the basis for choosing strategies and nursing orders. Several strategies exist that stem from scientific and practice disciplines. The principles of nursing practice include those strategies unique to the nursing profession.

Nursing orders are specified to give direction to the nurse, client, and others to achieve the expected outcomes. Nursing orders address the client's unique situation, as well as similar patterns of human responses. The nursing care plan is the tool used for documenting all plans for implementation.

Implementation, or the act of carrying out the nursing care plan, is addressed in Chapter 11. The importance of following the plan as written is stressed.

Critical Thinking Exercises BY ELIZABETH S. FAYRAM

1. Ms. Florence Simmons, 76 years old, was hospitalized for a hip replacement following a fractured femur. Ms. Simmons has had degenerative joint disease for many years. She has been transferred to an extended care facility for rehabilitation.

   Before surgery, Ms. Simmons lived in a second floor, walk-up apartment, which she paid for with social security and personal income. She was active in church and community groups, serving as a volunteer in the senior center and the local Red Cross chapter. Ms. Simmons had been walking and using public transportation to go to church, stores, and other activities.

   Ms. Simmons has made rapid progress while at the extended care facility. She is able to perform activities of daily living but has limited mobility. She uses a walker to walk short distances but is no longer able to climb stairs.

   As the Home Care Coordinator for the extended care facility, you meet with Ms. Simmons before her discharge to assist her in planning lifestyle changes compatible with her physical limitations.
   a. Identify what lifestyle changes are now necessary for Ms. Simmons to consider due to her physical limitations.
   b. Identify strategies that could be used with Ms. Simmons for discharge planning. Explain the advantages/disadvantages for each of these strategies.
   c. For one lifestyle change, develop actions Ms. Simmons plans to take as part of the discharge plan.

2. Mr. John Walker, 48 years old, comes to the health clinic for evaluation of hypertension following three elevated blood pressure readings at his place of employment. Mr. Walker reveals that he has resumed cigarette smoking after 4 months cessation and has recently separated from his wife. He watches his diet for fat and calories and is now playing racquetball two times per week. He is concerned about his blood pressure and is willing "to change my habits if it'll help." As his clinic nurse:
   a. Develop a nursing diagnosis and expected client outcomes.
   b. Select a strategy to meet one long-term expected outcome and state the rationale for its use in this situation.
   c. Write the short-term outcomes and nursing orders relevant to the long-term outcome and strategy.

3. You are the chairperson of the Program Planning Committee for a proposed senior citizens' day care center. The committee has identified one area of program planning to be regular exercise. The program, which the committee is to develop, will be based on the limitations of the participants, many of whom have impaired mobility and altered thought processes. Use the steps of the problem-solving process to develop a plan to meet the exercise needs of the participants at the day care center.

4. Explain how autonomy and individualization are incorporated into the planning component of the nursing process.

REFERENCES AND READINGS

American Nurses Association: *Standards of clinical nursing practice,* Kansas City, 1991, The Association.

American Nurses Association: *Standards: psychiatric–mental health nursing practice,* Kansas City, 1973, The Association.

Bailey JT and Claus KE: *Decision making in nursing: tools for change,* St. Louis, 1975, Mosby–Year Book.

Benner P and Wrubel J: *The primacy of caring: stress and coping in health and illness,* Redwood City, Calif, 1989, Addison-Wesley Nursing.

Betrus PA: Stress management. In Phipps WJ et al, editors: *Medical-surgical nursing: concepts and clinical practice,* St Louis, 1991, Mosby–Year Book.

Bloom B: *Taxonomy of educational objectives: the classification of educational goals. Handbook I: cognitive domain,* New York, 1956, David McKay.

Boehm S: Patient contracting. In Bulechek GM and McCloskey JC, editors: *Nursing interventions: essential nursing treatments,* Philadelphia, 1992, WB Saunders.

Bower FL: *The process of planning nursing care: nursing practice models,* St Louis, 1982, Mosby–Year Book.

Bradley JC and Edinberg MA: *Communication in the nursing context,* Norwalk, Conn, 1990, Appleton and Lange.

Brykcznski K: Health contracting, *Nurse Pract* 7:27, 1982.

Bulechek GM and McCloskey JC: *Nursing interventions: essential nursing treatments,* Philadelphia, 1992, WB Saunders.

Carpenito LJ: *Nursing diagnosis: application to clinical practice,* Philadelphia, 1992, JB Lippincott.

Friedman MM: *Family nursing: theories and assessment,* Norwalk, Conn, 1992, Appleton and Lange.

Gaut D: A theoretic description of caring as action. In Leininger MM, editor: *Care: the essence of nursing and health,* Detroit, 1988, Wayne State University Press.

Gillies DA: *Nursing management: a systems approach,* Philadelphia, 1989, WB Saunders.

Hamberger LK and Lohr JM: *Stress and stress management: research and applications,* New York, 1984, Springer.

Johnson BS, editor: *Psychiatric–mental health nursing: adaptation and growth,* Philadelphia, 1993, JB Lippincott.

Kinney C et al: Support groups. In Bulechek GM and McCloskey JC, editors: *Nursing interventions: essential nursing treatments,* Philadelphia, 1992, WB Saunders.

La Salle PC and LaSalle AJ: Small groups and their therapeutic forces. In Stuart GW and Sundeen SJ, editors: *Principles and practice of psychiatric nursing,* St Louis, 1991, Mosby–Year Book.

Leininger MM, editor: *Care: the essence of nursing and health,* Detroit, 1988, Wayne State University Press.

Mayeroff M: *On caring,* New York, 1971, Harper and Row.

Miller JF: *Coping with chronic illness: overcoming powerlessness,* Philadelphia, 1992, FA Davis.

Monat A and Lazarus RS: *Stress and coping: an anthology,* New York, 1977, Columbia University Press.

Neuman B: *The Neuman systems model,* Norwalk, Conn, 1989, Appleton and Lange.

Orem DE: *Nursing concepts of practice,* St Louis, 1991, Mosby–Year Book.

Peddicord HR: Behavior modification. In Stuart GW and Sundeen SJ, editors: *Principles and practice of psychiatric nursing,* St Louis, 1991, Mosby–Year Book.

Pender NJ: *Health promotion in nursing practice,* Norwalk, Conn, 1987, Appleton and Lange.

Phipps WJ et al, editors: *Medical-surgical nursing: concepts and clinical practice,* St Louis, 1991, Mosby–Year Book.

Pines AM and Aronson E: *Burnout: from tedium to personal growth,* New York, 1981, The Free Press.

Pohl ML: *The teaching function of the nursing practitioner,* Dubuque, 1981, Wm C Brown.

Ray MA: The development of a classification system of institutional caring. In Leininger MM, editor: *Care: the essence of nursing and health,* Detroit, 1988, Wayne State University Press.

Reakes JC: Behavioral approaches. In Johnson BS, editor: *Psychiatric–mental health nursing,* Philadelphia, 1993, JB Lippincott.

Redman BK: *The process of patient education,* St Louis, 1993, Mosby–Year Book.

Rorden JW: *Nurses as health teachers: a practical guide,* Philadelphia, 1987, WB Saunders.

Sampson EE and Marthas MM: *Group process for the health professions,* Albany, NY, 1990, Delmar Publishing.

Scandrett-Hibdon S: Cognitive reappraisal. In Bulechek GM and McCloskey JC, editors: *Nursing interventions: essential nursing treatments,* Philadelphia, 1992, WB Saunders.

Schaefer J: The interrelatedness of decision making and the nursing process, *Am J Nurs* 74:1852, 1974.

Schuring LT: Management of persons with problems of the ear. In Phipps WJ et al, editors: *Medical-surgical nursing: concepts and clinical practice,* St Louis, 1991, Mosby–Year Book.

Spradley BW: *Community health nursing: concepts and practice,* Glenview, Ill, 1990, Scott, Foresman.

Steckel SB: *Patient contracting,* New York, 1982, Appleton-Century-Crofts.

Steele SM and Harmon VM: *Values clarification in nursing,* Norwalk, Conn, 1983, Appleton-Century-Crofts.

Stuart GW and Sundeen SJ, editors: *Principles and practice of psychiatric nursing,* St Louis, 1991, Mosby–Year Book.

Sullivan EJ and Decker PJ: *Effective management in nursing,* Menlo Park, Calif, 1992, Addison-Wesley Nursing.

Sundeen SL et al: *Nurse-client interaction: implementing the nursing process,* St Louis, 1993, Mosby–Year Book.

Watson J: *Nursing: the philosophy and science of caring,* Boulder, Colo, 1985, Association University Press.

Whaley LF and Wong DL: *Nursing care of infants and children,* St. Louis, 1991, Mosby–Year Book.

Whitman NI et al: *Teaching in nursing practice: a professional model,* Norwalk, Conn, 1992, Appleton and Lange.

Yura H and Walsh MB: *The nursing process: assessing, planning, implementing, and evaluating,* Norwalk, Conn, 1988, Appleton and Lange.

CHAPTER 11

IMPLEMENTATION

Elizabeth S. Fayram

General Considerations

Implementation is the client and the nurse carrying out the plan of care. The nurse is responsible for client-focused, outcome-oriented nursing care as delineated in the plan. The primary focus of the implementation component is the provision of individualized, safe nursing care with a multifocal approach. Implementation of the plan involves completion of actions necessary to fulfill the expected outcomes as delineated in the plan. Actions may be carried out by the nurse, the client, family members, other health team members, or a combination of these. Implementation promotes client advocacy and coordination among team members.

Implementation of the plan is influenced by the model incorporated with the nursing process. Through the model's concepts relating to client, health, nursing, and environment, the model guides the nurse in the roles and actions performed with clients to improve, maintain, or promote their health.

This chapter begins with a discussion of the integration of previous components of the nursing process into the implementation component. Three categories of skills necessary for implementation are described. The three phases that comprise implementation are presented, including a description of nurse behaviors that occur in each phase. Documentation regarding the implementation component is explored. The guidelines for implementation are listed here and discussed at the end of the chapter.

1. The actions performed are consistent with the plan and occur after validation of the plan.
2. Interpersonal, intellectual, and technical skills are performed competently and efficiently in an appropriate environment.
3. The client's physical and psychological safety is protected.
4. Documentation of actions and client responses is provided in the health care record and care plan.

Integration of Nursing Process Components

Implementation incorporates aspects of previous components of the nursing process. Data collection continues, diagnoses are validated, and priorities and plans are reexamined. Assessment continues throughout implementation, providing further data about the concerns and strengths already identified or discovering new ones. Modifications of plans may be necessary before implementation proceeds. This is especially true when a period has elapsed between the nurse's contact with the client. For example, a nurse met 1 month ago with a single parent of a 6-week-old child. Before proceeding with the teaching plan regarding the need for immunizations that was agreed upon previously, the nurse reassesses the situation for changes that will make an impact on the implementation of the plan, such as the mother's concern about symptoms of a cold in the infant.

In other situations, such as in an emergency, the implementation component quickly follows the previous components (e.g., assessment, diagnosis, planning). An adult with a history of atherosclerotic heart disease who is complaining of chest pain is quickly assessed. The concerns of "alteration in comfort: pain" and "potential alteration in tissue perfusion: cardiopulmonary" require the nurse to quickly implement a plan. Actions by the nurse, based on the nurse's level of proficiency and experience, are quickly initiated.

Implementation Skills

The skills necessary to implement the plan are categorized as intellectual, interpersonal, and technical (Yura and Walsh, 1988). The nurse's ability to use these skills determines the success of implementation of the plan. Nurses' levels of proficiency are based on their knowledge, experience, and expertise (Benner, 1984). Novice practitioners need to attend to the steps or guidelines for these skills more specifically, whereas expert practitioners internalize the principles and can implement the skills with a more creative approach. In addition, clients' abilities to use these skills influence the extent of their participation and the outcome of the plan. Proficiency by other health team members in terms of these skills is also considered when involving others in the execution of the plan.

Intellectual skills involve the critical thinking skills of reasoning, decision making, priority setting, and problem solving. These skills are used by the nurse in reviewing a currently existing plan, as well as in determining how the plan is to be implemented. Decision making and priority setting are used as the nurse selects nursing actions or determines the timing of a procedure. The nurse's knowledge is used as the basis for scientific rationale for actions being implemented. Creativity and innovation are also intellectual skills used during this component of the nursing process. Observation skills are used by the nurse when collecting data regarding the client's reaction to implementation of the plan, as well as when assessing actual and potential concerns of the client. The client's ability to reason and understand are also considered when the nurse is actively involved in implementing strategies such as teaching/learning and problem solving.

Interpersonal skills are used during implementation by the nurse while communicating with the client and while collaborating with other health team members or members of other agencies (e.g., in making a referral). Interpersonal skills involve verbal and nonverbal communication techniques, including active listening, the provision of clear explanations, and support as feelings are expressed. These techniques convey a concern and respect for the client and are consistent with the purpose of the interaction. The nurse's ability to develop therapeutic nurse-client relationships influences the success of the implementation component. The client's interpersonal skills are considered and used, for example, in family dynamics or in consultation with health professionals.

Technical skills involve performing a procedure competently and safely. The focus in performing technical skills is usually with the individual client, such as in the provision of skin care or performance of passive range-of-motion exercises. Technical skills are also used while implementing a plan with a family or community. An example is the nurse assisting parents to learn the correct procedure to attach their infant to an apnea monitor. Technical skills the nurse uses with community clients include demonstrating cardiopulmonary resuscitation to a group and running a VCR to show a video to a community group. Clients' technical skills are often developed during implementation, such as self-administering an insulin injection or drawing blood from a Hickman catheter by a mother whose son is receiving chemotherapy.

Technical skills cannot be separated from intellectual and interpersonal skills. Intellectual skills related to technical skills include the nurse's knowledge of the principles and steps of the procedure, the expected outcomes, the possible complications, and the legal and ethical aspects of the procedure. The nurse uses decision making when determining the appropriateness of modifications to the procedure.

Interpersonal skills related to technical skills are used to offer support and instructions to the client, as well as to obtain data regarding the client's reactions. For example, before performing range-of-motion exercises, the nurse, through interaction, informs the client of the following:

1. Purpose of the action
2. Expected outcomes of the action
3. Client's role and responsibilities during the procedure
4. Equipment needed
5. Length of time the procedure will last
6. Sensations to be anticipated during the procedure
7. Amount of privacy that will be provided (Yura and Walsh, 1988)

Actions

Whether the nurse uses intellectual, interpersonal, or technical skills while implementing the plan, *actions* are being executed. The nurse is action oriented in teaching a family parenting skills, in supporting a client as the client ventilates feelings about adjustments in life after amputation of a leg, or in assisting a community with the planning process regarding home health services.

The actions of the nurse, as well as those of the client, are based on the model incorporated, the strategies selected, and the nursing orders developed as part of the plan. For example, Orem's Self-Care Theory of Nursing (1991) describes three nursing systems: wholly compensatory, partly compensatory, and supportive-educative. Nurse and client actions are influenced by which system is necessary at a particular point in time. A client requiring the supportive-educative system needs assistance in decision making, behavior control, or acquiring knowledge or skills. Actions used with this nursing system may include support, counseling, and teaching/learning, with active participation on the part of the client.

Strategies selected and the nursing orders included in the plan also influence the actions of the nurse and client. For example, when problem solving is the strategy selected with a group of adolescents, then actions taken by the group and the nurse are relevant to this strategy. The nurse facilitates problem solving by assisting the group to analyze the problem or to develop alternative solutions.

The model, strategies, and nursing orders also influence who carries out the actions of the plan. As described previously, the actions may be performed by the client, nurse, family members, or other health team members. During development of the plan, consideration is given to the skills necessary to carry out the actions, in terms of the client, the client's family members, other health team members, and the nurse. During implementation this consideration continues. The nurse determines when the client or the family members are ready to carry out the actions. The nurse still remains accountable for the actions carried out by the client and the family members, and facilitates the actions carried out by others.

Phases of Implementation

Implementation occurs in three phases: preparation, implementation, and postimplementation. The nurse's responsibilities for each phase are delineated below.

Preparation

The preparation phase of implementation involves preparing for the actual implementation of the plan. This phase consists of the following:

Knowledge of the plan
Validation of the plan
Knowledge and skills to implement the plan
Preparation of the client
Preparation of the environment

The nurse first becomes familiar with the established plan. The nurse may be familiar with the plan if he or she was involved in its development. The nurse can become familiar with the plan by listening to a verbal report or reading the written plan.

The plan is validated with the client and other health team members. By reviewing client records and using knowledge and experiences, the nurse determines whether the plan is still viable. Following are questions to consider regarding validity:

1. Is the plan relevant based on the client's status and concerns at this point in time?
2. Have priorities changed or remained the same?
3. Is the plan safe and based on sound rationale, including legal and ethical aspects?
4. Is the plan individualized?

Based on input from the client, other health team members, the client's record, and the nurse's knowledge and experiences, the nurse may decide that the plan needs to be revised. Modifications may be *temporary*, such as revising the time for implementation of the plan. A situation requiring temporary modification of the plan includes postponement of a teaching session when the client receives an unexpected visitor from out of town. A client's discomfort may also temporarily change priorities. Modifications to the plan may be *permanent*, for example, when the method of a procedure such as a dressing change is revised. In addition to time and method, modifications may include who is to implement the plan and where. If an elderly couple decides to have Meals on Wheels instead of going to the senior community center, validating the plan requires the nurse to be flexible enough to make the necessary changes when needed.

Another aspect of the preparation phase involves development of the nurse's knowledge and skills needed to implement the plan. If the nurse lacks the specific knowledge or skill, several options are available. The nurse may refer the plan to someone else, receive assistance from another nurse, read about the necessary knowledge or skill, or observe another nurse carry out the actions. The nurse should not attempt to implement actions without assistance when the nurse is inadequately prepared in knowledge and skill.

The nurse prepares the client for what will occur during implementation of the plan. The nurse explains the actions and the purpose, the expected sensations, the client's responsibilities, and the expected outcomes. Preparation of the client also involves providing privacy, preparing the client physically if necessary, such as positioning, and ensuring protection of the client's sense of modesty.

Before implementation of the plan, the nurse also

prepares the environment. The nurse obtains the resources necessary to carry out the plan, assembles the equipment needed for procedures and the audiovisual material for learning purposes, and gathers other members of the health team to assist with implementing the plan, if necessary. Other aspects of preparing the environment involve ensuring adequate lighting, considering seating arrangements, and minimizing distractions and interruptions by shutting doors, informing others where and how long the nurse will be involved with the client, turning down the volume of televisions or radios, and finding a quiet room for a group meeting.

Implementation

On completion of the preparation phase, the nurse carries out the plan with the client. The nursing care is client focused and outcome oriented, and meets the physical and psychological safety needs of the client. Skillful and efficient implementation of the plan enhances the provision of competent care. The nurse uses intellectual, interpersonal, and technical skills when providing nursing care.

Client-focused nursing care consists of being aware of the biophysical, psychosocial, and spiritual aspects of the client, and individualizing care. Examples are explaining a procedure thoroughly the first time the client experiences it, varying communication approaches according to age or cognitive level of the client, and allowing a newly formed group the time necessary to develop into the working phase of group development. Client-focused nursing care also involves the nurse acting in the role of client advocate, providing for active participation of the client, protecting client rights, and collaborating with other health care professionals.

Implementation of the plan is *outcome oriented.* Actions are consistent with the long-term and short-term expected outcomes of the plan. For example, the nurse implements the teaching and learning process as specified for counseling a pregnant teenager about nutrition. When appropriate, it is possible to meet several expected outcomes simultaneously. While assisting the client with a self-care deficit such as bathing or dressing, the nurse may also implement part of a teaching and learning plan. This uses time efficiently and focuses on the needs of the client.

The nurse provides for the *physical and psychological safety* of the client. Physical safety occurs when aseptic techniques are used, when assistance is obtained if necessary, and when the client is placed in a safe environment. Psychological safety and comfort are accomplished through interpersonal skills, for example, by explaining what is going to happen, holding an anxious client's hand during a procedure, and reinforcing the client's progress.

The nurse performs care *skillfully and efficiently.* Whether the actions involve intellectual, interpersonal, or technical skills, the nurse performs them competently. The competent nurse is more likely to enhance the client's progress toward the expected outcomes of the plan. Efficiency in implementing the plan by using time-management techniques allows more time for the nurse and client to interact or accomplish other outcomes. When the nurse performs actions skillfully and efficiently, the client's trust and confidence in the nurse's competence are enhanced, furthering the nurse-client relationship.

Through the development of the plan and its validation in the preparation phase, the client's role in carrying out the plan has been established. When the client is actively involved in creating and implementing the plan, the nurse's role shifts from provider of competent care to facilitator. The nurse ensures that safe and outcome-oriented care is provided. This is accomplished by adequate preparation, including thorough preparation of the client, and by being available to assist and support the client during implementation of the plan.

An important responsibility during implementation is the collection of data regarding the client's reactions to execution of the plan. These reactions include physical, psychological, social, and spiritual responses. During implementation of the plan the nurse focuses on the client, as well as on the specific procedure or teaching plan being implemented. For example, the nurse notes when a client is becoming tired, when family members show improved verbal communication with each other, and when group members react to alternative solutions to problems. These client responses may indicate the client's readiness to progress further with implementation of the plan or the need to modify the plan.

Postimplementation

When nursing actions are completed, the postimplementation phase begins. The first part of postimplementation involves *closure between the nurse and client* on the aspect of the plan being implemented. This includes summarizing what actions took place, clarifying information, answering questions, indicating follow-up with the client for evaluation or the implementation of other parts of the plan, and identifying the client's response to implementation of the plan.

Following implementation of the plan, the nurse leaves the client in a *safe, comfortable environment.* For example, the siderails are raised, curtains opened, and bedside table and call button are placed within easy reach. Any equipment or teaching aid that the nurse and client used is removed and disposed of properly. The nurse is then responsible for the *documentation of actions implemented and the client's response to the actions,* as well as *verbal communication to appropriate health team members,* to provide continuity and coordination of care.

Professional Nursing Roles

The nurse assumes a variety of roles during implementation of the plan. Professional nursing roles are practitioner, educator, researcher, collaborator, advocate, change agent, case manager, evaluator, and leader/manager. The plan, strategies, nursing orders, and model integrated into the nursing process influence the roles used by the nurse during implementation. The nurse's own philosophy, such as willingness to incorporate research findings into nursing practice, also determine the roles used.

A professional nursing role often used during implementation is that of educator, which is enacted when the teaching/learning strategy has been selected. The role of practitioner is also used frequently, for example, when the principles of nursing practice are being implemented. The case manager role involves coordinating client care of several health professionals in order to achieve desired outcomes. The nurse acts as a change agent when facilitating change in clients, such as those who are modifying lifestyle behaviors. Role modeling may be enacted when using therapeutic use of self as a strategy. Several roles may overlap and be enacted simultaneously, such as practitioner and advocate or collaborator, along with the role of leader/manager.

An important role of the nurse during implementation is that of client advocate. Being an advocate for a client involves a nurse-client relationship based on mutuality and respect. The client is an active participant in relation to health needs. The nurse as a client advocate protects client rights and keeps the client first in priority. It also involves speaking on behalf of a client and forming collaborative relationships with others in the health care system so that health needs of a client are met.

In the role of leader/manager during implementation, the nurse is involved in coordination and also delegation of client care. Coordination is a leadership/management activity that the nurse performs during implementation and during other components of the nursing process such as planning. The nurse is the one health professional who focuses on the client's whole response to the health situation. Therefore the nurse is responsible for coordinating the client's nursing care and other aspects of care needed, such as occupational therapy or counseling services in the community. While coordinating care, the nurse ensures that individuality is maintained, such as scheduling physical therapy to coincide with pain relief measures or referring to agencies with a sliding scale fee for those with limited income.

Coordination of care avoids duplication of effort and provides organized care so that the client's expected outcomes can be achieved. In providing effective client care, coordination requires frequent exchange of information among the nurse, client, and other health care members. Collaborative relationships and assertive communication techniques are used by the nurse when coordinating client care.

Delegation is another aspect of the role of leader/manager during implementation. *Delegation* is sharing responsibility, authority, and accountability with another health team member for actions performed with a client. At times it is necessary for the professional nurse to delegate certain actions to another health care member, such as another professional nurse or a licensed practical nurse, or to delegate from a primary nurse to an associate nurse.

The other health team member needs to be legally qualified to safely perform the actions. State laws, policies, job descriptions, educational preparation, and the health team member's strengths and limitations are used to guide the nurse regarding delegation of actions to another health team member. When a therapeutic nurse-client relationship is needed to accomplish the actions of the plan, delegation is not recommended. For example, clients who need to verbalize feelings or would benefit from encouragement and emotional support need a consistent professional caregiver.

Delegation works best if the actions are well defined. The nurse who is delegating to others provides the following:

- Clear objectives and instructions
- Checkpoints and follow-up
- An empathetic ear if problems arise (Vestal, 1987)

Guidelines to effective delegation involve selecting the right person to perform the actions and providing the health team member with sufficient instructions to carry out the actions with the client. Delegation requires an investment of time in preparing the health care member to perform the action. Instructions are to be as specific as possible. The other health care members need to know their exact responsibilities and accept the request. The nurse also needs to develop an effective means of communication involving such things as feedback, problem solving, and client responses when delegation is occurring (Wywialowski, 1993).

The nurse realizes that the actions done by another may not be performed exactly the same way. Proper selection and instructions can minimize inconsistency. The person to whom the action is delegated becomes accountable and responsible for the action. However, the nurse who delegates the action also retains responsibility and is accountable for the client's care (Sullivan and Decker, 1992).

Delegation allows the nurse to implement nursing care efficiently by using others to perform actions for which they are qualified. This provides the professional nurse with additional time for implementing other actions and accomplishing other components of the nursing process.

Documentation

Documentation of implementation involves the use of written records—the health care record and the care plan. The care plan is actually becoming a permanent part of the health care record in many agencies. Documentation describes the actions implemented by the nurse, client, or others to facilitate achievement of the client's expected outcomes. The client's response to the implementation of the plan is also recorded. Responses consist of biophysical, psychosocial, and spiritual behaviors. The progress the client is making toward meeting the expected outcomes is noted on the care plan to provide continuity of care with other health team members. Documentation also includes a description of the actions that were not implemented and why, such as when priorities change.

Recording in the client's health care record guides future care by providing additional data and a reference point for changes that may take place. Documentation also fosters greater individualization of care and reduction in the duplication of efforts. The health care record improves the quality of care when it is used as an evaluation tool to determine what actions were effective and could be used again in similar situations. In addition, the health care record provides the legal proof that care was or was not given.

To meet the purposes of documentation, various types of record systems have been formulated. In the traditional narrative or source format, nurses write notes for a given period or after each client contact. This format has been found to be ineffective because the narrative is usually unsystematic and includes information about several areas of concern in one paragraph. It becomes difficult to follow the progression of a concern during the course of the client's care.

Problem-Oriented Medical Record

To counteract the disadvantages of the unorganized narrative format, Weed (1970) developed the problem-oriented record. This multidisciplinary system consists of the following components:

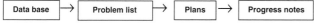

Data base → Problem list → Plans → Progress notes

The database consists of a history, physical examination, and laboratory data. The problem list is num-

bered and dated and is the first page of the client's health record. A plan for each problem is formulated and is numbered and titled according to the number and title in the problem list. The progress notes are the mechanism for follow-up on each problem. Progress notes consist of structured narrative notes, flow sheets, and a discharge summary. The narrative notes are structured using the SOAP format: subjective data, objective data, assessment, and plan (Iyer and Camp, 1991).

The problem-oriented record has been modified to incorporate the components of the nursing process. The nursing diagnoses give direction to the planning, implementation, and evaluation of nursing care and therefore are used in the recording system. Each relevant nursing diagnosis appears in the problem list or a separate nursing diagnosis list and is addressed in the care plan. The progress notes address a specific nursing diagnosis and include the actions implemented, the client's reactions, and any additional data pertinent to that particular nursing diagnosis. The status of the concerns and expected outcomes, as well as recommendations for continuation or modification of the original plan, is also recorded in the progress notes.

One format for writing progress notes oriented toward the nursing process is the SOAPIER method (Fischbach, 1991). It involves the following:

S	Subjective data	Client statements/interactions
O	Objective data	Nurse's observations and measurements
A	Analysis	Status of nursing diagnosis
P	Plan of care	Outcomes and actions planned
I	Implementation	Actions implemented
E	Evaluation	Client responses to actions/outcomes
R	Revision	Changes in plan when necessary

The entire format does not have to be used in every recording. An example of the SOAPIER method follows:

2/18/94   *Nursing diagnosis:* alteration in nutrition (more than body requirements)

S: I've lost 3 pounds. That's great! I really tried to watch the salt and I did my walking.

O: 3-lb wt loss in 2 weeks.

A: Remains 19% over ideal wt.

P: 1. Client will lose 1-2 lb per week until ideal wt reached.
    a. Continue with 1450 calorie, low-sodium diet.
    b. Weigh self 1/wk.
    c. Complete a 3-day food diary for next clinic visit in 1 month.
  2. Client will continue walking program at least 3×/wk for 30 min.

I: Discussed difficulties with diet.

E: Realizes that new nutritional patterns will be life-long. Plans to continue with the 1450-calorie, low-sodium diet.

Focus Charting

Focus charting, another common system of documentation, was developed from a nursing process perspective. The topic, or focus, of the documentation is a client concern or a change in status. The focus is often a nursing diagnosis, which ties the care plan and the progress notes together.

This system of documentation uses flowsheets and progress notes. The progress notes use the following format:

D Data	Subjective and objective information	
A Action	Immediate and/or future actions	
R Response	Client response to actions (Fischbach, 1991)	

This system provides a more positive approach than a "problem-oriented" system. It also is more adaptable to the use of nursing diagnoses as the focus of documentation.

Charting By Exception

The Charting By Exception system of documentation was developed by nurses to increase efficiency and reduce duplication and repetitiveness. It is an abbreviated documentation system where narrative notes are written for abnormal or significant findings. This system centers around clinical standards, protocols, and nursing/physician order flow sheets. The narrative notes, when written, usually use a SOAP(IER) format (Fischbach, 1991).

Computerized Documentation Systems

An increasing number of nursing organizations are using computerized information systems to facilitate documentation in terms of care planning and recording assessment data, actions, and client responses. Automated assessments, care plans, and progress notes benefit the nurse and the client by decreasing the time spent in documenting nursing care and revising care plans, increasing the accuracy and legibility of recordings, allowing immediate availability of the client record to other health team members, and providing efficient retrieval of information for the evaluation of care (Gillies, 1989).

Nursing Model–Oriented Documentation Systems

Nursing models also provide the framework for documentation systems. King (1981) has suggested that a Goal-Oriented Nursing Record be used when incorporating the Theory of Goal Attainment. This system documents both the process and outcomes in nurse/client situations. The Goal-Oriented Nursing Record has five major elements: database, problem list, goal list, plan, and progress notes. In this system goals or expected outcomes are recorded, as well as the methods and the process used to achieve them. Progress notes are written in the SOAP format.

The type of record forms and method of charting are determined by the agency. Nurses often have input into the design of chart forms and the method of charting used in the agency. The method chosen should foster efficiency, meet legal requirements, and be oriented toward the client's concerns and the selected nursing model within the nursing process.

When documenting implementation of the plan, the recording of actions and responses is done systematically, clearly, and accurately, no matter what type of record is used. Descriptions of behavior rather than labels are recorded. Attempts are made to avoid duplication of recording. Recording in a systematic, clear fashion benefits the client and the health care team.

Guidelines for Implementation

The guidelines describe the important elements necessary for the implementation component.

1. *The actions performed are consistent with the plan and occur after validation of the plan.* Before actions are implemented, the plan is validated. Validation determines whether the plan is still relevant, of immediate concern, based on sound rationale, and individualized. The nurse ensures that the actions being implemented, whether by the client, nurse, or others, are purposeful and outcome oriented. The actions during implementation are directed toward meeting the plan.

2. *Interpersonal, intellectual, and technical skills are performed competently and efficiently in an appropriate environment.* Nursing actions during implementation consist of interpersonal, intellectual, and technical skills. The nurse needs to be competent and able to efficiently perform these skills to carry out the plan. The nurse's self-awareness of strengths and limitations contributes to providing competent and efficient care while enacting the professional nursing roles.

3. *The client's physical and psychological safety is protected.* During execution of the plan, the client's physical and psychological safety is ensured by adequately preparing the client, performing skillful and efficient nursing care, applying sound principles, individualizing actions, and supporting the client during the actions. A caring attitude and protection of client rights also are aspects of psychological safety.

4. *Documentation of actions and client response is provided in the health care record and care plan.* Documentation in the health care record consists of a description of the actions implemented and the client's response to the actions. Actions not imple-

mented are also recorded, as well as the reason. In addition, documentation occurs on the care plan to provide continuity of care and to note the client's progress in meeting the expected outcomes.

Summary

Implementation involves the client, the nurse, and others to carry out the plan. Other components of the nursing process, such as assessment and planning, continue during this component. The nurse's ability to perform interpersonal, intellectual, and technical skills influences the effectiveness of the actions provided. Implementation consists of three phases: preparation, implementation, and postimplementation. In this chapter, the responsibilities and roles of the nurse, including client advocacy, coordination, delegation, and documentation during each phase of implementation were described.

Critical Thinking Exercises BY ELIZABETH S. FAYRAM

1. Janet is a new graduate working as a staff nurse on an adult medical unit. She is to be the primary nurse with Ms. Robinson, a newly diagnosed insulin-dependent diabetic. Janet and Ms. Robinson have planned a learning program; however, Janet has never implemented a diabetic learning program to this extent. Knowing Janet's limited expertise with a diabetic program, explain how Janet could ensure that Ms. Robinson's learning outcomes are achieved.

2. Describe how to ensure physical safety and psychological comfort in the following situations. In addition, explain the cultural and developmental factors to consider in each.
   a. Mike is a 3-year-old in the emergency department. You are to insert an intravenous line (IV) for hydration.
   b. Carmella is a 15-year-old in the emergency department who is to have a cast applied to her left leg for a fractured tibia.

3. You are a staff nurse on an inpatient rehabilitation unit during the day shift.
   Routine of the unit: All clients eat breakfast in the dining room at 7:30 AM (do not need to be dressed). Occupational therapy (OT) comes at 8:15 AM to work with clients on oral hygiene and dressing. Physical therapy (PT), OT, and speech therapy (ST) are scheduled from 9 to 11:30 AM. Lunch is at 11:30 AM. Afternoon therapies are from 1 to 4 PM. Medications are usually scheduled at 8 AM and noon.

   You have the following staff working with you today: a senior nursing student who will do total care for one client during the shift and a nursing assistant with 3 years of experience on the rehabilitation unit. You are assigned the following five clients:
   a. Allan—a 21-year-old paraplegic who is beginning to learn intermittent self-catheterization (every 4 to 6 hours). He uses a sliding board with assistance from two staff members for transfers.
   b. Bill—a 67-year-old client with a cerebrovascular accident (CVA) resulting in hemiplegia, aphasia, and dysphagia. He requires gastrostomy feedings every 4 hours and wears an external condom. Transfers are with maximum assistance of two staff members.
   c. Edwin—a 30-year-old, brain-injured client. He is disoriented and is frequently found in his wheelchair on the elevator or in another unit. He transfers with assistance of one staff member.
   d. Helen—a 64-year-old client with a right-sided CVA. She is impulsive and has left-sided paresis. She transfers with standby assistance. She is to be discharged in 3 days. She is on self-administered medications, for which she must ask at the appropriate times.
   e. Marie—a 59-year-old diabetic with a below-the-knee amputation of the right leg. She requires stump care, blood glucose monitoring before meals, and is on sliding scale insulin therapy. She transfers with the assistance of one staff member.
      1) Determine activities to be delegated to the student and the nursing assistant.
      2) Identify guidelines that influenced your decision.
      3) Explain how you would adequately prepare others to do the activities you have requested.
      4) Explain how you would evaluate the effectiveness of the delegation.

4. Ms. Johnson has brought her two children, ages 4 months and 2 years, to the well-child clinic. This is the first time the children have been seen at this clinic. When asked what her goal is for this visit, Ms. Johnson states, "I think they need some shots." When questioned further, Ms. Johnson states that Raymond, 2 years old, and Esther, 4 months old, have not received any immunizations before this visit. She says that the children are healthy and have just not needed to go to a doctor. You record the following measurements:

   Raymond: Height 33 in; Weight 29 lb; Temperature, Pulse, Respiration Rate (TPR) 97.7 (axillary), 90, 24

   Esther: Height 25 in; Weight 14 lb; TPR 98.2 (axillary), 126, 30

   The children receive their first series of diphtheria-tetanus-pertussis (DTP), oral polio, and *Hemophilus influenzae* type B vaccines. Raymond also receives a measles-mumps-rubella (MMR) vaccine. Ms. Johnson is given written instructions on immunizations including importance, side effects, and future schedule. Ms. Johnson makes an appointment to return in 2 months.
   a. Write a progress note for this clinic situation using the SOAPIER format.
   b. Write a progress note using focus charting's DAR format.
   c. List the advantages and disadvantages of using each of the above formats in this situation.

REFERENCES AND READINGS

Alfaro R: *Applying nursing diagnoses and nursing process,* Philadelphia, 1992, JB Lippincott.

American Nurses Association: *Standards of clinical nursing practice,* Kansas City, 1992, The Association.

Benner P: *From novice to expert: excellence and power in clinical nursing practice,* Menlo Park, Calif, 1984, Addison-Wesley.

Bradley JC and Edinberg MA: *Communication in the nursing context,* Norwalk, Conn, 1990, Appleton and Lange.

Bulechek GM and McCloskey JC: *Nursing interventions: essential nursing treatments,* Philadelphia, 1992, WB Saunders.

Burke L and Murphy J: *Charting by exception,* New York, 1988, John Wiley and Sons.

Fischbach FI: *Documenting care: communication, the nursing process, and documentation standards,* Philadelphia, 1991, FA Davis.

Gillies DA: *Nursing management: a systems approach,* Philadelphia, 1989, WB Saunders.

Iyer PW and Camp NH: *Nursing documentation: a nursing process approach,* St Louis, 1991, Mosby–Year Book.

Iyer PW et al: *Nursing process and nursing diagnosis,* Philadelphia, 1991, WB Saunders.

King IM: *A theory for nursing: systems, concepts, process,* New York, 1981, John Wiley and Sons.

Kron T and Gray A: *The management of patient care,* Philadelphia, 1987, WB Saunders.

Lampe S: *Focus charting,* Minneapolis, 1988, Creative Nursing Management.

Lampe S and Hitchcock A: Documenting nursing diagnoses using focus charting. In McLane A, editor: *Classification of nursing diagnoses: proceedings of the seventh conference,* St Louis, 1987, Mosby–Year Book.

Leddy S and Pepper JM: *Conceptual bases for professional nursing,* Philadelphia, 1993, JB Lippincott.

Orem DE: *Nursing: concepts of practice,* ed 4, St Louis, 1991, Mosby–Year Book.

Peplau HE: *Interpersonal relations in nursing,* New York, 1991, Springer.

Roy SrC and Andrews HA: *The Roy adaptation model: the definitive statement,* Norwalk, Conn, 1991, Appleton and Lange.

Soontit E: Installing the first operational bedside nursing computer system, *Nurs Management* 18:39, July 1987.

Sullivan EJ and Decker PJ: *Effective management in nursing,* Menlo Park, Calif, 1992, Addison-Wesley Nursing.

Sundeen SJ et al: *Nurse-client interaction: implementing the nursing process,* ed 5, St Louis, 1993, Mosby–Year Book.

Vestal KW: *Management concepts for the new nurse,* Philadelphia, 1987, JB Lippincott.

Weed LL: *Medical records, medical education, and patient care,* Cleveland, 1970, Case Western Reserve University Press.

Wilkinson JM: *Nursing process in action: a critical thinking approach,* Redwood City, Calif, 1992, Addison-Wesley Nursing.

Wong DL: *Whaley and Wong's essentials of pediatric nursing,* ed 4, St Louis, 1993, Mosby–Year Book.

Wywialowski E: *Managing client care,* St Louis, 1993, Mosby–Year Book.

Yura H and Walsh MB: *The nursing process: assessing, planning, implementing, and evaluating,* Norwalk, Conn, 1988, Appleton and Lange.

CHAPTER 12

EVALUATION

Janet W. Kenney

General Considerations

Evaluation is a planned, systematic process of *collecting, organizing, analyzing,* and *comparing* the client's health status with the desired expected outcomes, and *judging* the degree of client achievement of the outcomes. It is an ongoing, continuous, deliberate activity that involves the client, family, nurse, and other health care team members. Knowledge of health, pathophysiology, nursing intervention strategies, and evaluation methods is required for an effective evaluation. The Joint Commission on the Accreditation of Healthcare Organizations (JCAHO, 1990) defines evaluation as follows:

Analysis of collected, compiled, and organized data pertaining to important aspects of care or service. Data are compared with threshold (a pre-established level of performance) for evaluation and variations are judged . . . and problems or opportunities to improve care are identified.

Evaluation serves several purposes. The major purpose is to determine the client's progress in meeting the designated expected outcomes. Another important purpose is to judge the effectiveness of the nursing process components in assisting the client to achieve the expected outcomes. Evaluation is also used to determine the overall quality of care given to a group of clients, through quality improvement and total quality management programs.

The chosen nursing model is used to guide evaluation by identifying *what* to evaluate. The client's des-

ignated expected outcomes are based on the nursing model and thus serve to guide the evaluation. For example, if Orem's Self Care model is selected, the expected outcomes would identify the client's expected self-care skills. These skills would be compared with the client's response to nursing care to determine the client's progress during evaluation.

The Standards of Clinical Nursing Practice (ANA, 1991), which delineate six standards in the nursing process, state in Standard VI, Evaluation, that *"The nurse evaluates the client's progress toward attainment of outcomes."* The six measurement criteria designated to meet this standard are as follows:

1. Evaluation is systematic and ongoing.
2. The client's responses to interventions are documented.
3. The effectiveness of interventions is evaluated in relation to outcomes.
4. Ongoing assessment data are used to revise diagnoses, outcomes, and the plan of care, as needed.
5. Revisions in diagnoses, outcomes, and the plan of care are documented.
6. The client, significant others, and health care providers are involved in the evaluation process, when appropriate.

Nurses are accountable for designing effective care plans, implementing appropriate nursing actions, and judging the effectiveness of their nursing interventions. Unfortunately, systematic evaluation is often the most neglected part of the nursing process. Ideally, evaluation is an integral part of each component of the nursing process. The client's initial assessment serves as a baseline with which to compare changes in human responses and to determine the client's progress. The nursing diagnosis identifies the client's health concerns and directs the areas that will be evaluated. The client's expected outcomes are the criteria used to improve the client's health status. The client's current health behaviors are compared with the expected outcomes to determine the client's progress. During nursing implementation, the nurse appraises the client's response to the nursing orders and judges whether the plans are facilitating the client's progress. Based on the client's progress, the nurse may maintain, modify, or change the nursing care plan.

Both the client's progress and the nursing actions are considered in evaluation. In measuring the client's progress toward meeting the desired outcomes, the nurse also judges the effectiveness of the nursing care plan and the quality of care, and identifies ways to promote attainment of expected outcomes. These actions demonstrate accountability for nursing actions and practice. Accountability implies responsibility for one's behavior; it requires the ability to define, explain, and measure the results of nursing actions. Quality improvement enables nurses to demonstrate accountability for the quality of their practice to society. Without evaluation, nurses would not know whether the care they gave was effective or not; thus ineffective nursing actions might be continued. Evaluation helps the nurse identify nursing actions that are effective or ineffective, and also enhances the scientific foundation of professional nursing practice.

As nurses acquire increased clinical experience, their personal, experiential, and scientific knowledge expands. With increased proficiency, nurses constantly use these ways of knowing, along with their intuitive knowledge, in all forms of evaluation and as the basis for their practice.

Critical Thinking in Evaluation

Critical thinking is an integral aspect of the evaluation process. Evaluation involves many critical thinking skills such as application of knowledge, analysis, and synthesis. In addition, critical thinking involves identifying appropriate expected outcomes in relation to the nursing model and relevant indicators of those outcomes. Analyzing and comparing the client's responses, and judging the client's progress are also important skills. Critical thinking is also necessary to identify which components of the nursing care plan were effective and which need to be modified.

This chapter begins with a brief history of the development of evaluation in nursing. The difference

between the use of criteria and standards in evaluation is explained. Three major forms of evaluation—structure, process, and outcome—are described and illustrated, along with the differences between concurrent and retrospective evaluation. General characteristics of evaluation are presented, including who should evaluate, what should be evaluated, and when evaluation should occur. Broad guidelines for the evaluation component of the nursing process are listed below and discussed later in the chapter. Quality assurance programs and JCAHO standards for nursing care conclude this chapter.

Guidelines for Evaluation

1. The nurse reviews the client's expected outcomes and identifies relevant indicators to monitor changes in the client's health status.
2. The nurse continuously monitors, appraises, and reassesses the client's response to nursing actions.
3. The client's response to nursing actions is compared with the client's short-term outcomes to determine the extent to which these outcomes have been achieved (*ongoing evaluation*).
4. The client's progress or lack of progress toward achievement of long-term expected outcomes is determined (*concluding evaluation*).
5. The nursing care plan is reviewed to determine which actions were effective or ineffective in assisting the client's progress.
6. The nursing care plan is revised to reflect changes in the client's condition or when the short-term or long-term expected outcomes have not been adequately met.

Historical Perspective

In the last two decades, evaluation of health care delivery has changed hands and focus, sparked by the concerns of consumers and the government over increasing costs and inadequate services. In health care agencies, client evaluation was formerly the prerogative of physicians. With new legislation and interest among all health care providers, evaluation is now performed by each profession. In the 1970s the federal government created professional standard review organizations (PSROs) to monitor costs of health services, and the Joint Commission on the Accreditation of Hospitals developed guidelines to evaluate hospital services.

Traditionally nurses were evaluated by their supervisors. Characteristics such as clinical skills, organization, leadership, dependability, and punctuality were judged. These evaluations did not consider the effectiveness of nursing care or improvement in the client's health status. As the responsibility for evaluation was dispersed among health care professionals and agencies, nurses recognized the need to change their focus and improve their methods.

In 1990 the JCAHO reaffirmed the essential value of the nursing process in evaluation and required that this process be thoroughly documented in the care of all clients. The JCAHO also required that important aspects of care be identified and indicators developed to monitor the quality and appropriateness of these aspects of care. Currently, professional nurses use established standards of clinical nursing practice (ANA, 1991) and JCAHO standards to deliver quality care and to evaluate their ability to provide high-quality care. These standards guide evaluation of nursing care for both individual clients and groups of clients in health care agencies. Agency evaluation was formerly called *quality assurance* and involved nursing audits with standard guidelines. Currently, overall evaluation of hospitals and health care agencies is known as *Total Quality Management* (TQM) or *Continuous Quality Improvement* (CQI). The JCAHO defines CQI as follows:

An approach to quality management that builds upon traditional quality assurance methods by emphasizing the organization and systems (rather than individuals), the need for objective data with which to analyze and improve processes, and the ideal that systems and performance can always improve even when high standards appear to have been met.

Evaluation of nursing care is a complex task because it is extremely difficult to separate the unique contributions of nurses to client care from the overlapping functions of other team members. This difficulty makes it hard to evaluate the results of nursing actions. The activities unique to nursing must be identified and the results of nursing interventions evaluated. The profession continues to address these issues.

Criteria and Standards

Although the terms *criteria* and *standards* are often used interchangeably in evaluation, they have very different meanings. *Criteria* are measurable qualities, attributes, or characteristics that describe specific skills, knowledge, attitudes, or behaviors. They describe acceptable levels of performance by stating the expected behaviors of the client or nurse in the short-term outcomes or nursing orders. *Criteria may be written by individual nurses in care plans.*

Standards represent acceptable, expected levels of performance by nursing staff or other health team members. *Standards are established by authority, custom, or general consent.* Professions such as nursing have developed standards to improve the level of practice.

In 1973 the American Nurses Association (ANA, 1974) established the Standards of Nursing Practice, which described eight essential actions in the nursing process. In 1991 the ANA revised the original standards and delineated six Standards of Clinical Nursing Practice to reflect current practice. These standards are broad, general statements that describe how nurses should practice. Measurement criteria are listed for each of these six standards. Nursing standards describe quality nursing care and are used to guide nursing actions. They provide a frame of reference for judging the quality of nursing care. Most clinical specialty groups within the ANA have adopted and modified the generic standards to reflect clinical practice and teaching within the specialty. In some health care agencies, standards are often written for routine nursing procedures on specific units to guide nursing practice. The JCAHO (1990) defines standards as follows:

Patient-focused guidelines for care. Focuses on outcomes. Standards are guiding principles in caring for the patient. They provide the basis of information necessary to skillfully care for a patient with a disease or human response need.

Forms of Evaluation

Evaluation has been classified according to *what* is to be judged and *when*. There are three types of evaluation that describe what is to be evaluated: structure, process, and outcome. Each type has a different focus and criteria as defined below.

Structure—the physical facilities, equipment, services, and credentials of employees

Process—the *nursing actions* within each component of the nursing process, which include:

- *Adequacy*—the amount and quality
- *Appropriateness*—relevance to each component and the client situation
- *Effectiveness*—ability to facilitate client's expected outcomes
- *Efficiency*—conservation of time, energy, and resources of client, health team, and agency

Outcome—the changes in the *client's behaviors*, which include:

- *Physiological responses*—temperature, wound healing, neurological responses
- *Psychological responses*—appropriate affect, congruent verbal and nonverbal behaviors
- *Psychomotor skills*—infant care, wound dressing, colostomy irrigation, crutch walking
- *Knowledge*—about illness, including drugs, treatments, diet, and prevention
- *Abilities*—to resolve grief, perform activities of daily living, exercise

Within process and outcome types of evaluation, there are two forms, *concurrent* and *retrospective*, based on *when* the evaluation occurs:

Concurrent—"Review of process and outcome of patient care conducted during the patient's hospital stay" (JCAHO, 1990). Concurrent evaluation reflects review of present, ongoing nursing actions (process) or client behaviors (outcome) as they occur.

Retrospective—"Review of process and outcomes of patient care performed after the patient has been discharged ..." (JCAHO, 1990). It is the evaluation of nursing actions or client behaviors after services to the client have been discontinued.

Each of the three major forms of evaluation is presented separately. Table 12-1 describes the different purposes and sources of data, along with examples of evaluation.

Structure

The focus of structure evaluation is on the physical facilities, equipment, organizational pattern, staffing patterns, services provided, and the employees' qualifications for administrative and staff positions. The basic question addressed by this type of evaluation is whether the agency or institution has the necessary resources and policies to provide the services offered to the client population.

Most community agencies and organizations, including hospitals and health care centers, have established guidelines or policies describing the required facilities, equipment, administrative structure, and employee qualifications and responsibilities. The JCAHO (1990) also has specific standards that are used to evaluate hospitals periodically. Each state also has a health department that establishes acceptable standards for hospitals, health departments, long-term care facilities, and home health agencies.

Process

Process evaluation focuses on the nurse's activities. These activities are judged by (1) observing the nurse's performance, (2) asking clients what the nurse did, and (3) reviewing the nurse's notes in the chart. Process evaluation looks at each component of the nursing process and makes judgments about nursing care by asking the following questions:

Table 12-1	**Different Forms of Evaluation**	
Structure	**Process**	**Outcome**
Purpose		
Structure evaluation measures existence and adequacy of facilities, equipment, procedures, policies, and staffing to meet client's needs	Process evaluation measures adequacy of nurse's actions and activities in implementing each component of nursing process	Outcome evaluation measures changes in client's behavior in comparison with expected outcomes
Sources of data	*Concurrent*	*Concurrent*
Procedure manuals	Nurse demonstrates knowledge and performance of skills	Client demonstrates new knowledge, skills, and physiological and psychosocial improvement in health care
Policy statements	Client interviews of nursing care provided	
Position descriptions	Chart contains evidence of nursing actions performed	Client interviews to determine knowledge learned from nurse
Nursing care plans		
Orientation and in-service programs		
Staff educational credentials	*Retrospective*	*Retrospective*
Facilities and equipment available	Chart cites nursing procedures implemented, such as measuring vital signs and teaching	Chart cites evidence of changes in client's behavior, skills, and knowledge
Charting and Kardex	Client surveys	Client surveys
Staffing patterns		
Examples		
Staffing patterns are appropriate to patient acuity level	Nursing assessment is performed on admission to unit	Client's response to, and the outcomes of, nursing care, are documented in the chart
Orientation of nurses to unit covers relevant information	Nursing diagnoses are specified for each client	Client's abilities to manage care after discharge are documented
Standards of nursing practice are readily available	Nursing care is based on identified nursing diagnoses	

Was the nursing care *adequate?*
Were nursing actions *appropriate?*
Were nursing strategies *effective?*
Were nursing actions accomplished *efficiently?*

There are two forms of process evaluation: concurrent (during the nursing action) and retrospective (after the client has been discharged).

Concurrent process evaluation judges nursing performance as it takes place. The nurse is observed during a client interaction, or the client may be asked what the nursing actions were. For example, a nurse may be evaluated while giving an injection on use of the appropriate technique, or a nurse may be evaluated after instructing a client to determine whether specific topics were covered. In addition, the client's chart may be reviewed while the client is receiving services to determine whether appropriate nursing actions are charted. The JCAHO (1990) Standards for Nursing Care include concurrent process evaluation and are discussed at the end of this chapter. Some examples of concurrent process evaluation are as follows:

- Was each client's need for nursing care related to his or her admission assessed by a registered nurse?
- Was each client's nursing care based on identified nursing diagnoses?
- Does the nurse identify the client before giving medications?
- Is the consent form signed before the client's surgery?
- Are all procedures adequately explained to the client?
- Are all nursing actions properly performed?

Retrospective process evaluation judges nursing performance *after* services to the client have been discontinued. This evaluation, called a *nursing audit* or *chart review,* examines any aspect of nursing that should be documented in the client's chart and determines whether specific nursing actions were performed and documented. The audit is usually performed by trained clerks. The differences between concurrent and retrospective process evaluation are shown in Table 12-2. Examples of retrospective process evaluation are as follows:

- Were interventions identified to meeting the client's nursing care needs?
- Were the client's response to, and the outcomes of, care recorded?
- Were the abilities of the client to manage continuing care needs after discharge documented?
- Were the client's intake and output accurately recorded?
- Were a client history and nursing physical examination recorded?
- Were all medications and treatments signed?
- Were all relevant symptoms monitored on time?

Outcome

Outcome evaluation focuses on changes in the client's health status by comparing changes in the client's baseline health with the client's expected outcomes. Outcome evaluation is directly related to efforts to promote, maintain, and restore the client's health. During nursing interventions, the nurse appraises the client's health status for changes that indicate progress toward the expected outcomes. Examples of these changes are altered physiological

Table 12-2	Methods of Process and Outcome Evaluation
Process (Evaluation of Nurse)	**Outcome (Evaluation of Client)**
Concurrent	
Client: Ask client about actions performed by nurse.	*Client:* Observe client for changes toward improved health status through new knowledge, skills, or abilities. Observe client's physiological status or psychosocial affect and behaviors for signs of improvement.
Nurse: Observe nurse administering care, teaching, and examining client.	
Chart: Audit client's chart for documentation of appropriate nursing action, plans, and evaluation while client is receiving service.	
Retrospective	
Chart audit: Look for documentation of nursing actions: nursing history, client expected outcomes, nursing plans, and actions implemented, such as vital signs, medications given, and teaching performed, after client has been discharged from health service.	*Chart audit:* Look for documentation of changes in client's health status, knowledge, abilities, or skills. Physiological and psychosocial behavioral changes toward improved health would also be appropriate evidence, after client has been discharged from health service.

and psychological responses, acquired psychomotor skills, and increased knowledge and abilities. Outcome evaluation, though difficult, is the most meaningful way to judge the effectiveness of nursing interventions. The client's progress toward meeting the expected outcomes is evaluated by asking these and other related questions:

- Have the client's *physiological* and *psychological responses* improved?
- What *psychomotor skills* can the client perform?
- What specific *knowledge* has the client acquired?
- What *abilities* has the client developed?

There are also two forms of outcome evaluation: concurrent and retrospective.

Concurrent outcome evaluation judges the client's *present* health status, skills, knowledge, and abilities *before* services to the client are discontinued. The nurse measures the client's progress by comparing the client's initial database with the current health status in relation to the expected outcomes. This comparison can be done by observing the client directly or by examining the chart for documentation of client behaviors that indicate the client's health status, knowledge, or abilities. Usually outcome evaluations are individualized for each client; however, some hospitals have developed standardized expected client outcomes for specific diagnoses. Examples of concurrent outcome evaluation questions are as follows:

- Can the client demonstrate crutch walking correctly?
- Does the client relate to others appropriately?
- Can the client prepare and administer insulin accurately?
- Are the client's vital signs stable?
- Is the client's surgical wound healing properly?

Retrospective outcome evaluation judges the client's health status and behaviors as documented in the chart *after* services to the client have been discontinued. The chart is examined for documentation of the client's progress toward meeting the long- and short-term expected outcomes as a result of nursing intervention. The JCAHO (1990) incorporated some aspects of retrospective outcome evaluation in their guidelines. The following are examples of retrospective outcome evaluation questions:

- Was the client able to demonstrate activities of daily living?
- Was the client's attitude positive upon discharge?
- Was the client able to plan a diabetic daily menu?
- Did the client demonstrate appropriate bonding behaviors?

- Was the client's caregiver able to perform physical care activities?

Characteristics of Evaluation

Three major aspects of evaluation need to be considered in the nursing process: *Who* participates in the evaluation? *What* should be evaluated? *When* should evaluation occur? Evaluation always involves judgments based on knowledge and experience. The quality of health care is based on the values of those who participate in the evaluation. They determine what is important to evaluate and when to evaluate. Therefore the client, nurse, health team members, and agency all may be involved in evaluation.

Who participates in the evaluation? The Standards of Clinical Nursing Practice (ANA, 1991) criteria for evaluation require that *"The client, significant others, and health care providers are involved in the evaluation process, when appropriate."* This criteria identifies who participates in evaluating the client's response and progress in achieving the expected outcomes. Although other health team members may participate, the nurse is solely responsible for writing the evaluation data in the client's chart.

What should be evaluated? Ultimately, the client's responses to nursing interventions and the effectiveness of those interventions are evaluated in relation to the client's expected outcomes. The nurse may focus solely on the client's progress and achievement of specific outcomes, or the nurse may broaden the evaluation to include all aspects of the nursing process. In evaluating the nursing process, each component that contributed to the client's behavioral changes and progress is examined. This broad, comprehensive process evaluation includes judging the *adequacy*, *appropriateness*, *effectiveness*, and *efficiency* of each component. This type of evaluation may be part of the quality improvement program in a health care organization.

Some questions that the nurse may use to evaluate the effect of the nursing process in facilitating the client's progress toward achievement of expected outcomes are shown in the box on p. 201.

When should evaluation occur? Evaluation is a continuous process and includes both ongoing and concluding elements. Ongoing evaluation is the continuous judgment of the client's health status and progress in meeting short-term outcomes. It begins with the initial assessment, during which baseline data are collected for comparison at a later time. In the planning component, expected outcomes are identified for ongoing comparison with the client's health status. During interventions the nurse monitors, appraises, and reassesses the client's response. As data accumulate, the nurse identifies the client's

Questions to Evaluate the Effectiveness of the Nursing Process

Assessment

Adequacy

Was data collection comprehensive and multifocal?

Were sufficient data collected on client's health concerns?

Were data collected from a variety of sources?

Was client's record updated periodically?

Appropriateness

Were appropriate methods used for data collection?

Were data relevant to client's health concerns?

Were relevant data verified by others?

Effectiveness

Were there sufficient data to establish nursing diagnoses?

Efficiency

Were data collected in a systematic, organized manner using a nursing model?

Diagnoses

Adequacy

Were nursing diagnoses clear and concise?

Were *all* nursing diagnoses client-centered, specific, and accurate?

Did all nursing diagnoses include an etiological statement?

Were all client's health concerns identified?

Appropriateness

Were diagnoses relevant to the client and the agency?

Were diagnoses appropriate for nursing intervention?

Were diagnoses mutually agreed on by the client and nurse?

Were diagnoses appropriate to the resources and the timetable?

Effectiveness

Did nursing diagnoses accurately reflect data analysis?

Did nursing diagnoses guide client goals and objectives?

Did nursing diagnoses guide planning and interventions?

Planning

Adequacy

Were client objectives sufficient to achieve each goal?

Were there sufficient nursing orders to achieve each expected outcome?

Did the strategy and nursing orders clearly guide nursing interventions?

Were nursing plans clearly documented?

Appropriateness

Were client long-term outcomes appropriate to their respective diagnoses?

Were client short- and long-term outcomes prioritized appropriately?

Were short-term outcomes and nursing orders in a logical sequence?

Were plans realistic for the client, the setting, and the timetable?

Effectiveness

Was client agreeable to the plans?

Did plans facilitate the client's progress?

Was client satisfied with plans and progress?

Efficiency

Did plans use resources and team members efficiently?

Implementation

Adequacy

Were all plans implemented accordingly?

Were team members able to follow plans?

Were all resources available as needed?

Appropriateness

Were nurses able to implement nursing orders?

Were client's safety, privacy, and confidentiality maintained?

Were nursing actions realistic to achieve client expected outcomes?

Effectiveness

How did client respond to nursing actions?

Did nursing actions facilitate client's progress?

Were client's expected outcomes achieved within timetable?

Efficiency

Were nursing actions performed efficiently?

Were resources used economically?

Was client's energy expenditure minimized?

---

pattern or behavioral trend, and compares this with the initial database and the long-term expected outcomes and timetable. The nurse then judges the level of the client's progress toward achieving the expected outcomes. As the plan is implemented, the nurse evaluates the client's response to determine the effectiveness of the plan or the need to change the plan.

Ongoing evaluation may be performed by the nurse as frequently as every few minutes in a life-threatening situation, every hour, during every change of shift, or daily or weekly. Each contact with the client provides an opportunity to assess the client's signs, symptoms, and behaviors, and to evaluate the client's progress toward short-term outcomes. Is the client attaining the short-term outcomes and making progress toward the long-term expected outcomes? The frequency of evaluation depends on the client's condition or health status, the types of client changes expected, and the unit or agency policies. For example, an unconscious client in an acute care unit may need to be checked every 15 minutes for signs of change, whereas a home health client with a chronic disability may be evaluated on a weekly schedule.

While implementing nursing care, the nurse evaluates the effects of the nursing actions in achieving the plan and the client's progress toward attaining the expected outcomes. Ongoing evaluation compares the client's response with the actions in the plan and the client's progress toward achieving the outcomes. This serves as a basis for continuing, modifying, or changing the plans. For example, the nursing orders may state, "The client will discuss dietary likes and dislikes." The client's response: "Mr. Smith said he likes red meat and chicken but won't eat liver or seafood." The nurse charts the identified health concern, the short-term outcome that was evaluated, and the client's response, and interprets the degree of progress in meeting the outcome.

Concluding evaluation occurs after the client has met several short-term outcomes. The nurse judges the client's progress or lack of progress toward attainment of long-term expected outcomes. The nurse writes a summary of how well or to what degree the client has progressed toward attaining each expected outcome. Sometimes short-term outcomes or resources are insufficient to attain a long-term outcome, or the timetable for accomplishment is unrealistic. Occasionally the short-term outcomes may be met, but the client has not achieved the long-term expected outcome. For example, the outcome may state, "The client will modify his diet to lose weight." After achieving several short-term outcomes, the nurse's concluding evaluation may read, "The client can explain the reasons for weight loss and plan appropriate menus but lacks motivation to stay on the diet. Further counseling is needed." The concluding evaluation describes how well and to what degree the client has achieved the long-term expected outcome.

Revising the Nursing Care Plan

After comparison of the client's progress toward achieving the long-term expected outcomes, the nurse is responsible for revising the nursing care plan. The measurement criteria for evaluation in the Standards of Clinical Nursing Practice (ANA, 1991) clearly state the following:

Ongoing assessment data are used to revise diagnoses, outcomes, and the plan of care, as needed. Revisions in diagnoses, outcomes, and the plan of care are documented.

During both ongoing and concluding evaluation, the nurse judges the client's response to determine the effectiveness of the nursing care plan. The client may have achieved several objectives completely, partially, or not at all. The nurse compares the client's health status with the objectives and timetable and makes *one* of the following decisions:

1. Continue the plan as documented.
2. Reconsider the importance or priority of the short-term outcomes.
3. Modify the nursing actions, expected outcomes, or timetable.
4. Change the nursing diagnoses and care plan.

If the short-term outcomes were achieved, has the client met the long-term expected outcomes? If the outcome was met, has the nursing diagnosis been alleviated or resolved? If the client's health concern was alleviated, this is documented in the chart and further action is not required. However, if the concern is temporarily resolved, the nurse would continue to monitor the client's progress. If the outcomes are only partially met or not met at all, the nurse must reassess the client and evaluate the nursing care plan to determine the reason for the client's lack of progress. Some explanations for modifying or revising the nursing care plan include the following:

- The nursing diagnosis was inaccurate.
- The client's condition changed or new diagnoses occurred.
- The nursing orders were unrealistic (inadequate time or resources).
- The nursing orders overestimated or underestimated the client's capabilities.
- Additional data altered the client's health concern.
- Resources were unavailable or became available.
- Another nursing strategy may be more appropriate.

Guidelines for Evaluation

The guidelines describe the broad phases of the evaluation component. They presuppose the achievement of all the preceding components in the nursing process. Examples of individual, family, and community evaluations are shown on pp. 203 and 204. These examples reflect evaluations of selected short-term outcomes to meet a long-term outcome.

1. *The nurse reviews the client's expected outcomes and identifies relevant indicators to monitor changes in the client's health status.* Before implementing nursing actions, the nurse reviews the client's short-term and long-term expected outcomes. These criteria provide

Example of Individual Outcome Evaluation

Nursing Diagnosis: *Inability to maintain diabetic diet r/t lack of knowledge.*
Nursing Model: Orem's Self-Care model for supportive education of client.

Expected Outcome	*Ongoing evaluation* *Client's response*
Client will apply the ADA diabetic diet in menu planning and daily nutritional intake, as evidenced by:	
1. Accurately planning three daily menus, including snacks	Mr. G. stated he was unsure how to calculate carbohydrates (CHO). Mr. G. wrote accurate diabetic meal plans for 3 days, except CHO were excessive.
2. Recording all food and fluid intake at home for 3 days	Mr. G. recorded his meals but forgot his snacks. Mr. G.'s food intake was low in protein and high in CHO on 2 days.
	Minimal progress toward expected outcome

Example of Family Outcome Evaluation

Nursing Diagnosis: *Inadequate child safety precautions in the home.*
Nursing Model: Friedman's Structural Functional model to address family physical necessities.

Expected Outcome	*Ongoing evaluation* *Client's response*
Family will eliminate safety hazards to children from their home, as evidenced by:	
1. Identifying safety hazards in the home	Using a safety checklist, the family identified 8 of 12 safety hazards.
2. Removing or correcting safety hazards in the home	Family agreed to correct hazardous problems but had only eliminated 5 of 12 hazards. Stated they will work on the remaining hazards.
	Some progress toward expected outcome

indicators of what changes to observe and measure in the client to determine whether the nursing interventions are effective. If nurses do not know what changes to expect, they will not know if the client's condition is improving, nor if the nursing actions are effective.

2. *The nurse continuously monitors, appraises, and reassesses the client's response to nursing actions.* While implementing any nursing order, the nurse observes the client's current health status and response to nursing interventions. The nurse collects pertinent, specific client data related to the short-term and long-term expected outcomes. By reviewing the client's chart, the nurse notes changes in the client's condition as a result of nursing care. The results of blood studies, chest radiographs, urinalysis, and vital signs may be useful in evaluating the client's progress. The nurse also checks on the client's or family's compliance with the prescribed therapeutic regimen and tests. The client's understanding of information or care is also ascertained.

3. *The client's response to nursing action is compared with the client's short-term outcomes to determine the extent to which these outcomes have been achieved (ongoing evaluation).* The nurse judges the appropriateness of the nursing actions and their intended and unintended effects on the client and family. The nurse compares what the client is able to do with the short-term outcomes. The effectiveness of the nursing orders is determined by changes in the client's behavior.

Example of Community Outcome Evaluation

Nursing Diagnosis: *Increased incidence of veneral disease (VD) among teenagers in community.*
Nursing Model: Community as Client with teenagers as aggregate core.

Expected Outcome	*Ongoing evaluation* *Client's response*
The community and teenagers will be more informed about the causes and complications of VD, as evidenced by:	
1. Teenager's higher scores on VD exams	The mean test scores on VD exams increased from 65 to 85 in 1 year.
2. Parental survey on VD	Although there was only a 45% response rate, parent's mean score was 90 on VD survey.
The incidence of teenagers with VD will be reduced, as evidenced by: 1. Reduced teen annual morbidity statistics for gonorrhea, trichomoniasis, human papillomavirus (HPV), and syphilis	The teen incidence of gonorrhea, trichomoniasis, and HPV decreased slightly 2 years after the awareness program.
	Good progress toward expected outcomes

The client's statements and behaviors, such as physiological and psychological responses, skills, knowledge, and abilities, are written in the chart and in the evaluation column of the nursing care plan. Appropriate information from the family and health team members is also recorded. The nurse then judges whether and to what extent the client has progressed in achieving the short-term outcomes. The nurse decides whether these outcomes have been completely met, partially met, or not met at all. Based on this decision, the nurse also decides whether a change is needed in the plan of care.

4. *The client's progress or lack of progress toward achievement of long-term expected outcomes is determined (concluding evaluation).* To determine whether the client has met the expected outcomes, the nurse evaluates the client's response in meeting the short-term outcomes and judges whether the client's behavior shows progress toward the long-term expected outcomes. Is the client's response desirable and reasonable, considering the allotted time and situation? Have the client's needs, concerns, or potential concerns been resolved, and if so, to what extent? The nurse may gather evaluation data from the family, team members, and chart. The client's response, indicating progress or lack of progress toward the expected outcomes, is recorded in the chart and in the nursing care plan. Lastly, the nurse decides whether to revise the short- or long-term expected outcomes or the nursing orders.

5. *The nursing care plan is reviewed to determine which actions were effective or ineffective in assisting the client's progress.* It is important to determine whether the client's expected outcomes were achieved through specific nursing actions. Numerous other variables may have contributed to achieving the expected outcomes. The nurse cannot assume that the nursing actions contributed to each outcome, but must determine the effect of each action and try to identify other factors that might have promoted or hindered the effectiveness of the action.

6. *The nursing care plan is revised to reflect changes in the client's condition or when the short-term or long-term expected outcomes have not been adequately met.* Modification of the nursing orders or expected outcomes is the last phase in the evaluation process. If the outcomes were easily met, perhaps the nursing care plan is moving too slowly or at just the right pace. The client's behavior may show little or no change or change in the wrong direction. If the expected outcomes were only partially met or not met at all, the nurse must gather more information to determine what happened. At this point, the nurse may need to examine the adequacy, appropriateness, effectiveness, and efficiency of each component of the nursing process. Relevant questions that may be addressed were listed earlier in this chapter. The nurse considers the possible reasons why the orders or the short- or long-term expected outcomes were not achieved and then decides whether to reassess the client or revise

the care plan. New outcomes or nursing orders would be mutually established by the client and nurse, and written in the Kardex or chart and the nursing care plan.

Quality Improvement

A quality improvement (QI) program is an ongoing, systematic process to monitor, evaluate, and improve the level of health care services given to clients in an agency. The purpose of a QI program is to assure the public that there is a system to identify, evaluate, and correct nursing care problems. Monitoring important aspects of nursing practice serves to identify opportunities to improve client care. In health care agencies, these programs may be called *Total Quality Management* (TQM) or *Continuous Quality Improvement* (CQI). Quality improvement programs benefit both clients and health care agencies by identifying strengths of services and areas that could be improved.

The following five characteristics of monitoring and evaluation in QI programs were identified by Schroeder (1991:2):

1. A planned and organized approach is used.
2. Monitoring and evaluation are based on valid standards of care and practice.
3. The process is rigorous enough to produce usable results.
4. Staff nurses are involved in implementation.
5. Results are used to improve care and practice.

To structure and guide the monitoring and evaluation of QI programs in health care agencies, the JCAHO developed a 10-step process. This process emphasizes that monitoring must be based on systematic advanced planning; identification of client groups, services, and clinical activities; and an ongoing commitment to collect and use relevant clinical data for quality improvement.

The process recommended by JCAHO includes the following:

1. Assign responsibility.
2. Delineate the scope of care and service.
3. Identify important aspects of care and service.
4. Identify indicators related to the important aspects of care.
5. Establish thresholds for evaluation.
6. Collect and organize data.
7. Evaluate care.
8. Take action when opportunities for improvement or problems are identified.
9. Assess the effectiveness of actions.
10. Communicate relevant information to the organization-wide quality assurance committee (Joint Commission, 1989:13).

Monitoring, analyzing, and evaluating data, as well as identifying areas for improvement, must be implemented in a realistic manner with consideration for time requirements, staff capabilities, and resources available.

Evaluation of services is based on meeting established standards and criteria, related to the structure, process, and outcomes of health care delivery. According to the JCAHO (1990), every hospital must have defined *Standards of Care* that

describe a competent level of nursing care as demonstrated through the use of nursing process. Nursing process encompasses all significant actions taken by the nurse in providing care to all patients, and forms the foundation of all clinical decision making.

Standards of care define the client's expected outcomes and the nurse's approach to achieving them, both process and outcome. Previously, monitoring programs focused on process alone by monitoring tasks, procedures, or aspects of documentation. Currently, successful monitoring programs integrate process and outcome measures and involve those who deliver care in measuring and improving the quality of care. These programs examine the essence of the professional nurse's care and the essential outcomes patients must achieve. Careful monitoring and evaluation of practice must be required of all practitioners to find opportunities to improve delivery of health care.

To provide competent care, the JCAHO believes that nurses must assess appropriate patient information, and identify and prioritize patient needs in six areas: biophysical, biopsychosocial, environmental, self-care, educational needs, and discharge planning. In the *Accreditation Manual for Hospitals*, the JCAHO (1990) lists five broad standards for nursing care, each with numerous identifiers that are monitored, reviewed, and evaluated. The five broad standards and types of evaluation are as follows:

1. Patients receive nursing care based on a documented assessment of their needs (*process and outcome*).
2. All nursing staff members are competent to fulfill their assigned responsibilities (*structure*).
3. The nurse executive and other appropriate registered nurses develop hospital-wide patient care programs, policies, and procedures that describe how the nursing care needs of patients or patient populations are assessed, evaluated, and met (*structure and process*).
4. The hospital's plan for providing nursing care is designed to support improvement and innova-

tion in nursing practice and is based on both the needs of the patients to be served and the hospital mission *(structure and process)*.

5. The nurse executive and other nursing leaders participate with leaders from the governing body, management, medical staff, and clinical areas in the hospital's decision-making structures and processes.

The *structure* of the agency is evaluated by gathering information about existing policies, procedures, staffing patterns, and available equipment and resources. *Process* evaluation involves a random review of selected client's charts to determine whether procedures were carried out properly and documented.

Government agencies and the JCAHO require quality improvement reviews for continued funding and accreditation of the agency. These reviews usually involve an on-site visit by a team of evaluators who check that specific criteria and standards are being met. The evaluators gather data through direct observation of physical facilities and by reviewing written policies and records.

Summary

Evaluation is an ongoing, systematic, planned process of comparing the client's health status with the expected outcomes. Evaluation involves comparing the client's present responses with baseline behaviors to determine the client's progress in achieving the short-term and long-term expected outcomes. Judgments about the client's progress are made by analyzing and judging objective and subjective data by the nurse, client, family, and team members. If progress is insufficient toward attaining the expected outcomes, the client and nurse revise the plan of care. Health care agencies have implemented quality improvement programs to improve health care delivery. These programs have a direct influence on the nursing care provided as well as the data available for evaluation.

Critical Thinking Exercises BY ELIZABETH S. FAYRAM

1. Discuss why evaluation is often the most neglected component of the nursing process. Identify how evaluation could be improved when using the nursing process.
2. Compare and contrast how evaluation is performed with clients in two distinct clinical settings, such as the cardiac surgery ICU, well-child visits to a public health clinic, or depressed clients at a mental health outpatient program. Identify how a client's progress toward meeting expected outcomes is determined in each setting.
3. You are working with a teenage mother who has a 1-month-old, low birth weight infant. The nursing diagnosis is *High risk for altered parenting r/t lack of knowledge and*

parenting skills. One of the expected outcomes is: *The parent will develop parent-child attachment behaviors.* Describe how you would evaluate the outcome in this situation.
4. The client and the nurse have judged that the outcomes for one nursing diagnosis have not been achieved as planned. Identify possible reasons why the outcomes may not have been achieved.
5. You are interested in evaluating the effectiveness of the teaching and learning program for clients receiving outpatient hemodialysis. Identify several ways the teaching and learning program could be evaluated. Consider both ongoing and concluding aspects in your evaluation.

REFERENCES AND READINGS

Alfaro R: *Applying nursing diagnoses and nursing process: a step-by-step guide,* ed 2, Philadelphia, 1990, JB Lippincott.

American Nurses Association: Standards of nursing practice, *Am Nurse* 6:11, July 1974.

American Nurses Association: *Standards of clinical nursing practice,* Washington, DC, 1991, ANA Publications.

Barba M, Bennet B, and Shaw WJ: The evaluation of patient care through use of ANA's standards of nursing practice, *Superv Nurse* 9:42, Jan. 1978.

Deets C and Schmidt A: Process criteria based on standards, *AORN J* 26:685, 1977.

Deets C and Schmidt A: Outcome criteria based on standards, *AORN J* 27:657, 1978.

Deurr B and Staats K: Quality assurance program evaluation: a view from the unit base, *J Nurs Qual Assur* 2:1–11, 1988.

Dickson N: Quality assurance: do you measure up? *Nurs Times* 83(44):25, 1987.

Foglesong D: Standards promote effective production, *Nurs Manage* 18(1):24, 1987.

Goldmann RC: Nursing process components as a framework for monitoring and evaluation activities, *J Nurs Qual Assur* 4(4):17–25, 1990.

Hegyvary ST and Haussmann RK: *The relationship of nursing process and patient outcomes,* National League for Nursing Pub. 21–2194, 1987, NLN, p. 29.

Hover J and Zimmer M: Nursing quality assurance: the Wisconsin system, *Nurs Outlook* 26:242, 1978.

Iyer PW et al: *Nursing process and nursing diagnosis,* ed 2, Philadelphia, 1991, WB Saunders.

Joint Commission on the Accreditation of Healthcare Organizations: *Update on nursing services monitoring and evaluation,* Chicago, 1989, JCAHO.

Joint Commission on the Accreditation of Healthcare Organizations: *Accreditation manual for hospitals,* Chicago, 1990, JCAHO.

Joint Commission on the Accreditation of Hospitals: *Procedure for retrospective patient care audit in hospitals, nursing edition,* Chicago, 1973, JCAHO.

Kanar RJ: Standards of nursing practice assessed through the application of the nursing process, *J Nurs Qual Assur* 1(2):72, 1987.

Katz J: *Managing quality: a guide to monitoring and evaluating nursing services,* St Louis, 1992, Mosby–Year Book.

Kemp N: Monitoring the nursing process, *Nurs Focus* 4(8):1, 1983.

Law GM: Accountability in nursing: providing a framework, *Nurs Times* 79(40):34, 1983.

Leary CB: Use of nursing process to develop unit specific quality assurance plans, *J Nurs Qual Assur* 4(2):1–6, 1990.

Lillesand KM et al: Nursing process evaluation: a quality assurance tool, *Nurs Adm Q* 7(3):9, 1983.

Machie LCR et al: Quality assurance audit for the nursing process, *Nurs Times* 78(42):1757, 1982.

McHugh MK: Does the nursing process reflect quality care? *Holistic Nurs Pract* 5(3):22–8, 1991.

Mehmert PA: A nursing information system: the outcome of implementing nursing diagnoses, *Nurs Clin North Am* 22(4):943, 1987.

Patterson CH: Standards of patient care: the Joint Commission focus on nursing quality assurance, *Nurs Clin North Am* 23(3):625, 1988.

Pinnell NN: *The nursing process: theory, application, and related processes,* New York, 1986, Appleton-Century-Crofts.

Pulliam L et al: Computerized quality assurance monitoring: a collaborative project, *J Nurs Care Qual* 17(1):44–52, 1992.

Richards DA and Lambert P: The nursing process: the effect on patients' satisfaction with nursing care, *J Adv Nurs* 12(5):559, 1987.

Roeder MA: Patient care plans and the evaluation of nursing process, *Superv Nurse* 11:57, June 1980.

Roper N et al: Identifying the goals: the importance of assessment and evaluation in the nursing process, *Nurs Mirror* 156(24):22, 1983.

Runtz SE et al: Evaluating your practice via a nursing model: the Orem self-care model and the Peplau interpersonal process model, *Nurse Pract* 8(3):30, 1983.

Schmidt A and Deets C: Writing measurable nursing audit criteria, *AORN J* 26:495, 1977.

Schmidt A and Deets C: Responsibilities for audit criteria, *AORN J* 27:657, 1978.

Schroeder P: *Monitoring and evaluation in nursing,* Gaithersburg, Md, 1991, Aspen.

Smeltzer CH et al: Nursing quality assurance: a process, not a tool, *J Nurs Adm* 13(1):5, 1983.

Tucker SM et al: *Patient care standards: nursing process, diagnosis, and outcome,* ed 5, St Louis, 1992, Mosby–Year Book.

Wandelt MA and Ager JW: *Quality patient care scale,* New York, 1974, Appleton-Century-Crofts.

Watson A and Mayers M: Evaluating the quality of patient care through retrospective chart review, *J Nurs Adm* 6:17, March–April 1976.

Wilkinson JM: *Nursing process in action: a critical thinking approach,* Menlo Park, Calif, 1992, Addison-Wesley.

Zimmer MJ: Quality assurance for outcomes of patient care, *Nurs Clin North Am* 9:305, 1974.

Zimmer MJ: Guidelines for development of outcome criteria, *Nurs Clin North Am* 9:317, 1974.

Application of the Nursing Process to Practice

CHAPTER 13

NURSING PROCESS OF THE INDIVIDUAL CLIENT IN THE HOSPITAL

Linda J. Dries
Cathy D. Meade
Paula J. Christensen

The client in this case study is a 15-year-old girl (C.L.) who is facing knee surgery. She is an active participant in school sports, on the track team, is an avid runner, and has many friends. Her academic work is above average, and she hopes to get a college scholarship. She had a skiing accident that necessitates hospitalization and corrective surgery. She is concerned about activity limitations that the surgery will impose on her. In selecting a nursing model to guide the development of C.L.'s care plan, a critical analysis of the concepts of a model and its application to nursing practice are necessary. Recent emphasis has been placed on client participation and accountability for health care. A model that is congruent with this aspect of client participation is Orem's (1991) concepts of nursing practice, which provides a framework for self-care.

Orem's generalized model of nursing is composed of three major concepts. First, the type of assistance that the nurse can provide to the client may be focused on universal, developmental, or health deviation self-care requisites. Second, self-care deficits determine the relationship that is established between client and nurse. The central idea is that clients can benefit from the nurse, either through support/education, partial assistance with deficits, or total assistance. A self-care limitation is present when self-care demands are not within the capability of the client, and the nursing do-

main can help meet these demands. Last, nursing systems identify the qualities and capabilities of the nurse that can assist the client in maximizing self-care. Inherent in Orem's model is the recognition that a variety of factors may influence the establishment of this relationship, such as gender, age of client, knowledge competencies, previous hospital experiences, and values placed on health (Orem, 1991).

The first type of requisite refers to conditions common to all individuals that are related to basic human structure and functioning. The six *universal* self-care requisites are maintenance and balance of air, water, and food intake; rest/activity; elimination; solitude/social interaction; prevention of hazards; and promotion of human functioning and development. In our case example, hospitalization and surgery necessitate incorporation of these requisites into a plan of nursing care for C.L. The second type of requisite refers to *human development* processes that occur during an individual's life span—in the case of C.L., adolescence. *Health deviation* self-care requisites are reflective of conditions that develop abnormally. Such requisites represent structural or functional deviations that may exist in persons who are ill or injured (e.g., knee injury). When care is directed toward meeting these requisites, the likelihood for self-actualization and control over health is increased. All these requisites help initiate and foster the development of the nurse-client relationship (Orem, 1991). Self-care is the second major concept within Orem's model of nursing and delineates self-care activities as learned behaviors that may vary among individuals.

The authors wish to thank Jan Johnson, RN (SwedishAmerican Hospital, Rockford, Ill.) for her thoughtful review and suggestions about this case example.

Featuring the client in a central focus with rights and responsibilities makes Orem's model of nursing very appealing in a clinical setting. The concept of self-care implies that individuals can increase their competencies required for self-care in illness. Nurses have the responsibility and skills necessary in assisting clients to increase their self-care capabilities. At times, the nurse may provide and compensate totally for the client's self-care deficits, for example, immediately after surgery. In other instances, partially compensated care occurs when the nurse and client work together in increasing self-care abilities, such as during the recovery period as C.L. learns ambulation. A third variation of nurse-client relationships may be based on the supportive-educative system. This situation occurs when the client needs assistance in performing required care activities; for example, the nurse provides teaching, guidance, and support to C.L. as she copes with body image changes.

The following case study is guided by Orem's model of nursing and specifically focuses on self-care deficits that emphasize that individuals can benefit from nursing because health limitations are predictive of nursing requirements. When a self-care deficit exists in the client's knowledge, motivation, or skill, for example, as related to knee surgery, the nurse is uniquely qualified to assist in maximizing the client's self-care agency. The client's long-term expected outcome is to return to her previous level of self-care activities. The nursing process described in this chapter reflects 2 consecutive days of contact with C.L., starting with her morning admission (day of surgery).

The nursing process is organized into two sections. First the nursing assessment, analysis/synthesis, and nursing diagnoses for each of the 2 consecutive days are presented. Then the nursing plans, which include the expected outcomes, strategies, nursing orders, scientific rationale, and evaluation, are presented. Although plans for implementation are placed last, they are written after the initial assessment and are implemented and updated with each successive visit. The dates of each implementation are identified in the short-term outcomes, orders, and evaluations. The nursing plans—expected outcomes through evaluation—are written consecutively to show their interrelationship and sequence. They are placed at the end of the nursing process because they are ongoing and subject to revision, and because they demonstrate the continuity of the care plan.

DATA COLLECTION: Day 1—Preoperative, 1/15/94 (Day of Surgery: 0400)

Subjective data		Objective data
Interactions	**Observations**	**Measurements**
	From chart	**From chart (pre-op testing)**
	Client's initials: C.L.	Age: 15 years
	Reason for admission: Rt anterior cruciate and medial collateral ligament repair; right medial meniscectomy 1/15/94.	Urinalysis: color—yellow; clarity—clear; sp gr—1.031; pH—5.0; protein—neg; glucose—neg; acetone—neg; Hb—neg; WBC—none; RBC—none.
	No previous health concerns noted.	Complete blood count: WBC—8.0; RBC—5.67; Hb—17.1; HCT—50.8; MCV—90; MCH—30.2; MCHC—33.7 (All within hospital norms)
	No known allergies.	
	Lives with parents.	
	Religious preference: Protestant.	
	Insurance: Blue Cross/Blue Shield.	Chest x-ray: WNL.
	Surgical consent signed by mother.	Admission blood pressure: 110/70.
	Regular diet—no specific food preferences; drinks 8 glasses water or juice/day.	Admission TPR: 98.4° F, 90/min, 20/min.
	NPO after midnight.	Height: 5'3".
		Weight: 115 lb.
		Preop medications: Reglan 10 mg, Zantac 150 mg, together upon admission.
	From client	
Hi! Yeah, I'm C.L. and this is my mother.	Eye contact with nurse; smiles.	
Oh, pretty good.	Lying supine in bed with head of bed up.	
Well, my right knee hurts a lot (responding to questioning about how she feels).	Rt leg is in an immobilizer.	
	Rt knee is swollen.	
	Head is resting on pillow.	
	Looks down toward bed, and then up at nurse.	

DATA COLLECTION: Day 1—Preoperative, 1/15/94 (Day of Surgery: 0400)—cont'd

Subjective data		Objective data
Interactions	**Observations**	**Measurements**
	From client	
Yeah, I really like running. I like sports in general. I swim and bicycle, too. Then I like to watch football and basketball games with my friends.	Flat facial expression.	
I sure hope I'll be able to run again after the surgery. I love to be involved in sports.	Maintains eye contact.	
No, I'm not too sure what's going to happen tonight or tomorrow.	Uncovers legs; looks at knee; smiles at nurse.	Toes on both feet have capillary return when blanched <5 sec.
Oh, OK.		Flexes left knee 0°–135°.
No, I think I understand now.		Rt knee flexion unable to determine.
Sure. What do you want me to do?		Pedal pulses 3+
No, they (her feet and legs) don't tingle or anything.		Lungs clear to auscultation.
Yeah, it hurts a lot.		System assessment WNL.
OK, I'll see you.		
Thanks. Bye.		

Analysis/Synthesis of Data: Day 1

When Orem's concepts related to self-care are used, each universal self-care requisite is addressed and appropriate data are referred to. Supporting theories and concepts are included when appropriate.

Analysis/Synthesis

1. *Maintenance of sufficient air intake.* The data indicate adequate circulation to C.L.'s legs. Capillary return on toes <5 seconds. Pedal pulses 3+ bilaterally. Whaley and Wong (1991) cite the following normal measurements: (1) average systolic blood pressure for 15-year-old, 120 mmHg; (2) pulse for a person over 4 years of age, 55-90 beats per minute; (3) respiration, 18-19 per minute. When these norms are compared with C.L.'s vital signs, a tentative inference can be made regarding adequate intake of air. More readings of vital signs, other circulatory data, and her history of smoking are data needed for a conclusion to be made. Due to immobility and the effects of anesthesia, C.L. may have inadequate air exchange after surgery.

2. *Maintenance of sufficient intake of water.* A very tentative inference can be made of adequate water intake. Adolescents should take in 50 cc of water/kg body weight over a 24-hour period. C.L. should have approximately 2600 cc water/day (Whaley and Wong 1991). According

to her history, C.L. consumes 1900 cc water from her fluid intake alone. More data are needed, such as observations of the skin and mucous membrane conditions (Whaley and Wong, 1991). C.L. may have an inadequate intake of water postoperatively if intake decreases.

3. *Maintenance of sufficient food intake.* Data were not collected about C.L.'s eating habits. She is on a regular diet with no dietary restrictions. After midnight she will be NPO, which will alter her food intake. Her height and weight fall within the norms given by Malasanos and others (1991) for her age (height range: 59.5-68.1 inches; weight range: 89.5-150.5 lb). The calorie intake for C.L.'s age is 2000 to 2400 calories/day according to Whaley and Wong (1991). The sources of her nutrition are data gaps at this time.

4. *Adequate elimination processes and excrements.* Minimum data on elimination were obtained. The values of the urinalysis fell within the norms given by the hospital. Urinary excretion can be considered adequate, but data gaps exist about patterns of excretion as to difficulties experienced previously and bowel output.

5. *Maintenance of balance between activity and rest.* Exercise requirements vary according to the individual's health status and age. Sports help to contribute to growth and development by increasing heart rate, respirations, and muscle tone (Whaley and Wong, 1991). Data collected

indicate that the client had regular exercise before her knee injury. Malasanos and others (1991) indicate that the normal range of motion of the knee is 0° to 135° flexion. However, due to leg immobility, flexion information on rt leg is not available. A tentative inference of inadequate exercise can be made at this time, especially in anticipation of upcoming surgery. No data were obtained regarding rest and sleep patterns. Teenagers vary in sleep and rest requirements.

6. *Maintenance of balance between solitude and social interaction.* The data obtained indicate that C.L. is involved in activities with other people. Orem discusses the importance of bonds of affection, love, and friendship; social warmth and closeness; and individual autonomy. More data need to be collected regarding C.L.'s family and friends in meeting these needs. C.L. is friendly and warm toward the nurse. Observations of the number of visitors, cards, and phone calls that C.L. will have, as well as how she responds to these, are important data to obtain.

7. *Prevention of hazards to human life, functioning, and well-being.* Orem describes this requisite as including awareness of potential hazards and knowledge of preventive measures to avoid or minimize their effects. C.L. will have hazards to her functioning. One specific hazard is her lack of understanding of the events surrounding her surgery and the outcome. She is also concerned about activity limitations.

8. *Promotion of human functioning and development within the individual's potential and desire to be normal.* Orem describes the elements of this requisite as having a realistic self-concept, fostering human development, and acting to maintain and promote the integrity of human structure and function. Some data indicate that the client is striving to maintain and promote her physical integrity. Data indicate that C.L. has been concerned about her health and tries to maintain a

physical fitness level. She states she is involved in social activities with friends. Erikson (1968) discusses the developmental task of this age as identity versus identity confusion. The adolescent essentially restages each of the previous stages of development in reestablishing a separate autonomy. Much data are needed from C.L. to ascertain her stage of development and sense of identity. Sundeen and others (1989) describe self-concept as the aspects of the self that the individual is aware of. Self-concept includes the individual's feelings, values, and beliefs that influence behavior. Self-ideal is the standard by which one judges one's own behavior, including goals, aspirations, and values one would like to achieve. After surgery the nurse needs to explore the impact of surgery and its effects to better assess C.L.'s self-concept.

Considering the previous review of universal self-care requisites, the following strengths and health concerns are identified:

Strengths

1. Adequate intake of air
2. Adequate urinary excretion
3. Desire to promote human functioning
4. Desire to be normal in relation to peer group

Health concerns

1. Potential alteration of intake of air, water, and food
2. Inadequate activity
3. Hazards to human functioning
4. Decreased self-concept

Because of the concerns listed, C.L. has a therapeutic self-care demand and health-deviation self-care requisites. Her desire and ability to promote her own human functioning, plus assistance from health care professionals, place her in a supportive-educative nursing system at this time.

NURSING DIAGNOSIS: Day 1—Preoperative, 1/15/94 (Day of Surgery)

Date	Diagnoses	Priority
1/15/94	1. Hazards to human functioning related to upcoming surgery and lack of knowledge concerning surgery	1
1/15/94	2. Potential alteration of air, water, and food intake related to upcoming surgery	2
1/15/94	3. Decreased self-concept related to alteration in role of active sportsperson	3
1/15/94	4. Inadequate activity related to right knee injuries and upcoming surgery	4
1/15/94	5. Potential alteration in bowel elimination related to immobility	5

DATA COLLECTION: Day 1——Preoperative, 1/15/94 (Day of Surgery)—cont'd

Subjective data		Objective data
Interactions	**Observations**	**Measurements**

From 7-3 report from nurse

C.L. has been sleeping since she got back,
until 1500.
She has been using PCA pump.
Circulation checks have been WNL: capillary
return <5 seconds on toes of both feet;
pedal pulses present bilaterally.
Ice bag is on her rt knee.
Rt leg is in a bon joy brace.

Vital signs are stable; next due at 1600.
She's been taking a little ice and 7-Up by
mouth with no problem.
Yes, she has voided.
No drainage noted through dressing.

From chart

Postop orders:
Clear liquids, advance to regular diet.
I and O.
Elevate rt leg on pillow.
Ice on rt knee.
Bed rest.
Tylenol, gr X q4h prn for T 101° PO.
PCA order: 1 mg morphine sulfate with delay
10 minutes. Initiate basal rate of 1 mg/hr
from 2200-0600.
Toradol 60 mg bolus.
Toradol 30 mg q6h scheduled D/C after PCA
stopped.
Vicodin 1 q3h PO prn, start after PCA D/C.
IV: D_5NS at 75 ml/hr.
Vital signs q4h.
Preop med given upon admission to OR at
0730.
Returned from surgery at 1200.
Client sleeping most of time since 1200.
Tolerating cl liq PO sm amts.
IV infusing according to schedule.

TPR: 98.4°, 76, 18 (preop)
        99°, 72, 16 (postop)
BP: 108/60 (preop)
       110/68 (postop)
PCA pump morphine 11 mg (7-3)
I & O (7-3)
  I: IV (surg): 500 ml
      IV (unit): 225 ml
      PO: 100 ml
  O: 500 ml (urine)

From client

Hi, not so good right now. I've been
pressing my PCA button.
I had to use the bedpan a while ago and
that was hard to do—but I did go.
Uh-huh. I can feel it. OK (in response to
telling C.L. to let me know if she has any
tingling or numbness of rt leg).
I see (in response to telling C.L. about the
possible postop complications of
decreased sensation, discomfort, and
decreased circulation secondary to
surgery).
Yeah, they showed me earlier (in response
to nurse asking if she knew how to cough
and deep breathe [CDB] and use incentive
spirometry [IS]).
I'll try (in response to nurse informing C.L.
about the need to CDB q2h while she is
on bedrest to increase air intake).
OK (in response to nurse encouraging her to
rest now)

From client

Lying supine in bed with head of bed (HOB)
up 15°.
Rt leg elevated on two pillows.
Bon joy brace on rt leg.
No drainage noted through dressing.
Rt toes warm to touch.
Wriggled rt toes when asked.
Facial skin and arms warm, dry, and pinkish.
Lips pink and moist.
Flat facial affect.
Eye contact with nurse.

Took five deep breaths and coughed (CDB)
when nurse requested her to do so.

Environment:
  C.L. using incentive spirometry (IS)
    10–15 cycles q1h.
  Mother at bedside.
  Call light within C.L.'s reach.
  Bedside table within reach.
  Glass of clear liquid and ice chips on
    bedside table.
  Television on low volume.
  Roommate in bed watching television.

From client

Capillary return when rt toenails blanched
<5 sec.
Vital signs at 1600
  BP: 106/66
  TPR: 99°, 76, 18

(Nonproductive cough)

Continued

DATA COLLECTION: Day 1—Preoperative, 1/15/94 (Day of Surgery)—cont'd

Subjective data		Objective data
Interactions	Observations	Measurements
Later I need to use the bedpan again. Thanks. I'm better now. It still hurts, but not as much. Oh, that's enough.	Used trapeze with ease when bedpan was placed under buttocks. Urine deep amber and clear. IV infusing into lt hand at 75 ml/hr (D_5NS). HOB up 30° for supper. Drank all broth and juice and ate gelatin by herself.	Voided 350 ml urine
That's better. When will I be able to get this thing out [referring to IV]? Oh, OK (in response to "probably tomorrow" from nurse).	Mother assisted C.L. in reaching items on supper tray. Visited each other during meal. Overheard mother updating C.L. on dad's and brother's activities. C.L.'s facial expression indicated interest. Pillows resituated to provide more support for rt leg. New ice bag applied to rt knee for 24 hr. CDB (IS) incentive spirometry 10 times when nurse initiated. Mother remained at bedside until 1900.	Oral intake: 575 cc (supper)
Later No, no tingling or numbness. It's just a constant aching most of the time. Now it's starting to pound. I can't get comfortable. I'm going to press my button for pain. Could I have some more 7-Up, too?	Rt toes warm to touch and move freely. C.L. grimaces. HOB to 10° elevation. Turned to lt side. Lungs clear to auscultation. Skin on back moist and warm. No redness on back or hips. IV infusing on schedule. CDB (IS) incentive spirometry 10 times on request of nurse. Nonproductive coughs. Skin warm and dry.	Vital signs at 2000 BP: 110/70 TPR: 98.6°, 72, 16. Oral intake: 120 ml 7-Up
Later	C.L. lying supine wth eyes closed. Relaxed facial muscles. Body in alignment. Rt leg elevated with ice bag to rt knee.	PCA pump: morphine 15 mg 3-11) I & O (3-11) I: 600 ml (IV) 695 ml (PO) O: 350 ml urine

Analysis/Synthesis of Data: Day 1

Orem's concepts of universal self-care requisites are addressed individually.

Analysis/Synthesis

1. *Maintenance of sufficient intake of air*. C.L.'s intake of air has been threatened because of surgery and immobility. Phipps and others (1991) state that the ef-

fects of both anesthesia and immobility impair adequate intake of air. According to the norms given by Malasanos and others (1990) and the implementation of preventive postoperative measures suggested by Phipps and others (1991), and by Ferrell (1986), data indicate that this self-care requisite is being met now but remains a potential health concern.

2. *Maintenance of sufficient intake of water*. Data indicate that intake of water has been threatened because

of surgery and inability to take fluids in volume by mouth. Phipps and others (1991) state that fluid volume depletion manifests itself with the following symptoms: poor skin turgor, dry mucous membranes, low blood pressure, tachycardia, increased respiration, decreased vein filling, weight loss, low urine output, and increased specific gravity. Phipps and others (1991) and Ferrell (1986) provided the rationale for plans for implementation that were initiated regarding threatened intake of water (IV replacement, clear liquid diet). According to the data, C.L. does not exhibit symptoms of fluid volume deficit and is participating in the implementation of plans to prevent inadequate intake of water (drinking fluids and receiving IV fluids), and is therefore maintaining sufficient intake of water. This self-care requisite remains a potential health concern.

3. *Maintenance of sufficient intake of food.* Williams (1990) states that adequate protein intake is of prime importance postoperatively because of the loss of protein from tissue breakdown and loss of plasma proteins. Essential amino acids are necessary for wound healing. The goal is to reach 60 gm protein daily. One liter of 5% dextrose solution contains 50 gm sugar and 200 calories. According to the above information, compared with the data, C.L. is not maintaining sufficient intake of food. Progressing from a clear liquid diet to a regular diet should be done as soon as C.L. can tolerate it. Overall eating habits remain a data gap.

4. *Adequate elimination processes and excrements.* Phipps and others (1991) state that intake of fluids exceeds output for about the first 48 hours after surgery. This is due to the loss of fluid in surgery, insensible fluid loss, vomiting, and increased secretion of antidiuretic hormone (ADH). The client should be expected to void within 6 to 8 hours after surgery. Data indicate that C.L. has voided within the recommended time and that her fluid intake does exceed her fluid output. According to the above data and norms for the postoperative client, C.L. is maintaining adequate urinary output (1/15/94: 7-3, 3-11: I, 2120 ml; 0, 850 ml). Phipps and others (1991) state that bowel patterns are altered after surgery because of the stress response, anesthesia, use of narcotics, and immobility. Even on a clear liquid diet and IV replacement, a client should have bowel movements if peristalis is present. C.L. has not had a bowel movement at this time. Bowel function remains a potential health concern. Further data need to be obtained in regard to bowel function, such as usual bowel function habits.

5. *Maintenance of balance between activity and rest.* Phipps and others (1991) and Ferrell (1986) indicate that early activity and ambulation are beneficial for increasing alertness, morale, ventilation, muscle tone, and peristalsis; facilitating voiding and wound healing; and decreasing venous stasis. Adequate rest is necessary for an accurate perception of pain and events surrounding recovery from surgery. Quadriceps-setting exercises began on the unaffected side, along with upper extremity strengthening exercises. According to the data, C.L. has had minimum activity and interrupted rest periods related to pain. Therefore an imbalance exists between activity and rest.

6. *Maintenance of balance between solitude and social interaction.* Data indicate minimum interactions with others at this time (except with C.L.'s mother), because of C.L.'s need for rest and her sedation from the anesthesia and analgesics. Data gaps remain concerning visitors, and cards and phone calls from friends and other family members.

7. *Prevention of hazards to human life, functioning, and well-being.* Data indicate that C.L. is more aware of potential hazards (e.g., CDB for adequate air exchange and importance of moving in bed to maintain skin integrity) and is participating with preventive measures cooperatively. Because of the surgery, this remains a health concern at this time.

8. *Promotion of human functioning and development within the individual's potential and desire to be normal.* Data obtained reflect biophysical health promotion at this time because of the recent surgery and actual and potential changes in biophysical health. C.L. needs assistance in promoting aspects of human functioning. C.L. responds to positive feedback of participating in self-care activities and her progress.

According to the previous review of universal self-care requisites, the following strengths and health concerns are identified:

Strengths

1. Adequate intake of air
2. Adequate intake of water
3. Adequate urinary excretion
4. Cooperative in actively participating in methods to decrease hazards to human functioning

Health concerns

1. Potential alteration of intake of air and water
2. Inadequate intake of food
3. Potential alteration of bowel elimination
4. Inadequate activity
5. Hazards to human functioning

In view of the concerns listed, C.L. continues to have a therapeutic self-care demand and health-deviation self-care requisites. Because of her recent surgery and inability to maintain most universal self-care requisites and therapeutic self-care demands without assistance, C.L. is in a wholly compensatory nursing system.

No incongruencies in the data were identified.

NURSING DIAGNOSIS: Day 1—Postoperative, Day of Surgery

Date	Diagnoses	Priority
1/15/94	1. Hazards to human functioning related to surgery and lack of knowledge concerning surgery.	3
1/15/94	2. Potential alteration of air, water, and food intake related to surgery (anesthesia, NPO/cl liq status).	1
1/15/94	3. Decreased self-concept related to alteration in role of active sportsperson.	5
1/15/94	4. Inadequate activity related to right knee injuries and upcoming surgery.	2
1/15/94	5. Potential alteration in bowel elimination related to immobility.	4

DATA COLLECTION: Day 2—Day after Surgery, 1/16/94

Subjective Data	Objective Data	
Interactions	Observations	Measurements

1/16/94 Evening

From 7-3 report from nurse

She's had a good day today. C.L. is doing quad-setting exercises on unaffected leg, and she's done them every couple of hours.

She sleeps well with basal PCA. Started her on a soft diet this morning, and she's tolerating it well. I tried to get her out of bed this afternoon. She had pain and tensed up, so she couldn't get into the chair. She had quite a few visitors today, so she's pretty tired and has been sleeping off and on.

From chart

New orders: Out of bed in chair at least tid.
   Tolerating regular diet well
Vital signs stable (see Measurements)

C.L. starts on continuous passive motion (CPM) machine
0-45° tolerance qid (2 hr session)
Washed self except for back in AM.
IV running at TKO (42 ml/hr).

Circulation checks

Warm rt foot; can move rt roes
Pedal pulses bilaterally 3+
Capillary refill <5 sec on toes

From chart

Vital signs: BP: 106/68-112/74; T: 98.4-99°;
   P: 68-76; R: 12-18

PCA pump morphine 13 mg (11-7)
I & O (11-7)
   I: 600 ml (IV)-400 cc (PO)
   O: 400 ml urine
PCA pump morphine 14 mg (7-3)
I & O (7-3)
   I: 336 ml (IV)-1005 ml (PO)
   O: 450 ml urine

From client

I'm doing OK. I had a hard time trying to get out of bed, though. Guess I didn't do well.

Yeah, I pressed pain button. Oh, OK (in response to waiting half an hour, then getting up into a chair).
Are these exercises to keep my good leg strong? That's what I thought.
Yeah, I remember some of the possible complications.
Well, bad circulation, pneumonia, funny feeling in my leg.
That's why you have me do all this—like breathing and coughing, and the exercises on my left leg, keeping my leg up, isn't it?
OK (in response to suggestion to rest now).

Later
Oh, boy, here we go!
OK (in response to instruction on how I will support her leg while turning her body and holding rt leg for her).

From client

Looks at nurse and smiles.

C.L. focuses eyes on rt leg.
Rt toes warm to touch.

Wriggles rt toes when requested.
Rt leg elevated on two pillows.
Ice bag to rt knee.
No drainage noted through dressing.

Environment
   Two plants and one vase of flowers at
      bedside; several cards on bedside stand.
C.L. helped herself to move rt side of bed
   by sliding her body across mattress with
   support of her arms.
Nurse supported rt leg.
Blank facial expression.
Looked at rt leg while standing.

From client

Vital signs at 1600:
   BP: 110/72
   TPR: 98.4°, 76, 16
Capillary return <5 sec when rt toe-nails
   blanched
Pedal pulses 3+ bilaterally

Subjective Data	Objective Data	
Interactions	**Observations**	**Measurements**
Yeah, I'm OK.	Took a few deep breaths upon instruction.	
	Stood on lt leg and pivoted to chair at side of bed.	
	Sat in chair using arms to support herself as she sat.	
Well it's OK now. It felt bad for a second.	Rt leg elevated on pillow on second chair.	
Thanks.	Bedside tray with supper placed in front of C.L.	
Later	C.L. had eaten two thirds of food on tray.	Oral intake: 450 ml (supper)
I need to use the commode. Then I'm ready to go back to bed.	Lifted herself up and pivoted to commode.	Voided 500 ml urine
	Assisted back to bed.	
It was easier this time.	Nurse held rt leg while C.L. stood on lt leg	
My pain is better today.	and pivoted. CDB (IS) incentive spirometry	
It hurts less.	10 times on request.	
The doctor told me today that I should be able to run again.	Smiled at nurse.	
Sure, that makes me happy. The track team means a lot to me.		
At least I know it'll be OK sometime.		
I can still be the timekeeper until I can run. That way I can still be with my friends.		
Yeah, they gave me most of these—and those flowers.	Pointed with rt hand to flowers.	
The rest are from my relatives.	Rt leg elevated on two pillows.	Pedal pulses 3+
Maybe if I work hard at exercising I'll be able to run sooner!	Rt foot warm to touch.	PCA pump: morphine 15 mg (3-11)
	Hair groomed, wearing own nightgown.	I & O (3-11)
See you later.	Drank <240 ml 7-Up.	I: 336 ml (IV), 690 ml (PO)
		O: 500 ml urine

Analysis/Synthesis of Data: Day 2

Orem's concepts of universal self-care requisites are addressed individually.

Analysis/Synthesis

1. *Maintenance of sufficient intake of air.* According to data and norms given in analysis/synthesis for day 2, C.L. is maintaining adequate air intake. VS stable. C.L. coughs on her own and it is a nonproductive cough. Circulation checks of legs WNL. This still remains a potential health concern because of her decreased mobility and inactivity.

2. *Maintenance of sufficient intake of water.* According to the norms given in the last analysis/synthesis regarding intake of water, C.L. is meeting this health care requisite. This requisite also remains a potential health concern because of her surgery.

3. *Maintenance of sufficient intake of food.* Data show that C.L. has started eating a soft diet and is tolerating it. According to the projected ideal intake of food and calories given in analysis/synthesis day 2, C.L. has a greater chance to meet the requirements now that she is eating solid foods. Data gaps exist regarding the nutritional value of the food she is eating. This is a potential health concern.

4. *Adequate elimination processes and excrements.* C.L.'s intake still exceeds her output, which was stated as a norm for postoperative clients in the last analysis/synthesis on 1/16/94 (11-7, 7-3, 3-11: I—2755 ml, O—1350 ml). Bowel function remains a potential health concern and a data gap.

5. *Maintenance of balance between activity and rest.* According to the data, C.L.'s activities are increasing. She is now up in the chair and transfers from bed to chair with help. She states she has more uninterrupted periods of sleep. The activities recommended in the discussion of analysis/synthesis day 2 have been implemented. This remains a health concern until C.L. is more mobile independently.

6. *Maintenance of balance between solitude and social interaction.* Data indicate that C.L. is having more contact with friends and family. A data gap still exists with respect to the quality of these relationships and

how they satisfy C.L.'s needs and can be of assistance to her during her recovery.

7. *Prevention of hazards to human life, functioning, and well-being.* Data indicate that C.L. is aware of these hazards and is cooperating in preventive measures to decrease the potential of complications developing. C.L. coughs and deep breathes, uses incentive spirometry, eats more, exercises the unaffected leg with encouragement, and shows more interest in social interactions. Continued monitoring of these measures is needed until C.L. is more independently mobile and able to get up.

8. *Promotion of human functioning and development within the individual's potential and desire to be normal.* The norms given in analysis/synthesis day 1 regarding adolescent development compared with these data support C.L.'s concern with her self-concept and relation to peers. This remains a health concern and will require greater focus because C.L.'s role will be altered for an extended period.

The following list represent C.L.'s strengths and health concerns at this time:

Strengths

1. Adequate intake of air
2. Adequate intake of water
3. Adequate urinary excretion
4. Social interaction with significant other people

Health concerns

1. Potential alteration of air, food, and water
2. Potential alteration in bowel elimination
3. Inadequate activity
4. Hazards to human functioning
5. Altered self-concept

According to the concerns identified, C.L. still has a therapeutic self-care demand and health-deviation self-care requisites. Because C.L. remains somewhat dependent on others to maintain universal self-care requisites and therapeutic self-care demand, she is in a partly compensatory nursing system.

No incongruencies in the data were identified.

NURSING DIAGNOSIS: Day 2—Day after Surgery

Date	Diagnoses	Priority
1/15/94	1. Hazards to human functioning related to upcoming surgery and lack of knowledge regarding surgery (resolved 1/16/94).	5
1/15/94	2. Potential alteration of air, water, and food intake related to surgery (anesthesia, NPO/cl liq status)	2
1/15/94	3. Decreased self-concept related to alteration in role of active sportsperson	3
1/15/94	4. Inadequate activity related to right knee injuries and upcoming surgery	1
1/15/94	5. Potential alteration in bowel elimination related to immobility	4

Plans for diagnoses 1, 2, 3, and 5 are given on the following pages. Initial plans for diagnosis 4 are included in plans for diagnosis 2. A more detailed plan is needed regarding increasing C.L.'s activity and discharge planning.

As of the day after surgery, C.L. is not able to return to her previous level of functioning. Therapeutic self-care demands are still present; for example, C.L. needs to learn crutch walking on day 3. However, as C.L.'s recovery progresses and the nurse continues to assist her to increase self-care capabilities, it is anticipated that C.L. will begin to achieve more independence and a sense of well-being.

PLANS FOR IMPLEMENTATION

Nursing diagnosis 1: Hazards to human functioning related to upcoming surgery and lack of knowledge (1/15/94).
Long-term expected outcome: The client will decrease hazards to human functioning by increasing knowledge of upcoming surgery by (1/17/94).

Short-term expected outcomes	Nursing orders	Scientific rationale	Evaluation
1. Client will name the sequence of events leading to surgery by 1/15/94.	1a. Nurse and client will discuss previous experiences the client has had with surgery on 1/15/94.	1a. Teaching/learning strategy by Redman (1993). Principle of learning: new learning is based on previous knowledge experience (Whitman, 1992).	**Criteria statement:** Client will cite sequence of four events leading to surgery as noted in 1c. Nurse implemented orders la-1d 1/15/94

PLANS FOR IMPLEMENTATION—cont'd

Nursing diagnosis 1: Hazards to human functioning related to upcoming surgery and lack of knowledge (1/15/94).
Long-term expected outcome: The client will decrease hazards to human functioning by increasing knowledge of upcoming surgery by (1/17/94).

Short-term expected outcomes	Nursing orders	Scientific rationale	Evaluation
	1b. On 1/15/94 the nurse will use open communication techniques, such as: Open-ended questions and statements Clarifying statements Summary statements.	1b. Principles of teaching: Good nurse-learner rapport is important. Teaching requires effective communication.	**Ongoing evaluation** Client responded that she understood the sequence of events on 1/15/94. Short-term outcome met 1/15/94.
	1c. Nurse will explain the events leading to surgery on 1/15/94. Injection in AM To holding area and then surgery Return to room about 4 hr later.	1c. Increase C.L.'s sense of physical control and knowledge to promote powerfulness of client (Dennis, 1991).	
	1d. Nurse will ask C.L. if she understands the sequence of events on 1/15/94.	1d. Evaluation is an integral part of learning (Redman, 1993).	
2. Client will state changes in activity level surgery by 1/16/94	2a. Nurse will discuss with C.L. and C.L.'s mom their knowledge of the purpose of surgery by 1/15/94.	2a. Principles of teaching and learning: New learning is based on previous knowledge and experience (Whitman, 1992). Planning time for teaching and learning requires special attention. Physical and mental readiness is necessary for learning.	**Criteria statement** Client will name at least three changes in activity, as noted in 2b postop. 1/15/94 Orders 2a-2d implemented. **Ongoing evaluation** C.L. and C.L.'s mom indicated general knowledge of surgery and need for crutches, limits on activity, and feelings about it. Short-term outcome met.
	2b. Nurse will review the effects of surgery on human functioning: Bon joy brace to immobilize rt knee in mild flexion. Use of crutches 2 days postop, non-weight-bearing. Walk with crutches 6–8 wk postop. Hospitalized for 3–4 days. Nurse will state that some differences may occur because of physician's individual practice.	2b. Principles of medical-surgical (orthopedic) nursing practice strategy: Immobilization of the right knee joint allows for healing of traumatized tissue (Ferrell, 1986). Exercises facilitate strengthening of muscles around traumatized tissue (Ferrell, 1986). Knowledge of what to expect after surgery increases the client's sense of physical control and powerfulness (Dennis, 1991).	

Continued

Nursing diagnosis 1: Hazards to human functioning related to upcoming surgery and lack of knowledge (1/15/94).
Long-term expected outcome: The client will decrease hazards to human functioning by increasing knowledge of upcoming surgery by (1/17/94).

Short-term expected outcomes	Nursing orders	Scientific rationale	Evaluation
	2c. Nurse will ask C.L. and her mother to state changes in activity level on 1/16/94.	2c. Effective learning requires active participation of the learner. Evaluation is an integral part of learning (Redman, 1993).	**Concluding evaluation:** Long-term outcome met 1/16/94. C.L. increased her knowledge regarding surgery and the main effects surgery will have on her.
	2d. Nurse and client will discuss the client's feelings about altered functioning on 1/17/94.	2d. A positive body image is particularly important to the adolescent (Murray and Zentner, 1993).	

Nursing diagnosis 2: Potential alteration of air, water, and food intake related to upcoming surgery 1/15/94.
Long-term expected outcome: The client will decrease the degree of alteration of air, water, and food intake by using preventive postoperative measures by 1/16/94.

Short-term expected outcomes	Nursing orders	Scientific rationale	Evaluation
1. Client will state three possible postop problems on 1/15/94.	1a. Nurse will ask C.L. what she knows about possible problems caused by surgery on 1/15/94. 1b. On 1/15/94 the nurse will use open communication techniques to discuss postop problems as: Decreased air intake and circulation. Decreased sensation. Discomfort. Decreased physical activity. Decreased food and water intake.	1a. Teaching-learning strategy by Redman (1993). Principle of learning: new learning is based on previous knowledge and experience. 1b. Principle of teaching: Teaching requires effective communication. Principles of medical-surgical (orthopedic) nursing practice strategy. These are considered possible problems after surgery due to the effect of anesthesia and immobility on general body systems. The possible decrease in circulation, sensation, and discomfort in the right leg is related to swelling of tissue as a response to surgical intervention (Phipps et al., 1991).	**Criteria statement:** Client will state three of the possible problems as noted in 1b. Order 1b was implemented on 1/15/94. C.L. acknowledged information given to her. Orders 1a and 1c were implemented on 1/15/94. **Ongoing evaluation** C.L. able to state two problems on 1/15/94; short-term outcome not met 1/15/94.
	1c. Nurse will ask C.L. to state three of the possible occurrences mentioned above on 1/15/94.	1c. Principles of learning: Effective learning requires active participation of the learner. Evaluation is an integral part of learning.	Short-term outcome met on 1/15/94 when C.L. was able to state three possible problems postop.
2. Client will name three preventive measures for possible postop problems on 1/1/5/94.	2a. Nurse will discuss preventive measures for possible postop problems on 1/15/94. CDB (IS) every 2 hours.	2a. Principle of teaching: Teaching requires effective communication. Principles of nursing practice. To increase ventilation of lungs and facilitate removal of secretions (Phipps et al, 1991).	**Criteria statement:** Client will name three of the preventive measures as listed in 2a.

Nursing diagnosis 2: Potential alteration of air, water, and food intake related to upcoming surgery 1/15/94.
Long-term expected outcome: The client will decrease the degree of alteration of air, water, and food intake by using preventive postoperative measures by 1/16/94.

Short-term expected outcomes	Nursing orders	Scientific rationale	Evaluation
Order 2a partially implemented 1/15. C.L.	Elevate rt knee on pillows.	To facilitate venous return and decrease swelling (Ferrell, 1986).	Order 2a partially implemented 1/15. C.L. acknowledged nurse's information.
	Positioning for comfort and analgesics.	To decrease pain and increase comfort.	
	IVs and clear liquid diet as tolerated to regular diet as tolerated.	Fluid is lost during surgery and must be replaced. ADH is stimulated post trauma. GI function slowed (Phipps et al, 1991).	
	Out of bed within 1 day. Ambulatory within 2 days.	Increases morale, alertness, ventilation, muscle tone, and peristalsis. Facilitates healing and voiding. Decreases pain and venous stasis.	
	2b. Nurse will ask C.L. to name four of the above preventive measures on 1/15/94.	2b. Principles by Redman: Effective learning requires active participation of the learner. Evaluation is an integral part of learning.	Order 2b not implemented 1/15 because of client's health status. Order 2b implemented 1/16. **Ongoing evaluation** C.L. identified three preventive measures. Short-term outcome met on 1/15/94.
3. Client will participate in at least four postop preventive measures by 1/15/94.	3a. Nurse will demonstrate CDB on 1/15/94. 3b. C.L. will demonstrate the above on 1/15/94.	3a. Learning may occur through imitation (Whitman, 1992). 3b. Effective learning requires active participation of the learner. Repetition strengthens learning.	**Criteria statement:** Client will participate in at least four of the following preventive measures as noted in 3c.
	3c. Nurse will provide necessary equipment and monitor their effectiveness for the following preventive measures on 1/15/94. Elevate rt leg on pillows. Ice bag to rt knee. Position rt leg for comfort. Administer analgesics per physician order as needed via PCA. IVs and clear liquid diet as tolerated to regular diet.	3c. Nurse is responsible and accountable for the client's physical safety and well-being postoperatively (Phipps et al, 1991). (See rationale for each preventive measure in short-term outcome 2.)	Order 3a and 3b done 1/15/94. C.L. showed nurse how to CDB. Order 3c done 1/15 and 1/16/94. Order 3d implemented 1/15 and 1/16/94. I and O maintained by nurse. Order 3e implemented 1/15 and 1/16/94. Short-term outcome met.
	3d. Nurse will monitor intake and output postoperatively 1/15/94 and as needed.	3d. Physiological changes due to surgical intervention and anesthesia interfere with usual intake and output (Phipps et al, 1991).	**Concluding evaluation** Long-term outcome met (needs monitoring until C.L. is more mobile) 1/16/94. C.L. is knowledgeable of possible postop occurrences and preventive measures and is actively participating with postop care.
	3e. Nurse will initiate use of measures in 3c when appropriate.	3e. Health restoration and maintenance are the responsibility of the nurse (Phipps et al, 1991).	

Continued

PLANS FOR IMPLEMENTATION—cont'd

Nursing diagnosis 3: Decreased self-concept related to alteration in role of active sportsperson 1/15/94.
Long-term expected outcome: The client will accept a realistic self-concept considering her role change by 1/18/94.

Short-term expected outcomes	Nursing orders	Scientific rationale	Evaluation
1. Client will verbalize at least two feelings regarding loss of function by 1/18/94.	1a. Nurse and client will discuss C.L.'s perception of the loss of function from surgery on 1/17/94.	1a. Strategies of therapeutic use of self, problem solving, and principles of medical-surgical nursing practice. Client reaction to a temporary or permanent loss depends on the client's perception of the loss.	**Criteria statement** Client will verbalize at least two feelings, such as sadness, anger, neutrality, frustration, pleasure, and joy on 1/17/94.
	1b. Nurse will ask C.L. how and what she feels regarding the loss of function of her rt leg on 1/16 or 1/17.	1b. Nurse needs to facilitate ventilation of feelings regarding loss (Phipps et al, 1991). In adolescence, the body acts as a source of acceptance or rejection by others (Murray and Zentner, 1993). Problem identification step of problem-solving process (Bower, 1982).	Orders not implemented because of dates not yet occurring. C.L. is anxious to get back to sports. She feels frustrated by inactivity. Nurse supported C.L. in her feelings.
	1c. Nurse will accept and support C.L.'s response in 1b on 1/16 and 1/17.	1c. Nurse needs to support client in all phases of body image change (Murray and Zentner, 1993).	
	1d. Nurse will ask C.L. to think about coping methods on 1/17, to be discussed on 1/18.	1d. Active participation by the learner promotes learning (Pohl, 1981). Generation of options of problem solving (Bower, 1982).	Short-term outcome met.
2. Client will state three ways she can cope with altered body function by 1/18/94.	2a. Nurse and C.L. will discuss possible ways of coping with altered body function on 1/18/94 such as: Take care of own body. Participate in diversional activities. Learn to use crutches and increase mobility to the best of her ability within limits. Ask family to arrange home to allow C.L. increased mobility. Ask friends to carry books for her at school. Plan to continue being timekeeper for track team. Initiate social contact with friends.	2a. Identification of options in problem-solving process (Ford et al, 1979). Nurse is responsible for health promotion (Phipps, 1991). Nurse needs to participate in supporting the client with all aspects of changed body image.	**Criteria statement** Client will name three of the coping methods identified in 2a. Short-term outcome not met.

PLANS FOR IMPLEMENTATION—cont'd

Nursing diagnosis 3: Decreased self-concept related to alteration in role of active sportsperson 1/15/94.
Long-term expected outcome: The client will accept a realistic self-concept considering her role change by 1/18/94.

Short-term expected outcomes	Nursing orders	Scientific rationale	Evaluation
	2b. Nurse and client will discuss the feasibility of each possible coping measure on 1/18/94.	2b. Analyzing alternatives in problem-solving process (Bower, 1982). Increasing C.L.'s sense of physical, psychological, and environmental control and knowledge to promote powerfulness (Dennis, 1991).	
	2c. C.L. will choose at least three ways she will cope with altered body function on 1/18/94.	2c. Increasing sense of powerfulness Making the decision in the problem-solving process (Bower, 1982). A positive body image is built or reconstructed through encouragement of movement and activities (Murray and Zentner, 1993).	
3. Client will exhibit at least two signs of acceptance of altered body function by 1/18/94.	3a. Nurse will ask and encourage C.L. to initiate use of at least two coping measures by 1/18/94. 3b. Nurse will monitor and evaluate the use of coping measures by 1/18/94.	3a. Increase C.L.'s sense of physical, psychological, and environmental control and powerfulness. 3b. Nurse is responsible for promotion of health (Phipps et al, 1991). Evaluation is an integral part of teaching.	**Criteria statement** Client will participate in at least two of the coping measures listed in criteria statement for short-term outcome 2 by 1/18/94. Orders not implemented because of dates not yet occuring. Short-term outcome not met.
	3c. Nurse will give positive reinforcement to C.L. for using coping measures by 1/18/94.	3c. Nurse needs to participate in and support the client with all aspects of changed body image (Murray and Zentner, 1993).	**Concluding evaluation** Long-term outcome not met.

Nursing diagnosis 5: Potential alteration in bowel elimination related to immobility 1/15/94.
Long-term expected outcome: The client will resume normal pattern of bowel elimination by 1/17/94.

Short-term expected outcomes	Nursing orders	Scientific rationale	Evaluation
1. Client will identify (state) decreased bowel function as a possible complication of surgery and immobility by 1/15/94.	1a. Nurse will ask the client if she knows of any bowel changes that might occur as a result of surgery and immobility. 1b. According to C.L.'s response, the nurse will explain to C.L. the possible complication of altered bowel function on 1/15/94. 1c. Nurse will ask C.L. to acknowledge information given above on 1/15/94.	1a. Teaching-learning strategy by Whitman (1992): new learning is based on previous learning and experience. 1b. Principles of medical-surgical nursing practice strategy: anesthesia and immobility decrease peristalsis and therefore potentially alter bowel function (Phipps et al, 1991). 1c. Evaluation is an integral part of teaching.	**Criteria statement** Client verbally states or acknowledges that bowel function is a possible complication by 1/16/89. Short-term outcome not met.

Continued

PLANS FOR IMPLEMENTATION—cont'd

Nursing diagnosis 5: Potential alteration in bowel elimination related to immobility 1/15/94.
Long-term expected outcome: The client will resume normal pattern of bowel elimination by 1/17/94.

Short-term expected outcomes	Nursing orders	Scientific rationale	Evaluation
2. Client will participate in the assessment of bowel function by 1/16/94.	2a. Nurse will ask C.L. if she has felt any need to move her bowels or any "rumbling" in lower abdomen or passed any flatus ("gas") since surgery on 1/15/94.	2a Subjective data are an important source regarding bowel function (Phipps et al, 1991).	**Criteria statement** Client will answer questions and position body to facilitate data collection of bowel function upon request on 1/16/94. Short-term outcome not met.
	2b. Nurse will use the following physical assessment techniques to collect data about bowel function on 1/16/94. Inspection Auscultation Palpation Percussion	2b. Physical assessment techniques used to identify distention, bowel sounds, bowel segments, and fluid, gas, and solid elements in bowel (Malasanos et al, 1990).	
3. Client will participate in three measures to stimulate bowel function by 1/16/94.	3a. Nurse will ask C.L. to identify three ways to promote bowel function on 1/16/94.	3a. Whitman's (1992) learning principle: new learning is based on previous learning and experience. Learning needs must be assessed.	**Criteria statement** C.L. lists three ways to promote bowel movement.
	3b. According to the above response, the nurse will identify measures to increase bowel activity on 1/16/94. Fluids to 2000–3000 cc per day. Maximum safe physical activity. Fruit juice intake. Mild laxative. Stool softeners.	3b. Development of concepts is a part of learning. These measures increase fluid volume in bowel and stimulate peristalsis (Phipps et al, 1991).	Client will participate in three measures listed in order 3b on 1/18/94. Short-term outcome not met.
	3c. Nurse will encourage C.L. to participate in the first three measures above if needed on 1/16/94.	3c. Nurse is responsible for health promotion and maintenance (Phipps et al, 1991).	**Concluding evaluation** Long-term outcome not met.

REFERENCES AND READINGS

Bower FL: *The process of plannng nursing care: nursing practice models,* St. Louis, 1982, Mosby–Year Book.

Dennis KE: Empowerment. In Creasia JL and Parker B, editors: *Conceptual foundations of professional nursing practice,* St. Louis, 1991, Mosby–Year Book.

Edelman C and Mandle C: *Health promotion throughout the life span,* ed 2, St Louis, 1990, Mosby–Year Book.

Erickson EH: *Identity, youth and crisis,* New York, 1968, WW Norton.

Ferrell J: *Illustrated guide to orthopedic nursing,* ed 3, Philadelphia, 1986, JB Lippincott.

Jones D, Lepley M, and Baker B: *Health assessment across the life span,* New York, 1984, McGraw-Hill.

Malasanos L et al: *Health assessment,* ed 4, St Louis, 1990, Mosby–Year Book.

Murray RB and Zentner JP: *Nursing assessment and health promotion through the life span,* ed 5, Englewood Cliffs, NJ, 1993, Prentice-Hall.

Orem DE: *Nursing: concepts of practice,* ed 4, New York, 1991, McGraw-Hill.

Phipps WJ, Long BC, and Woods NF: *Medical-surgical nursing: concepts and clinical practice,* ed 4, St Louis, 1991, Mosby–Year Book.

Redman B: *The process of patient education,* ed 7, St Louis, 1993, Mosby–Year Book.

Stuart GW and Sundeen SJ: *Principles and practice of psychiatric nursing,* ed 4, St Louis, 1991, Mosby–Year Book.

Sundeen SJ et al: *Nurse-client interaction: implementing the nursing process,* ed 4, St Louis, 1989, Mosby–Year Book.

Whaley L and Wong D: *Nursing care of infants and children,* ed 4, St Louis, 1991, Mosby–Year Book.

Williams SR: *Essentials of nutrition and diet therapy,* ed 5, St Louis, 1990, Mosby–Year Book.

Whitman NI et al: *Teaching in nursing practice: a professional model,* Norwalk, Conn, 1992, Appleton and Lange.

CHAPTER 14

NURSING PROCESS OF THE INDIVIDUAL CLIENT IN THE COMMUNITY

Elizabeth S. Fayram

Model for Assessment

The client in this community-based case study is F.N., a 38-year-old black woman who has been coming to an urban clinic for control of hypertension. She has come to the clinic monthly for 4 months. Although she is taking antihypertensive medications, her blood pressure remains elevated.

The Roy Adaptation Model (1991) is incorporated into the nursing process for this case study. This model is used for a variety of reasons: the nurse's philosophy and past experiences, the client situation, and the focus of the model. The goal of nursing according to Roy is to promote adaptation. The nurse has observed that many of the clients coming to the urban clinic, including F.N., require the nurse's assistance to promote adaptation. In addition, the model views clients holistically, with all dimensions addressed within the four adaptive modes. These adaptive modes are physiologic, self-concept, role function, and interdependence. The adaptation level is influenced by the focal, contextual, and residual stimuli present, and the response is either adaptive or ineffective.

Nursing activities as specified by Roy (1991) occur in six steps:

1. Assess behavior in each of the four adaptive modes.
2. Determine stimuli for ineffective behaviors.
3. Formulate nursing diagnoses.
4. Set goals.
5. Select interventions that will change the stimuli affecting adaptation.
6. Evaluate.

In this case study, data are collected and then analyzed according to the four adaptive modes. A judgment is made concerning the adaptive response. If responses are found to be ineffective, the stimuli affecting the behavior are identified and the nursing diagnoses are formulated. The Roy Adaptation Model (1991) and the NANDA classification system (Carpenito, 1992) provide guidance for the development of nursing diagnostic statements. Plans, including expected outcomes, strategies, and nursing orders, are developed to influence the stimuli for the nursing diagnoses. Evaluation completes the process.

The nursing process is organized into two sections. First, the assessment, analysis/synthesis, and nursing diagnoses are presented for each of two visits. This is followed by plans for each nursing diagnosis, consisting of expected outcomes, strategies, nursing orders, scientific rationale, and evaluation. Although the plans are placed last, they are initiated, implemented, and evaluated concurrently with the assessment visits. They are placed in the second section because they are ongoing and subject to revision, and demonstrate the continuity of the nursing process.

DATA COLLECTION: Visit 1—2/4/94

Subjective data	Objective data	
Interactions	**Observations**	**Measurements**
	From chart	**From chart**
	Client's initials: F.N.	Age: 38 yr.
	Reason for clinic appointment: hypertension. First seen at clinic 10/18/93. Chief complaint 10/18/93: headaches on awakening. Hypertension diagnosed.	Blood pressure: 10/18/93 (sitting): 210/124(right) 208/120(left) 11/15/93 (sitting): 186/112(right) 182/104(left) 12/13/93 (sitting): 184/102(right) 186/108(left) 1/10/94 (sitting): 168/96(right) 170/98(left)
	Separated from husband. Lives with four children in an apartment. Receives public assistance. Met with social worker on 11/15/93 and 1/10/94; marital difficulties discussed.	Height: 5'4" Weight 10/18/93: 163 lb
	ECG 10/18/93: Left ventricular hypertrophy.	Urinalysis 10/18/93: Color: yellow Opacity: clear Specific gravity: 1.018 pH: 6.9 Glucose: neg Protein: neg RBC: neg WBC: neg
	Eye exam 10/18/93: Arteriolar narrowing.	Serum electrolytes 10/18/93: Sodium: 138 Potassium: 4.2 1/10/94: Potassium: 3.7
		Complete blood count 10/18/93: WBC: 7.8 RBC: 4.6 Hgb: 13.4 Hct: 42.3
		Medications: Prazosin (Minipress) 1 mg tid Propranolol (Inderal) 120 mg bid Hydrochlorothiazide (Hydrodiuril) 50 mg bid Potassium chloride 10 mEq tid
From client during clinic visit		
Hi. Sure, I can answer some questions.	Eye contact with nurse, arms crossed, not smiling. Sitting on chair next to desk.	
I'm feeling better but my pressure's still up.		BP (sitting): 162/96(right) 158/94(left) Weight: 162 lb.
I'm still having problems with my husband. That's probably why it's up.	Looking out window, speaking softly.	
Too much water in me makes the pressure go up, I guess.		
My father had high blood pressure. My brother does too.	Eye contact.	

DATA COLLECTION: Visit 1—2/4/94—cont'd

Subjective data	Objective data	
Interactions	**Observations**	**Measurements**

Subjective data (Interactions)	Objective data (Observations)	Measurements
I guess I've had it since I was 25.		
No, I was never given pills before.		
I take my pills with my meals. Boy, I don't like the way the potassium tastes!	Smiles.	
I guess I shouldn't eat that chicken from the take-out restaurant.	Shakes head.	
I know I'm supposed to stay away from salty foods.		
You mean I can't put salt on my food? Food doesn't taste good without it.		
I know my weight isn't good for my pressure. What can I do to lose weight?	Shifting around in chair.	
I eat when I'm upset.		
I've gained too much weight. Oh, about 20 pounds in the last year.	Abdomen obese; overall distribution of weight even.	
I'm not trying very hard to lose weight.		
I eat snacks. Oh, cookies and cake, mostly. I can't remember everything I've eaten in the last 3 days. At work I eat chicken or hamburger and fries from the take-out place.	Black skin with reddish tone; clean, neat, tight clothes; small amount of make-up, perfume, and jewelry; nails short with polish.	
At home I have eggs, bacon, bread, cheese. I want to lose weight. Can you give me a diet? I think I look good at about 135 pounds.		
Write down everything I eat for 3 days? Yeah, I can do that. Even all the snacks!	Nods head, smiling.	
No, I'm not having any more of those headaches.		
I really don't exercise. I work 6 days a week as a sales clerk at a resale shop.		
No, I've never smoked.	Sitting on exam table.	Pulse: 84/min Respirations: 20/min
I do get short of breath when I climb a flight of stairs.	Breath sounds regular and quiet; no use of accessory muscles. Pulses strong; extremities warm.	
I drink a lot of pop. I'm always thirsty.	Moist mucous membranes; skin shiny; no dependent edema in lower extremities.	
I go to the bathroom a lot with this water pill. Oh, about 10 or 12 times a day.		
Sometimes my rings get tight when my fingers get puffy.	Holds out hands to show tightness of rings on fingers.	
I'm getting a divorce soon, in about 3 weeks. I'm hoping he'll finally be convinced it's over and leave me alone.	No eye contact, shifting around on table; voice tone louder.	
I've been married 21 years.		
Yeah, I guess you could say I have a lot of stress.	Nods head.	
I have some friends at work and neighbors to talk to. I can't tell them everything.		

| Subjective data | | Objective data | |
Interactions	Observations		Measurements
Yes, I guess you could say I have a lot of stress.	Nods head.		
I have some friends at work and neighbors to talk to. I can't tell them everything.			
Yes, I did talk to the social workers. It helped to talk to someone. I told her I'd come back when I needed to.	Nods head.		
Well, my weight and getting my pressure down. I think those are the most important things right now.	Eye contact.		
I used to get more exercise. Hard to find the time now.			
Well, walking, I guess. My daughter would probably go with me. We could go before dinner.			
Sure, I'll try it. If it'll help my pressure and my weight, it's worth a try.	Nods head.		

Analysis/Synthesis of Data: Visit 1

The four adaptive modes identified by Roy (1991) are addressed in this analysis with reference to appropriate data. Supporting theories, norms, and standards are also included. The adaptive or ineffective responses are identified. Stimuli influencing an ineffective adaptive response are also identified and classified as focal, contextual, and residual when possible.

Analysis/Synthesis
Physiologic Mode

1. *Oxygenation.* Data indicate an ineffective adaptive response in the oxygenation pattern. Blood pressure measurements ranging from 158/94 to 210/124 are elevated (Bates, 1991). According to Bullock and Rosendahl (1992), F.N.'s diastolic pressure readings of 112, 120, and 124 are considered to be severely elevated. Diastolic blood pressure between 96 and 102 is moderately elevated. Based on the Joint National Committee on Detection, Evaluation, and Treatment of High Blood Pressure, hypertension is classified by stages (Johannses, 1993). F.N.'s blood pressure measurements have fallen from Stage IV (BP greater or equal to 210/120) to Stage II (BP 160 to 179/100 to 109) with treatment thus far.

F.N. has previously experienced headaches on awakening, which can be a symptom of hypertension (Phipps, 1991). Pulse (60) and respiratory rates (20) are within normal limits (Bates, 1991). F.N. describes symptoms of dyspnea on exertion, indicative of respi-

ratory or cardiovascular difficulty (Phipps, 1991). Other data include normal values in the complete blood count (Corbett, 1992), quiet and regular breath sounds without the use of accessory muscles at rest, skin with reddish tones, strong pulses and warm extremities, and no dependent edema in the lower extremities. Edema is present in the fingers, indicating fluid retention or circulatory congestion (Bates, 1991). Contextual stimuli contributing to the ineffective response include many of the risk factors of hypertension (Bullock and Rosendahl, 1992): family history, black female, diet high in sodium and calories, limited exercise, and stress from relationship with husband.

Other stimuli include a history of hypertension since age 25, which was not treated with medications. There is a data gap in regard to other methods of blood pressure control used in the past. Positive stimuli include no history of smoking, and taking medications prescribed to help control hypertension regularly. Elevated blood pressure over a period of about 13 years has contributed to changes within the cardiovascular/pulmonary systems: left ventricular hypertrophy, arteriolar narrowing in retina, dyspnea on exertion, and edema in upper extremities (Bullock and Rosendahl, 1992). The effect of propranolol on the cardiovascular system has affected the pulse rate, which is in the lower limits of normal (Bates, 1991). One effect of the beta-adrenergic blocking agents is slowing of the heart rate (Karch, 1992).

2. *Nutrition.* The nutritional pattern data indicate ineffective adaptation. F.N.'s weight of 163 lb is 20% over the ideal weight for her height (5 ft, 4 in); there-

fore she is considered to be obese (Dudek, 1993). Appearance indicates an obese abdomen. Data regarding eating patterns are limited but indicate that F.N. eats take-out food and snacks regularly, uses salt on food, and is not presently trying to lose weight. Contextual stimuli include F.N.'s inadequate knowledge of foods included in a low-sodium, low-calorie diet, eating when under stress, financial limitations, and limited exercise. Cultural influences on F.N.'s diet are unknown. Positive stimuli are indicated by F.N.'s request for a diet and assistance in losing weight.

3. *Elimination.* No data have been obtained about intestinal elimination. Data regarding urinary elimination include normal urinalysis (Corbett, 1992) and frequent urination. The prescribed diuretic (hydrochlorothiazide) contributes to frequent urination (Karch, 1992). Effective adaptation is occurring in the urinary elimination pattern.

4. *Activity and rest.* Physical activity is limited. A data gap exists as to how much exercise F.N. gets at work. An exercise program should consist of 20 to 60 minutes of exercise at least three times per week (Allan, 1992). The focal stimulus contributing to the ineffective adaptation of activity is time for exercise. A factor that could affect F.N.'s ability to exercise involves her dyspnea on exertion. Data gaps include F.N.'s attitude toward exercise and environmental factors. F.N. indicated a willingness to try an exercise program. Data gaps regarding motor function and rest are present, and no inference about these items can be made at this time.

5. *Protection.* Data on protection indicate effective adaptation. The skin has reddish tones and is warm to the touch. Mucous membranes are moist. White blood cell count is within normal limits (Corbett, 1992). Data are limited regarding condition of skin (e.g., lesions), hair, nails, perspiration, sensation, and immunizations. A stimulus that may contribute to the development of ineffective skin integrity involves edema of the fingers and tight rings, and is an area to continue to assess (Bates, 1991).

6. *The senses.* Minimal data have been obtained regarding the senses. An eye exam on 10/18/93 indicated arteriolar narrowing. No other data have been obtained regarding the senses. Data on pain also are limited. F.N. experienced headaches in the past. Headaches are a symptom of hypertension and did occur while F.N.'s hypertension was considered to be severe (Bullock and Rosendahl, 1992). No inference regarding adaptation of the senses can be made at this time.

7. *Fluid and electrolytes.* Data regarding fluid and electrolytes include the measurements obtained in the urinalysis, such as specific gravity (1.018), and serum sodium (138 mEq/L) and potassium levels (4.2 mEq/L), which are within normal limits (Corbett, 1992). An abnormal finding, edema in the fingers, indicates ineffective adaptation regarding fluids. Focal stimuli include ingestion of foods high in sodium and the use of salt on food. The presence of left ventricular hypertrophy limits the pumping action of the left ventricle, causing fluid to back up into the lungs and eventually into the systemic circulation (Phipps, 1991). Further assessment is necessary before determining whether this is a stimulus. A contextual stimulus is the use of a diuretic that can deplete sodium and potassium. The use of a potassium supplement (potassium chloride) has contributed to the effective adaptation of electrolyte levels. A data gap exists on the type and volume of fluids the client drinks.

8. *Neurological function.* Minimum data have been collected for this pattern. F.N.'s ability to answer questions indicates that the client is alert and oriented (Bates, 1991). Data have not been obtained regarding the cranial nerves or sensory and motor evaluation. A tentative inference is made that neurological function is adaptive.

9. *Endocrine system.* The only data on endocrine functioning are the urinalysis (glucose: neg) and the presence of adipose tissue. More data are needed regarding temperature changes, menstrual cycle, and sexual development before an inference can be made.

Self-Concept Mode

1. *Physical self.* Physical self includes body sensation and body image (Buck, 1991). Data are limited on body sensation but include statements that F.N. is "feeling better" and is not experiencing headaches presently. Data regarding body image center mainly around weight and include statements of a 20-pound weight gain within the past year, a desire to lose weight, and an ideal weight of 135 pounds. According to Dudek (1993), F.N.'s perception of ideal weight is within normal limits for a woman of medium frame. Grooming is adaptive as observed by F.N.'s appearance in neat, clean clothes and the wearing of a small amount of make-up, perfume, jewelry, and nail polish. A temporary inference is made that F.N. is adapting in regard to physical self.

2. *Personal self.* Buck (1991) includes self-consistency, self-ideal, and the moral-ethical-spiritual self as components of the personal self. No data have been collected on the personal self. This is a data gap.

Role Function Mode

F.N. is a 38-year-old woman, separated from her husband, who lives with her four children. F.N.'s developmental stage as defined by Erikson (1963) is generative adult, which involves generativity versus stagnation. Tasks included in this stage involve a satisfying marriage relationship, aiding the development of children, managing a home, meeting the needs of aging parents, and interdependence with others beyond the spouse. Data indicate that F.N. has the primary role of mother and provider for four children. She also has the role of sales clerk and is a recipient of public aid. F.N. has been married 21 years but is in the process of a divorce. She expresses a desire to terminate the marriage relationship. Friends include those at work and neighbors.

Data gaps are present regarding the development of the children, responsibilities for aging parents, and the exact nature of the relationships with co-workers and neighbors. Successful adaptation within this stage results in productivity and accepting responsibility with affection. A data gap exists regarding stimuli such as social and cultural norms, role models, knowledge of expected roles, and rewards and cooperation F.N. receives from the roles she has assumed (Nuwayhid, 1991). Due to the data gaps, an inference is deferred.

Interdependence Mode

The interdependence mode is divided into two components: significant others and support systems (Tedrow, 1991). Significant others are four children. A data gap exists regarding F.N.'s relationship with the children. F.N. is seeking a divorce from her husband of 21 years, who cannot be considered a significant other at this time. F.N. expresses difficulty with her husband. More specific data about the relationship with the husband are needed. Support systems include friends at work, neighbors, and the social worker at the clinic. F.N. does state that she cannot tell her friends everything. Another support system is the public assistance this family receives. A data gap exists about other family members.

According to Sato (1984), the black culture relies heavily on family as a support system. Another cultural factor affecting this mode is the underutilization of health care services by blacks. It is not clear whether F.N. and her children use the health care system on a regular basis or only when a crisis or illness occurs, such as the headaches F.N. experienced.

More data need to be obtained and considered when planning care with F.N. From the minimal data, a temporary inference of ineffective adaptation of this mode is made. The focal stimulus affecting this mode is the difficult relationship with F.N.'s husband. Data gaps regarding the stimuli include F.N.'s expectations of relationships, her nurturing abilities, and interactional skills (Tedrow, 1991).

Considering the previous review of the adaptive modes, the following strengths and concerns are identified:

Strengths

1. Adaptive response in seeking assistance for weight loss
2. Adaptive response in urinary elimination pattern
3. Adaptive response in willingness to implement an exercise program
4. Adaptive neurological response
5. Adaptive response in the physical self pattern
6. Adaptive response in use of support systems in the interdependence mode

Health concerns

1. Ineffective adaptive response in oxygenation pattern
2. Ineffective adaptive response in nutrition pattern
3. Ineffective adaptive response in activity pattern
4. Potential ineffective adaptive response in skin integrity pattern
5. Ineffective adaptive response in fluid pattern
6. Potential ineffective adaptive response in role function mode
7. Ineffective adaptive response in interdependence mode

NURSING DIAGNOSIS: Visit 1

Date	Diagnoses	Priority
2/4/94	1. Altered health maintenance (blood pressure control) related to excessive intake of sodium and calories, lack of exercise, and ineffective stress management.	1
2/4/94	2. Alterations in nutrition, more than body requirements, related to knowledge deficit (low calorie, sodium), eating patterns, financial limitations, and limited exercise.	2
2/4/94	3. Inadequate physical activity related to lack of providing time for exercise.	3
2/4/94	4. High risk for impairment of circulatory integrity of fingers related to fluid excess and tight rings.	6
2/4/94	5. Fluid volume excess related to excessive sodium intake.	4
2/4/94	6. High risk for ineffective role transition related to coping with change in marital status.	7
2/4/94	7. Ineffective interdependence related to stress from relationship with husband.	5

Subjective data	Objective data	
Interactions	**Observations**	**Measurements**

From client during clinic visit

Interactions	Observations	Measurements
I'm doing much better, I think.	Sitting in waiting room: smiles when name called; erect posture, coordinated gait.	

	Sits on exam table	Weight: 160 lb
		BP (sitting):
		  152/94(right)
		  156/98 (left)
		Pulse: 84/min
		Respirations: 20/min

I'm walking a lot. Yesterday we walked about 25 minutes. Usually three times a week for about 20 or 30 minutes. I like it.		
I was tired after the first day. No, no trouble breathing.	Eye contact. Extremities warm. No edema in lower extremities. Quiet, regular respirations.	
I think it helps me relax.		
I go to bed about 10:30 and get up at 6:30. I don't have trouble sleeping.		
Yeah, I wrote it all down for 3 days. I'm eating three meals a day, but I eat too many sweets. I usually eat with my kids or a friend at work. I snack at work when there's no customers.	Looking away, swinging legs.	
I've been cutting back on my salt. I might have salt when I eat things I fix for my kids that I put salt in.	Able to remove rings from fingers.	Pitting edema (+1) in fingers.
Yeah, I had a list of foods high in salt. I think it got lost.		
Yeah, I could use more information on that. Sure, I'll answer some more questions first. My BM's once a day. Soft, brown. No pain or bleeding.		
No bad smell or urine infections.		
No diabetes in my family. No, no thyroid changes. Heat and cold don't bother me.		
I had my first period when I was 12 years old. Lasts about 5 days. No, no problem.		
No, I don't check my breasts. Don't know how.	Shrugs shoulders.	
No, I don't wear glasses. I can see all right.	No squinting.	
I'm a Christian. The Lord has helped me get through this time with my husband.	Direct eye contact.	
It takes a lot to get me mad. I don't usually stay mad for long.	Looking down at hands in lap.	
It's hard for me to say something to someone. I guess I'm a kind-hearted, good person. At least, I try to be.	Looking up, smiling.	
My kids are great. I tell them they have to try hard. They do real well in school. They don't always understand they have to wait for things. You can only stretch a dollar so far. They have everything they need. I don't think kids should have everything they want.	Continues to smile.	Four children: Ages 9, 12, 14, 17.
They don't want me to go out with friends. They want me to stay home. I need to get out, too.	Louder tone of voice.	
I don't know what it would be like to date again after 20 years of being married.		
Sometimes I can't talk to others. I don't trust them with my feelings. I've been hurt too many times before. Some people just like to gossip. Most of the time I just keep my feelings inside.	Leans forward.	
I would like to better myself, but I do what I can and I'm all right for now.	Eye contact.	
My kids and my faith are the most important things in my life. We all help each other.		
I don't like taking money from public aid. But I work, and it's too hard to make the dollar stretch when you have four kids.		
My husband's hardly ever worked since we've been married. I always worked. I'm used to it.		
The nurse and client then reviewed the 3-day food diary for foods high and low in sodium and for factors influencing an increased caloric intake.		

Analysis/Synthesis of Data: Visit 2

Previous analysis is still applicable and is integrated for comparison when appropriate. Roy's four adaptive modes are addressed.

Analysis/Synthesis
Physiologic Mode

1. *Oxygenation.* F.N.'s blood pressure remains elevated (156/98) at Stage I (BP 140-159/90-99) (Johannsen, 1993). Data within normal ranges include a pulse of 84/min, quiet and regular respirations 20/min, warm extremities, and no edema in the lower extremities (Bates, 1991). Pitting edema (+1) is present in the fingers but has improved in that F.N. is able to remove her rings. Though progress has been made, the oxygenation pattern remains in an ineffective adaptive response. Stimuli contributing to more effective adaptation are that F.N. is trying to reduce sodium intake, and the implementation of an exercise program. The exercise program has increased her relaxation level and is being tolerated (no shortness of breath).

2. *Nutrition.* F.N. has lost 3 pounds in 2 weeks. The food diary was reviewed for eating patterns: eating times, eating companions, and snacking habits; food quantity and quality; foods high and low in sodium; activity level; and food-related cues. F.N. states that she is attempting to reduce sodium intake but continues to cook with it. She has received information about high-sodium foods in the past but has misplaced the written information. Her nutritional pattern remains an ineffective adaptive response. A positive stimulus is the establishment of an exercise program, which will influence caloric expenditure (Carpenito, 1992). Other positive stimuli include F.N.'s attempt to reduce sodium intake, the recognition that she eats too many sweets, and the interest in obtaining information about high-sodium foods.

3. *Elimination.* Data obtained about intestinal elimination indicate effective adaptation (Servonsky, 1991). Minimal data on urinary elimination have been collected, such as normal smell and no urinary tract infections. The urinary elimination pattern remains in adaptation.

4. *Activity and rest.* F.N. has established a walking program, which she does three times a week for 20 or 30 minutes. Data indicate that F.N. is tolerating the exercise program and has not developed shortness of breath or fatigue. Reasons for varying the length of time F.N. exercised were not explored. Data regarding motor function include F.N. walking with erect posture and coordinated gait and the ability to sit on the exam table, swing legs, and shrug shoulders. Motor function from the data is considered to be within normal limits (Bates, 1991). Data regarding rest indicate that F.N. does not have difficulty sleeping and sleeps for 8 hours, which is within normal limits (Roy, 1991).

The activity and rest pattern is in adaptation but will need to be supported, especially in the area of activity.

5. *Protection.* Minimal data have been collected. Extremities remain warm, and no edema is present in the lower extremities. Edema is still present in the fingers but has decreased. Effective adaptation of skin integrity has been maintained.

6. *The senses.* Again, a data gap remains. The only additional data are that F.N. is not squinting, does not wear glasses, and states she can see "all right." No additional data have been obtained about headaches or the other senses. No inference regarding adaptation of the senses is made at this time.

7. *Fluid and electrolytes.* Limited data have been collected for this pattern. Fluid volume excess continues to be present but to a lesser degree. The 3-day food diary was reviewed for foods high and low in sodium. Stimuli contributing to the reduction in fluid retention is F.N.'s attempt to reduce sodium intake (Phipps, 1991). Further analysis of the 3-day recall will yield additional data in regard to sodium, fluid, and potassium intake.

8. *Neurological function.* F.N. continues to be alert and oriented, responding when her name is called, and answering questions appropriately, demonstrating short- and long-term memory (Bates, 1991). Additional data regarding motor function is described in the activity and rest pattern. A data gap remains regarding cranial nerve and sensory evaluation. An inference is made that neurological function is adaptive.

9. *Endocrine system.* Additional data have been obtained regarding family history of diabetes, thyroid disorder, menstrual cycle, and breast self-exam. Specific data such as symptoms of diabetes were not explored. The endocrine pattern is adaptive (Phipps, 1991). However, F.N. acknowledges a lack of knowledge to perform a breast self-exam.

Self-Concept Mode

1. *Physical self.* Data continue to be limited regarding body sensation and image. F.N. indicates that she is "doing much better" and is more relaxed since initiating an exercise program. Other relaxation techniques were not explored. Physical self is in adaptive response.

2. *Personal self.* Data have been obtained regarding self-consistency, self-ideal, and moral-ethical-spiritual components. Data regarding self-consistency include F.N.'s description of herself as a kind-hearted, good person who does not get mad easily. F.N. does not like to receive public assistance but has accepted the need to do so. Nonverbal communication also adds data involving self-consistency: F.N. speaks freely about herself and uses direct eye contact, appropriate tone of voice, and facial expressions (Buck, 1991). Data regarding self-ideal are limited. Her statement that she would like to better herself is unclear and nonspecific. The statement, "I do what I can and I'm all right for

now," indicates that F.N. accepts her self-concept presently. The third component, the moral-ethical-spiritual self, includes the client's belief system and morals (Buck, 1991). Data indicate a strong spiritual belief that gives F.N. strength to cope with difficult situations, such as the relationship with her husband. Stress from the marital relationship remains a data gap, as are the methods of stress management F.N. uses. Other beliefs center around the children: valuing education and meeting children's needs but not necessarily all material desires. From the data obtained, an inference is made that F.N.'s personal self is adaptive.

Role Function Mode

Additional data have been obtained on F.N.'s role as a parent. From statements such as "my kids are great," a tentative conclusion is made that F.N. is satisfied in her role as parent of four children. She identifies them as one of the most important things in her life. Another role is that of sales clerk. Little additional data have been provided. F.N. is in a role transition at this time because of changes in her marital status. She has begun to discuss dating, expressing some anxiety about dating after 20 years of marriage. There also is a concern between F.N. and the children about her visiting with friends. This may be an area of conflict. Further assessment is needed. Based on F.N.'s satisfaction with her roles, the role function mode is adaptive. However, there is a potential ineffective adaptation regarding role transition and role conflict.

Interdependence Mode

Significant others continue to be the four children. Main support systems are friends and religion. F.N. states that she has difficulty expressing feelings to others and keeps them inside. A factor influencing friends as a support system is the conflict between F.N. and the children regarding her visiting friends. Financial support is obtained through employment and public assistance. Financial support from F.N.'s husband is not provided. Health promotion practices continue to be a data gap ex-

cept for the data indicating that F.N. does not perform breast self-exam. The focal stimulus is lack of knowledge. No additional data have been obtained about the relationship with F.N.'s husband. It is difficult to conclude whether this continues to be a problem. Interdependence continues to be an area of concern with the possibility of inadequate support systems for dealing with stress and her relationship with her husband.

The following are F.N.'s strengths and health concerns at this time:

Strengths

1. Adaptive response in nutrition pattern with a 3 lb weight loss in 2 weeks and an attempt to reduce sodium intake
2. Adaptive response in elimination pattern
3. Adaptive response in activity and rest pattern
4. Adaptive response in protection
5. Adaptive response in neurological function
6. Adaptive response in endocrine pattern
7. Adaptive response in self-concept mode
8. Adaptive response to roles as parent and employee
9. Adaptive response to interdependence with children, religion, and financial support

Health concerns

1. Ineffective adaptive response in oxygenation pattern
2. Ineffective adaptive response in nutrition pattern
3. Ineffective response in fluid pattern
4. Potential ineffective adaptive response in role function (role transition and role conflict)
5. Potential ineffective adaptive response in interdependence mode (emotional support)
6. Ineffective adaptive response to health maintenance practices (breast self-exam)
7. Ineffective adaptive response in interdependence mode (relationship with husband)

Plans for diagnoses 1, 2, 3, and 7 are given on the following pages. Initial plans for diagnosis 5 are included in diagnosis 2. Potential diagnoses (4, 6, 8, and 9) and diagnosis 10 would be dealt with at a later time and are not included.

NURSING DIAGNOSIS: Visit 2

Date	Diagnoses	Priority	Resolved
2/4/94	1. Altered health maintenance (blood pressure control) related to lack of knowledge of high-sodium foods, excessive intake of calories, and ineffective stress management.	1	
2/4/94	2. Alteration in nutrition, more than body requirements, related to knowledge deficit, eating patterns, and financial limitations.	2	
2/4/94	3. Inadequate physical activity related to lack of providing time for exercise.		2/18/94
2/4/94	4. High risk for impairment of circulatory integrity of fingers related to fluid excess and tight rings.	5	
2/4/94	5. Fluid volume excess related to excess sodium intake.	3	
2/4/94	6. High risk for ineffective role transition related to coping with change in marital status.	8	
2/4/94	7. Ineffective interdependence related to stress from relationship with husband.	4	
2/18/94	8. High risk for role conflict related to restricted time with friends.	7	
2/18/94	9. High risk for ineffective stress management related to inadequate emotional support system.	6	
2/18/94	10. Alterated health maintenance (breast self-exam) related to knowledge deficit.	9	

PLANS FOR IMPLEMENTATION

Nursing diagnosis 1: Altered health maintenance (blood pressure control) related to lack of knowledge of high-sodium foods, excessive intake of calories, and ineffective stress management (2/4/94).

Long-term expected outcome: Client will achieve blood pressure control by 4/1/94.

Short-term expected outcomes	Nursing orders	Scientific rationale	Evaluation
1. Client will state four risk factors contributing to hypertension by 2/4/94.	1a. Nurse will ask client what risk factors lead to development of hypertension on 2/4/94.	*Content:* Control of hypertension *Strategy:* Teaching/learning 1a. New learning is based on previous learning (Whitman, 1992).	**Criteria statement** Client will state four risk factors contributing to hypertension: Family history Racial predisposition Sodium intake Increased weight Stress Lack of exercise Nurse implemented orders 1a-c on 2/4/94.
	1b. Nurse and client will discuss additional risk factors unknown to client on 2/4/94.	1b. Teaching requires effective communication (Rorden, 1987). Risk factors include family history, racial predisposition, sodium intake, increased weight, stress, and lack of exercise (Bullock and Rosendahl, 1992).	
	1c. Client will state risk factors applicable to her hypertension on 2/4/94.	1c. Active participation is part of effective learning (Redman, 1993). Adult learners are motivated to learn when the information is applicable (Knowles, 1984).	**Ongoing evaluation** Client was able to state four risk factors: stress, sodium, weight, lack of exercise. Short-term outcome met.
2. Client will state two effects of hypertension on the body by 2/4/94.	2a. Nurse and client will discuss definition of hypertension on 2/4/94. 2b. Using audiovisual aids, nurse will explain how vasoconstriction influences pressure within blood vessels on 2/4/94. 2c. Nurse will explain that (1) The higher the pressure, the greater the likelihood of organ damage. (2) Hypertension is usually symptomless. (3) There are various consequences of hypertension on blood vessels and organs in the body on 2/4/94.	2a. New learning is based on previous knowledge (Whitman, 1992). 2b. Audiovisual materials involve the learner actively, focus the learner's attention, and aid memory (Rorden, 1987). 2c. The possibility of organ damage increases as the pressure increases (Bullock and Rosendahl, 1992). Individuals with hypertension are usually without symptoms until hypertension has progressed (Bullock and Rosendahl, 1992). Complications of hypertension include heart and kidney failure, stroke, and blood vessel changes in the eye (Bullock and Rosendahl, 1992).	**Criteria statement** Client will state two effects of hypertension on the body: Heart failure Kidney failure Stroke Blood vessel changes in the eyes Plan not implemented, due to other priorities and time constraints. Short-term outcome not met. Nurse and client have agreed to implement this short-term outcome on 3/18/94.
	2d. Client will discuss concerns regarding development of complications on 2/4/94.	2d. An effective nurse-client relationship fosters expression of concern (Sundeen, 1993).	

Continued

PLANS FOR IMPLEMENTATION—cont'd

Nursing diagnosis 1: Altered health maintenance (blood pressure control) related to lack of knowledge of high-sodium foods, excessive intake of calories, and ineffective stress management (2/4/94).

Long-term expected outcome: Client will achieve blood pressure control by 4/1/94.

Short-term expected outcomes	Nursing orders	Scientific rationale	Evaluation
3. Client will name four measures used to control hypertension by 2/4/94.	3a. Nurse and client will discuss reaching blood pressure 140/90 or less on 2/4/94. 3b. Nurse will ask client to state any control measures she is knowledgeable of on 2/4/94. 3c. Nurse will explain control measures not stated by client on 2/4/94.	3a. Outcomes serve as guides to evaluate progress (Redman, 1993). 3b. New learning is based on previous knowledge (Whitman, 1992). 3c. Control measures include low-sodium diet, weight control, medications, exercise program, reduction in caffeine, and stress management (Phipps, 1991).	**Criteria statement** 1. Client will name four measures used to control hypertension: Low-sodium diet Weight control Exercise program Medications Reduction in caffeine Stress management. 2. Client will state the individualized outcome of BP less than 140/90, indicating a controlled blood pressure level. 3. Client will state that blood pressure control is a lifelong process.
	3d. Nurse will explain that blood pressure control is a lifelong concern and that control measures should be continued on 2/4/94. 3e. Using open-ended questions, nurse will encourage client to express feelings about the difficulties following the control measures.	3d. Hypertension is not curable but is controllable (Phipps, 1991). 3e. About 50% of clients with hypertension do not follow through with their prescribed regimens (McEntee and Peddicord, 1987).	**Ongoing evaluation** Client identified five control measures: medications, low-sodium diet, weight control, stress reduction, and exercise program. Further explanation and clarification is necessary (e.g., low-sodium diet). Short-term outcome not met. Nurse and client plan to continue with this outcome on 3/18/94, emphasizing lifelong control and difficulties client is experiencing with control measures. **Concluding evaluation** Long-term outcome not achieved. F.N.'s blood pressure is decreasing but remains elevated. This plan, along with plans 2, 3, 5, and 7, should continue to be implemented to control hypertension.

Nursing diagnosis 2: Alteration in nutrition, more than body requirements, related to knowledge deficit, eating patterns, and financial limitations (2/4/94).

Long-term expected outcome: Client will improve nutritional status by decreasing caloric and sodium intake and achieving ideal weight by 6/15/94.

Short-term expected outcomes	Nursing orders	Scientific rationale	Evaluation
1. Client will state three factors that lead to increased caloric intake by 2/18/94.	1a. Nurse will explain factors that lead to increased caloric intake on 2/18/94: Eating patterns Food quantities Food quality Activity levels Food-related thoughts Food-related cues 1b. Client will discuss with nurse each factor in relation to own diet (time, place, financial considerations) on 2/18/94.	*Content:* Nutrition *Strategy:* Teaching/learning 1a. Factors contributing to an increased caloric intake stem from emotions, eating habits, and energy expenditure. Refer to nursing order 1a (Crist, 1992). 1b. Active participation by the learner facilitates learning (Redman, 1993).	Orders 1a-d were implemented on 2/18/94. Food diary was reviewed. Factors contributing to increased caloric intake include eating patterns (snacking), food quality (high fat), previous sedentary activity level, and eating when under stress. **Ongoing evaluation** Client was able to state four factors leading to increased caloric intake. Short-term outcome met.
	1c. Nurse and client will review the 3-day food diary on 2/18/94 in regard to factors listed in 1a. 1d. Client will state three factors that most likely lead her to increase caloric intake on 2/18/94.	1c. Active participation by the learner facilitates learning (Redman, 1992). 1d. Evaluation is a part of the teaching/learning process (Redman, 1993).	
2. Client will select three strategies to use to decrease caloric intake by 2/18/94.	2a. Client will discuss with nurse strategies used in past to lose weight on 2/18/94. 2b. Nurse and client will discuss strategies to decrease caloric intake safely by 2/18/94. Substituting non-food-related activities Small, frequent meals Cue elimination (eating only in one room) Reducing food quantity Increasing activity while decreasing calories Thinking positively about food intake (i.e., self-care) Including high-quality foods (e.g., protein, vitamin, minerals) Using self-help groups 2c. Client will select at least three strategies to use to decrease caloric intake on 2/18/94.	2a. New learning is based on previous knowledge and experience (Whitman, 1992). 2b. A variety of strategies is available to decrease caloric intake (Dudek, 1993). 2c. Active participation by the learner facilitates learning (Redman, 1993).	Orders 2a-c not implemented because of time constraints. Nurse and client have agreed to implement these orders at the next visit on 3/18/94.

Continued

PLANS FOR IMPLEMENTATION—cont'd

Nursing diagnosis 2: Alteration in nutrition, more than body requirements, related to knowledge deficit, eating patterns, and financial limitations (2/4/94).

Long-term expected outcome: Client will improve nutritional status by decreasing caloric and sodium intake and achieving ideal weight by 6/15/94.

Short-term expected outcomes	Nursing orders	Scientific rationale	Evaluation
3. Client will state five high-sodium foods consumed in her diet by 2/18/94.	3a. Nurse and client will discuss factors that lead to high-sodium intake by 2/18/94: Eating foods high in sodium Salting food when cooking and at the table Dislike of taste of foods without sodium 3b. Nurse and client will discuss ways to decrease sodium intake on 2/18/94. 3c. Nurse and client will review a written list of foods that have a high-sodium content on 2/18/94.	3a. Factors contributing to a high-sodium intake are listed in 3a (Dudek, 1993). 3b. Factors leading to ingestion of a high-sodium diet can be modified by choice of foods and elimination of the use of sodium (Dudek, 1993). 3c. The use of written information and discussion reinforce learning (Rorden, 1987).	Orders 3a-d implemented by nurse and client out of sequence due to client's interest in high-sodium foods. All three factors contributed to client's high-sodium intake. **Ongoing evaluation** Client was given written list of foods high in sodium. The client was able with help to identify foods in 3-day food diary that were high in sodium. She stated she was going to reduce her sodium intake by eliminating foods high in sodium and refraining from cooking with sodium and using it at the table. F.N. will try to use more spices and herbs in cooking instead of sodium, but she was unsure how her children would react.
	3d. Client will identify foods from high-sodium list that she eats regularly on 2/18/94.	3d. Active participation by the learner facilitates learning (Redman, 1993).	Short-term outcome met but needs further support and evaluation at future visits.
4. Client will plan 3 days of menus, incorporating a 1390-calorie, low-sodium diet by 3/18/94.	4a. Nurse and client will discuss foods and daily requirements of the food guide pyramid, using a handout from the American Dietetic Association on 3/18/94. 4b. Nurse and client will discuss the reason to consume 1390 calories/day on 3/18/94.	4a. Basic knowledge of nutrition is necessary before client can plan menus. 4b. Caloric requirement for a 1 lb weight loss per week is determined by the formula: Ideal body weight in pounds $\times$ 14 minus 500 ($135 \times 14 - 500 = 1390$) (Dudek, 1993).	**Criteria statement** 1. Client will plan 3 days of menus, incorporating a 1390-calorie, low-sodium diet, using the food guide pyramid. 2. Client will state financial consideration and palatability of diet for family. **Ongoing evaluation**
	4c. Client will plan 3 days of menus using low-calorie and low-sodium handouts as a guide by 3/18/94. 4d. Nurse and client will review menu plan for calorie and sodium content, financial considerations, and palatability by the client and family members on 3/18/94.	4c. Active participation by the learner is necessary for effective learning (Redman, 1993). 4d. Evaluation is a part of the teaching/learning process (Redman, 1993).	Orders 4a-d were not implemented at this point. Plan to be implemented at next visit.

Nursing diagnosis 2: Alteration in nutrition, more than body requirements, related to knowledge deficit, eating patterns, and financial limitations (2/4/94)
Long-term expected outcome: Client will improve nutritional status by decreasing caloric and sodium intake and achieving ideal weight by 6/15/94

Short-term expected outcomes	Nursing orders	Scientific rationale	Evaluation
5. Client will lose 1 to 2 lbs per week until ideal weight is reached.	5a. Nurse and client will discuss proper weight loss of 1 to 2 lbs per week on 3/18/94. 5b. Nurse and client will discuss how new nutritional patterns are lifelong on 3/18/94. 5c. Nurse and client will discuss importance of continuing exercise program while decreasing calories on 3/18/94. 5d. Client will weigh self weekly beginning 3/18/94.	5a. Safe weight loss is 1 to 2 lb per week (Crist, 1992). 5b. Ability to maintain ideal weight, once achieved, requires continuation of new nutritional patterns (Crist, 1992). 5c. Exercise aids in weight loss by increasing caloric requirements of the body (Carpenito, 1992). 5d. Client will be able to note progress.	**Criteria statement** 1. Client will state that safe weight loss should be 1 to 2 lb per week. 2. Client will record weight on a weekly basis. 3. Client will lose 1 to 2 lb per week until ideal weight is reached. Orders for short-term outcome will be implemented after implementation of nursing orders 2a-c and 4a-d.
	5e. Client will complete a 3-day food diary by 5/13/94. 5f. Nurse and client will review progress with eating changes, problems, and acceptance on 5/13/94.	5e. Evaluation is an integral part of teaching/learning process (Redman, 1993). 5f. Evaluation provides for review of progress and modifications necessary (Redman, 1993).	**Ongoing evaluation** Weight between 2/4/94 and 2/18/94 did decrease by 3 lbs, is an appropriate weight loss. Client attributed loss to trying to reduce sodium intake and starting an activity program. She was encouraged by the weight loss and wanted to continue to work on it. **Concluding evaluation** Long-term outcome not met, but client's awareness of nutritional status has increased. Nurse and client agreed to continue to work on implementing the plan.

Nursing diagnosis 3: Inadequate physical activity related to lack of providing time for exercise (2/4/94).
Long-term expected outcome: The client will increase physical activity by 2/18/94.

Short-term expected outcomes	Nursing orders	Scientific rationale	Evaluation
1. Client will verbalize benefits of a regular exercise program by 2/4/94.	1a. Nurse will ask client to explain the benefits that occur from exercising regularly on 2/4/94. 1b. On 2/4/94, the nurse and client will discuss benefits of a regular exercise program: Cardiovascular functioning Weight loss/control Relaxation	*Content:* Activity *Strategies:* Teaching/learning and problem solving. 1a. New learning is based on previous knowledge (Whitman, 1992). 1b. Regular exercise benefits cardiovascular functioning and will increase energy output, aiding in weight loss/control (Allan, 1992). When an enjoyable exercise program is initiated, relaxation may also be a benefit.	**Criteria statement** Client will state two benefits of a regular exercise program. Refer to 1b. Nurse and client implemented orders 1a-c on 2/4/94. **Ongoing evaluation** After implementation of plan, client stated that a regular exercise program would help reduce her blood pressure pressure and weight. Short-term outcome met.

Continued

PLANS FOR IMPLEMENTATION—cont'd

Nursing diagnosis 3: Inadequate physical activity related to lack of providing time for exercise (2/4/94).
Long-term expected outcome: The client will increase physical activity by 2/18/94.

Short-term expected outcomes	Nursing orders	Scientific rationale	Evaluation
	1c. Client will state two benefits of a regular exercise program on 2/4/94.	1c. Active participation fosters learning (Redman, 1993).	
2. Client will select an exercise program based on interest and time constraints by 2/4/94.	2a. On 2/4/94, nurse and client will discuss different types of exercise programs: Swimming Walking Bicycling	2a. A variety of exercise programs are available that provide moderate exercise (Allan, 1992). Programs mentioned by the nurse will be of low cost because of financial limitations of client.	Nurse and client implemented orders 2a-e. **Ongoing evaluation** Client selected walking. Time for exercise was before dinner. Enjoyment was enhanced by asking client's daughter to accompany her. Short-term outcome met.
	2b. Client will explain time constraints in present schedule on 2/4/94.	2b. Active participation is a part of effective problem solving. The first step is accurate identification of the problem (Sullivan and Decker, 1992).	
	2c. Nurse will discuss time commitments of an exercise program (3 times/week, 30 min duration) on 2/4/94.	2c. Exercise, to be of benefit, should be performed 3 times/week for at least 30 min (Allan, 1992).	
	2d. Client, with nurse's assistance, will analyze possible exercise options according to enjoyment and scheduling on 2/4/94.	2d. Problem solving includes determining possible solutions and analyzing consequences. The nurse is the facilitator, guiding client in the process (Sullvan and Decker, 1992).	
	2e. Client will select one type of exercise program and the time to do it for next 2 weeks on 2/4/94.	2e. Next step of problem-solving process is selection of a specific alternative by client (Sullivan and Decker, 1992).	
3. Client will implement selected exercise program 3 times/week, increasing to 30 min by 2/18/94.	3a. Client will select one type of exercise program to implement on 2/4/94.	3a. Problem solving includes selection of one alternative (Sullivan and Decker, 1992).	**Criteria statement** 1. Client will implement selected exercise program 3 times/week, increasing to 30 min duration.
	3b. Nurse and client will discuss precautions to take when implementing exercise program on 2/4/94. Begin slowly. Include 5 min of warm-up and 5 min of cool-down exercises. Watch for activity intolerance: shortness of breath, light-headedness, pain, fatigue.	3b. Activity intolerance can be prevented by beginning an exercise program slowly and including warm-up and cool-down exercises. Symptoms of activity intolerance should be assessed (Allan, 1992).	2. Client will state effects of the exercise program. Refer to 3d. 3. Client will state whether problems exist with scheduling of exercise program. **Ongoing evaluation** Client implemented exercise program from 2/4/94 to 2/18/94

PLANS FOR IMPLEMENTATION—cont'd

Nursing diagnosis 3: Inadequate physical activity related to lack of providing time for exercise (2/4/94).
Long-term expected outcome: The client will increase physical activity by 2/18/94.

Short-term expected outcomes	Nursing orders	Scientific rationale	Evaluation
			Ongoing evaluation
	3c. Client will perform the exercise program 3 times/week, increasing to 30 min if tolerated by 2/18/94.	3c. Implementation is the next step of problem-solving process (Sullivan and Decker, 1992).	Client states that she is walking, which is the exercise she selected. Frequency is usually 3 times/week for 20-30 min. Greater clarification should be obtained with F.N., such as reason why duration varies from 20-30 min. Client could write down dates and times of exercising for a more accurate evaluation.
	3d. Client will monitor the effects of exercise program by 2/18/94: symptoms of activity intolerance, relaxation and enjoyment.	3d. Evaluation is an integral part of problem-solving process (Sullvan and Decker, 1992).	Client stated the effects of exercising were tiredness the first day, no shortness of breath, and greater relaxation. No specific mention is made regarding pain or light-headedness. Client did state that she "likes it," indicating enjoyment.
	3e. Nurse and client will evaluate outcome of implementation of exercise program on 2/18/94: frequency, duration, enjoyment, time problems, and effects.	3e. Evaluation is an integral part of problem-solving process (Sullivan and Decker, 1992).	No information was obtained regarding whether time difficulties occurred. This should be specifically addressed when evaluating this program. F.N. was able to "usually" find 3 days/week to implement exercise program. Short-term outcome partially met.
			Concluding evaluation
			Client implemented an exercise program, so her physical activity has increased. Long-term expected outcome met. This pattern will need continued monitoring in terms of frequency and length of exercise, as well as support.

Continued

PLANS FOR IMPLEMENTATION—cont'd

Nursing diagnosis 7: Ineffective interdependence related to stress from relationship with husband (2/4/94).
Long-term expected outcome: Client will increase stress management techniques by 5/13/94.

Short-term expected outcomes	Nursing orders	Scientific rationale	Evaluation
1. Client will list two personal reactions to stress from relationship with husband by 3/18/94.	1a. Nurse will use open-ended statements and questions when discussing stressors and responses.	*Content:* Stress/adaptation *Strategies:* Stress management and teaching/learning 1a. Open-ended statements and questions facilitate communication (Sundeen, 1993).	
	1b. Nurse will explain what stressors are and the body's response by 3/18/94.	1b. First state in stress management and according to Hamberger and Lohr (1984) involves education (e.g., nature of stress).	
	1c. Client will identify two personal reactions to stress from relationship with husband by 3/18/94.	1c. Stressors affect different people in different ways (Phipps, 1991).	Orders not implemented because of other priorities. Short-term outcome not met.
2. Client will choose two coping strategies to use to manage stress by 3/18/94.	2a. Client will describe coping strategies she currently uses to deal with stress from relationship with husband on 3/18/94.	2a. Assessment of coping strategies currently used is a component of stress management (Scandrett-Hibdon, 1992).	**Criteria statement** Client will select two coping strategies to use to manage stress. Refer to nursing order 2c.
	2b. Nurse and client will discuss effectiveness of methods client currently uses to manage stress on 3/18/94.	2b. Learning needs of the client must be determined (Redman, 1993).	Orders not implemented because of other priorities. Short-term outcome not met. Orders to be implemented at next visit.
	2c. Nurse will explain a variety of coping strategies available to manage the stress reaction on 3/18/94: Relaxation techniques Assertiveness training Problem solving Biofeedback	2c. Stress management involves a variety of coping strategies that can be used by individuals (Phipps, 1991). Refer to nursing order 2c.	
	2d. Client will react to each coping strategy on 3/18/94.	2d. Client is an active participant.	
	2e. Client will select two coping strategies to use for stress management on 3/18/94.	2e. Client is an active participant in the selection of coping strategies, fostering motivation, and learning (Redman, 1993).	
3. Client will use the selected coping strategies on a regular basis by 5/13/94.	3a. Nurse will explain how each strategy is used correctly on 3/18/94.	3a. Learning occurs through imitation (Rorden, 1987).	**Criteria statement** 1. Client will demonstrate correct use of each coping strategy selected.
	3b. Client will practice with nurse each technique selected on 3/18/94 and 4/15/94.	3b. Effective learning requires active participation by the learner.	2. Client will state frequency each technique has been used to manage stress.
	3c. Client will implement one strategy at a time on 3/18/94 and 4/15/94.	3c. Learning is broken down into small steps to facilitate learning and achievement (Redman, 1993).	Orders not implemented. Short-term outcome not met.

PLANS FOR IMPLEMENTATION—cont'd

Nursing diagnosis 7: Ineffective interdependence related to stress from relationship with husband (2/4/94).
Long-term expected outcome: Client will increase stress management techniques by 5/13/94.

Short-term expected outcomes	Nursing orders	Scientific rationale	Evaluation
	3d. Nurse and client will evaluate the technique according to use, ability to perform, and usefulness at managing the stress on 5/13/94.	3d. Final stage of stress management is application of coping strategies to an actual stressor and evaluation of that application (Hamberger and Lohr, 1984).	Orders to be implemented at a future date. **Concluding evaluation** Long-term outcome not met.

REFERENCES AND READINGS

Allan JD: Exercise program. In Bulechek GM and McCloskey JC, editors: *Nursing interventions: essential nursing treatments,* Philadelphia, 1992, WB Saunders.

Bates B: *A guide to physical examination and history taking,* Philadelphia, 1991, JB Lippincott.

Buck MH: The personal self. In Roy SrC and Andrews HA, editors: *The Roy adaptation model: the definitive statement,* Norwalk, Conn, 1991, Appleton and Lange.

Buck MH: The physical self. In Roy SrC and Andrews HA, editors: *The Roy adaptation model: the definitive statement,* Norwalk, Conn, 1991, Appleton and Lange.

Bullock BL and Rosendahl PP: *Pathophysiology: adaptations and alterations in function,* Philadelphia, 1992, JB Lippincott.

Carpenito LH: *Nursing diagnosis: application to clinical practice,* Philadelphia, 1992, JB Lippincott.

Corbett JV: *Laboratory tests and diagnostic procedures with nursing diagnoses,* Norwalk, Conn, 1992, Appleton and Lange.

Crist JK: Weight management. In Bulechek GM and McCloskey JC, editors: *Nursing interventions: essential nursing treatments,* Philadelphia, 1992, WB Saunders.

Dudek SG: *Nutrition handbook for nursing practice,* Philadelphia, 1993, JB Lippincott.

Erikson E: *Childhood and society,* New York, 1963, WW Norton.

Fink JW: The challenge of blood pressure control, *Nurs Clin North Am* 16:301, June 1981.

Foster SB and Kousch D: Adherence to therapy in hypertensive clients, *Nurs Clin North Am* 16:331, June 1981.

Gerber AM et al: Socioeconomic status and electrolyte intake in black adults: The Pitt County study, *Am J Public Health* 81:1608, Dec. 1991.

Gullickson C: Client-centered drug choice: an alternative approach in managing hypertension, *Nurse Pract* 13:30, Feb. 1993.

Hamberger LK and Lohr JM: *Stress and stress management: research and applications,* New York, 1984, Springer.

Hochenberry B: Multiple drug therapy in the treatment of essential hypertension, *Nurs Clin North Am* 26:417, June 1991.

Johannsen JM: Update: guidelines for treating hypertension, *Am J Nurs* 93:42, March 1993.

Johnson MN et al: Psychological stress and blood pressure levels in black women, *J Nat Black Nurs Assoc* 1:41, Fall 1986–Winter 1987.

Karch AM: *Handbook of drugs and the nursing process,* Philadelphia, 1992, JB Lippincott.

Knowles M: *The modern practice of adult education: from pedagogy to andragogy,* Chicago, 1984, Follett Publishing.

MacDonald MB et al: Lifestyle behaviors in treated hypertensives as prediction of blood pressure control, *Rehab Nurs* 13:82, March-April 1988.

McEntee MA and Peddicord K: Coping with hypertension, *Nurs Clin North Am* 22:583, Sep. 1987.

Nakagawa-Kogan H et al: Self-management of hypertension: predictors of success in diastolic blood pressure reduction, *Res Nurs Health* 11:105, April 1988.

Neighbors HW: Seeking professional help for personal problems: black Americans' use of health and mental health services, *Community Ment Health J* 21:156, Fall 1988.

Nuwayhid KA: Role transition, distance and conflict. In Roy SrC and Andrews HA, editors: *The Roy adaptation model: the definitive statement,* Norwalk, Conn, 1991, Appleton and Lange.

Phipps WJ et al: *Medical-surgical nursing: concepts and clinical practice,* ed 4, St Louis, 1991, Mosby–Year Book.

Plawecki HM et al: Compliance and health beliefs in the black female hypertensive client, *J Nat Black Nurs Assoc* 2:38, Fall 1987–Winter 1988.

Pohl ML: The teaching function of the nursing practitioner, Dubuque, Iowa, 1981, William C. Brown.

Powers MJ: Profile of the well-controlled, well-adjusted hypertensive patient, *Nurs Res* 36:106, March-April 1987.

Redman BK: *The process of patient education,* ed 7, St Louis, 1993, Mosby–Year Book.

Rorden JW: *Nurses as health teachers: a practical guide,* Philadelphia, 1987, WB Saunders.

Roy SrC: *Introduction to nursing: an adaptation model,* Englewood Cliffs, NJ, 1984, Prentice-Hall.

Roy SrC and Andrews HA: *The Roy adaptation model: the definitive statement,* Norwalk, Conn, 1991, Appleton and Lange.

Sato MK: Major factors influencing adaptation. In Roy SrC, editor: *Introduction to nursing: an adaptation model,* Englewood Cliffs, NJ, 1984, Prentice-Hall.

Scandrett-Hibdon S: Cognitive reappraisal. In Bulechek GM and McCloskey JC, editors: *Nursing interventions: essential nursing treatments,* Philadelphia, 1992, WB Saunders.

Scandrett-Hibdon S and Uecker S: Relaxation training. In Bulechek GM and McCloskey JC, editors: *Nursing interventions: essential nursing treatments,* Philadelphia, 1992, WB Saunders.

Servonsky J: Elimination. In Roy SrC and Andrews HA, editors: *The Roy adaptation model: the definitive statement,* Norwalk, Conn, 1991, Appleton and Lange.

Sullivan EJ and Decker PJ: *Effective management in nursing,* Redwood City, Calif, 1992, Addison-Wesley Nursing.

Sundeen SJ et al: *Nurse-client interaction: implementing the nursing process,* ed 5, St Louis, 1993, Mosby–Year Book.

Tedrow MP: Overview of the interdependence mode. In Roy SrC and Andrews HA, editors: *The Roy adaptation model: the definitive statement,* Norwalk, Conn, 1991, Appleton and Lange.

Whitman NI et al: *Teaching in nursing practice: a professional model,* Norwalk, Conn, 1992, Appleton and Lange.

CHAPTER 15

NURSING PROCESS OF THE FAMILY CLIENT
Application of Neuman's Systems Model

Joanne R. Cross*

The community health nurse is working with the Ross family. This blended family consists of a married couple, Jim and Mary, both of whom have been formerly married, and their older children. Jim's 15-year-old son, Jim, Jr., and Mary's children, Danny, 23, and Mary, 20, reside in the home. The focus of this family nursing process is on Danny, who has Hodgkin's disease, and the stressors and family interactions related to his care.

The Neuman (1990) Systems Model, which is applicable to a family, was chosen to guide the nursing process in working with this family. In Neuman's model, the family is viewed as an open system in constant interaction with the environment. Successful transactions with the environment reflect adjustment to that environment by the family. Neuman's model was chosen because the major components of this model are stress and reaction to stress, and this family is experiencing various stressors related to illness. Family stressors during illness and ways in which the family copes with stressors are also addressed by Neuman's model. Stressors are defined as follows:

Intrafamily stressors occur within the family unit—the individual interactions among family members. These interactions can be within the biological, psychological, sociological, developmental, and spiritual realms. They may include actual or potential stress problems, cop-

ing mechanisms, lifestyle changes, physical problems, strengths and weaknesses, general mood, and decision-making processes, among other factors.

Interfamily stressors occur between the family and the immediate or direct external environment. Examples include interaction with other families such as in-laws, neighbors, ex-spousal relationships, friends and community groups such as church and school groups, and work environments.

Extrafamily stressors occur between the family and the distal or indirect environment (political and social issues or support and other groups).

The process of interaction and adjustment within the family relies on the "lines of defense," which are biological, psychological, sociocultural, developmental, and spiritual in nature. The interaction and impact of each of these realms must continually be considered as they impinge on the family's stress points (Story and Ross, 1986). If a stressor breaks through the normal line of defense, the equilibrium is disturbed and a whole range of responses occurs. In addition, internal resistance factors (lines of resistance) are activated that attempt to stabilize and return the client or family to normal functioning.

Stressors not only create reactions within the client (individual or family), but also create strong emotional fields between the client and other extrapersonal forces. Nursing interventions can begin at any point at which a stressor is suspected or identified,

*Revisions in fourth edition by J.W. Kenney.

and can be introduced at primary, secondary, or tertiary levels of prevention. Neuman's model facilitates attainment and maintenance of the highest possible level of function and addresses primary, secondary, and tertiary levels of care. This model guides the modes of nursing intervention for each level and focuses on returning the client to a previously healthy state. For a review of Neuman's major concepts, see Chapter 2.

In this nursing process of the family, the five nurse visits are presented sequentially, along with assessment data, analysis and synthesis of the data, and the list of nursing diagnoses for each visit. Then five nursing plans, which include expected outcomes, nursing orders, scientific rationale, and evaluation, are described. The plans are presented last because they are ongoing and subject to revision, and demonstrate the continuity of the entire nursing process. However, the nursing plans are initiated, implemented, and evaluated concurrently with the assessment visits.

Data Collection: Preliminary information

Jim and Mary have been married for 3½ years. The Ross family genogram is shown in Fig. 15-1 and explained on the following page. Jim's wife Jill died 5 years ago, and his son Jim Jr. lives with Mary and him. Mary is divorced from her first husband Bill. They had two children, Danny, 23, and Diane, 20, who are currently living with Jim and Mary. Danny is divorced and estranged from his ex-wife Lois, who lives in Florida with their 2-year-old son. Danny has Hodgkin's disease and is currently undergoing a course of chemotherapy treatment.

Source of referral:
John Shell, M.D.
Medical Oncology Unit
Sycamore Medical Center

Communication with collaborating agency:
Oncology unit at Sycamore Medical Center where Danny is a client

October 14, 1993: Information received from Dr. Shell, Danny's oncologist, in a phone conversation:

1. Diagnosed in February 1993. Stage IIIB Hodgkin's disease. Initial symptoms were night sweats, inguinal lymph node enlargement, severe lower back pain, and hematuria.
2. No response to MOPP,* first-line therapy.
3. Has had four courses of ABVD therapy (Adriamycin, bleomycin, vinblastine, and dacarbazine [DTIC].
4. Is in remission (not sure yet if complete remission). Lymph nodes and bone lesions have resolved.
5. If present therapy eventually fails, several other courses of therapy can be tried.
6. Not concerned about back pain; bone scan was negative.
   a. Received radiation therapy to this area in February 1993.
   b. Discontinued Dilaudid because he felt Danny was becoming too dependent on it.
7. Physician feels that right now Danny is coping with his disease well psychologically.
8. Since Danny has been feeling better, Dr. Shell has had no contact with the family (stepfather called him often during early phase of illness).

*MOPP = acronym for combination of nitrogen mustard, vincristine (Oncovin), procarbazine hydrochloride, and prednisone (Porth, 1986).

Genogram

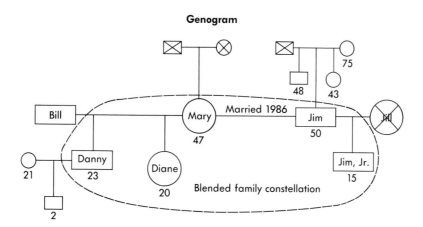

Figure 15-1 Ross family genogram.

Biographical Data and Initial Contact

Name	Age (yr)	Sex	Education	Occupation	Introductory data
Danny	23	M	Dropped out of high school in senior year	Unemployed	Impaired member—has Hodgkin's disease, is recently divorced, and has 2-year-old son who lives with his ex-wife
Jim	50	M	Working toward master's degree in business	Salesman for large insurance company	Stepfather of Danny and Diane; father of Jim, Jr.
Mary	42	F	Did not finish high school	Housewife; grooms, breeds, and shows poodles	Mother of Danny and Diane; stepmother of Jim, Jr.
Jim, Jr.	15	M	Freshman in high school	Not applicable	Stepbrother of Danny and Diane
Diane	20	F	High school graduate	Unemployed; assists mother with grooming of poodles	Sister of Danny, stepsister of Jim, Jr.

DATA COLLECTION: Visit 1—October 22, 1993

Setting: Nurse talked with client in hospital room at Sycamore Medial Center where he had been since October 18 to receive chemotherapy. No other clients were present in the three-bed room. Data were received verbally from client, by observation of nurse, and from the chart.

Subjective data	Objective data
Interactions	**Observations and measurements**

Biological data (from client)	
Hi, Joan. I'm doing a little better today. My doctor says I will probably be getting these drugs for 6–8 more months. He says he thinks I am starting remission, and if I can live for 5 years, I will probably not get the cancer back. If this drug stops working, there is one other drug they can try, and if that doesn't work, I've had it.	Client lying in bed. Head of bed slightly raised. Bedcovers covering him up to waist. Danny appeared well nourished and of normal weight. Skin was pale. No alopecia was noted. Hair was shiny and neatly combed. Eyes alert. Wearing a clean pair of striped pajamas.
I get sick with this drug but not as bad. They give me THC† (like "joints"), and they let me smoke "joints" while I'm getting therapy. It makes me feel like I'm in a different place, and I don't mind the nausea as much. I still get the shakes, but if I can get my mind on something else, that helps, even if it's just tapping my fingers. I'm usually sick for 3–5 hr after getting the drug.	Client takes THC 7.5 mg every 4 hr when receiving chemotherapy (chart) Client demonstrated by tapping fingers on bedside stand. Smiled and rolled his eyes.
I ate supper last night after getting therapy in the late afternoon and kept it down. I just eat light foods.	
They've really messed up my veins. It's hard to find a good one any more. My doctor says they might have to start putting it in my neck or legs. I don't want them to do that. I'm afraid that will really hurt.	Both arms appeared "black and blue" at injection sites.
I still get tired easily.	
My doctor says I should not get a job yet. I can feel fine for a while and then get sick again and would have to quit a job.	Smoked filtered cigarettes continously throughout interview.
Still gets sweats but no bleeding from UT‡ now.	Smoked 4 cigarettes/hr.
Denies any itching of skin.	Sat up, showed part of back that was affected (midlumbar).

DATA COLLECTION: Visit 1—October 22, 1993—cont'd

Subjective data	Objective data
Interactions	**Observations and measurements**

Started having symptoms in January 1993—sweats, bleeding from kidney, lower back pain. "I was very sick. I couldn't stand or sit without severe pain."

They did a lot of tests and finally diagnosed it as cancer. At first they thought I would only live about 5 months.

For the past 2 months I have been receiving one drug as an outpatient 1 day every month, and then 2 weeks later, 5 days of DTIC* in the hospital.

From chart (also from physician)

Feb–Aug: received MOPP§ chemotherapy, which caused severe nausea and vomiting. This therapy was then found to be ineffective.

Received radiation therapy to coccygeal area in Feb '93, which helped to relieve pain.

Sociological data

I quit high school 3 weeks before graduation in 1988. That was really a mistake. I would like to get my high school diploma.

Looked wistfully out the window but sounded hopeful.

I was married for 2 years and got divorced in February '91. I have a 2-year-old son who lives with my ex-wife in Florida.

I worked as a machinist in a brush company repairing $5000 machines. It was a very responsible job, and I learned a lot. I also had a job laying pipes for a construction company.

I would really like to get a job now, but I would have to give up my Social Security. Then I might get really sick again and have to quit.

Sat up, looked alert, and gestured with hands.

I'm just now starting to receive Social Security and Medicaid. I have not been able to work since December. I have been receiving General Relief funds.

I have friends who really help. One friend in particular I see about every day. He sort of inspires me to do things that I didn't think I could still do. We play pool or ping-pong, ride cycles, or just go drink beer.

Smiled and looked contented.

My mother and stepfather have been married for 3½ years. I didn't approve of him, but since I have been sick I feel differently. He has really shown that he cares about me and has helped me financially.

My real dad lives in Florida. We're pretty close; I talk with him on the phone every 2 weeks. I'm going to visit him for 3 weeks in February. I haven't had a vacation in the past year, and my mom and stepdad think I should go for my birthday.

Psychological data

I felt really bad when Mike and Larry, my roommates on the oncology unit, died. It really makes you think about your life.

Sad expression on face while looking out window.

I started with the GED program at Montgomery County Vocational School twice to get my high school diploma but had to quit both times. I need a more structured classroom setting and help. I have difficulty doing everything on my own.

My goal is to become an electrical engineer.

I wouldn't mind working as an orderly at a hospital or as a pharmacy aide.

I like my physician very much and I think he is very competent.

My marriage seemed to be a disaster from the beginning, but we had a beautiful child. My son looks just like me, a really nice-looking kid. I still love my wife. That really messes up my head. During my marriage I drank a lot, wrecked my new car 3 times, quit a good job, and didn't do what I should have for my family. I guess I still had wildness in me.

Smiled broadly.

Voice sounded regretful.

I cope by trying to have a cheerful attitude. I pretend in my mind that I don't have cancer. I usually manage to have a good mental attitude.

He spoke cheerfully and appeared "high spirited."

It is difficult for me to have a close relationship with a woman. When I tell them about my condition they back away. I know it's because they don't want to get hurt.

His outward appearance throughout the interview was cheerful and friendly.

Continued

DATA COLLECTION: Visit 1—October 22, 1993—cont'd

Subjective data	Objective data
Interactions	**Observations and measurements**

Spiritual data

I've been going to the Church of the Nazarene on Main Street. I really like that church. I used to be Catholic, but I didn't believe in everything the Catholic Church teaches. Now I just say I'm a Christian.	
I have never believed in divorce. My mom and dad were divorced after being married 22 years, and I didn't think that was right. It was really hard for me when my wife wanted a divorce.	Sad expression on face; hands folded behind neck, cradling his head.

†THC = Delta-9-tetrahydrocannabinol.
‡UT = Urinary tract.
§MOPP = Acronym for combination of nitrogen mustard, vincristine (Oncovin), procarbazine hydrochloride, and Prednisone (Porth, 1986).
*DTIC = Dacarbazine.

Analysis/Synthesis: Visit 1—October 22, 1993

The central focus of the Neuman model is on the family's relationship during stress and their reaction to stressors and factors of reconstitution. In assessing the client, the various types of stressors—intrapersonal/family, interpersonal/family, and extrapersonal/family—are considered. The illness has not only penetrated the normal line of defense but also threatens the very core of Danny himself, as well as the family structure.

Intrapersonal/Intrafamily Stressors

According to Neuman, the balance and harmony within this family have been disrupted because of Danny's life-threatening illness, Hodgkin's disease, Stage IIIB. Initially, biological stressors and the lines of defense are analyzed. In this disease, the malignant proliferation of abnormal histiocytes replaces the normal cellular elements within the lymph nodes. The disease causes painless enlargement of the lymph nodes in one site and then spreads to other nodes throughout the body. This neoplastic process may spread to other organs such as the spleen, liver, ureters, bowel, bone marrow, and the bones themselves (Suddarth, 1991). Pain occurs if a nerve or nearby structure is infiltrated or compressed.

Hodgkin's disease is often classified in four stages according to the extent the disease has spread in the body. In Stage III, groups of nodes are involved, both above and below the diaphragm. The stages are subdivided into groups: A, no general symptoms, and B, presence of symptoms such as weight loss, fever, and night sweats (Suddarth, 1991; LeBlanc, 1978).

Normal line of defense invaded; physical integrity compromised. Danny's initial symptoms were night sweats, inguinal lymph node enlargement, severe lower back pain, and hematuria. His back pain and hematuria could have been caused by infiltration of the neoplasm into bone and urinary tract structures. After radiation therapy to his lower back and chemotherapy, the pain was relieved and the hematuria subsided. He still suffers from night sweats and fatigue. His energy integrity is compromised. The fatigue is probably due to anemia caused by decreased erythrocytes. Both Hodgkin's disease itself and chemotherapy can cause abnormal erythrocyte destruction and production (Suddarth, 1991).

An additional factor that could be affecting Danny's energy level is inadequate nutrition. He seems to be coping fairly well with the nausea and vomiting associated with chemotherapy by using THC and marijuana, and diverting his thoughts elsewhere. (THC is the major psychoactive compound in cannabis sativa, the hemp plant that is the source of marijuana. Cannabis is a psychotropic agent that causes altered consciousness and a dreamlike state.) A nutritional assessment should be done because one of the symptoms of Hodgkin's disease is anorexia (Suddarth, 1991). Data are also needed about other symptoms Danny may be having associated with his disease process or the effects of chemotherapy.

Another stressor involving the physical line of defense is the apparent collapse of Danny's arm veins due to frequent IV infusions. In summation, there are two nursing concerns in relation to Danny's energy and resistance level: he is at high risk for nutritional deficiencies, and he has reduced venous access resulting from repeated IV infusions.

There is a data gap in information about Danny's prognosis. He may be experiencing an objective remission in response to his current chemotherapy. LeBlanc (1978) defines *objective remission* as regression of the disease and *complete remission* as the return to normal function, with no physical, biochemical, or roentgenographic evidence of disease. According to Suddarth (1991), late-stage patients treated with combined chemotherapy had an arrest rate greater than 70% in 1980.

Other intrapersonal stressors affecting Danny's well-being, as well as that of the family, are in the developmental and psychosocial realms. Danny seems to be working through the developmental tasks in two of Erikson's stages, identity versus role confusion, and intimacy versus isolation (Eshleman, 1988). A major event in the *ego identity stage* is emancipation from parents. When a young adult develops a chronic illness, he or she often has to resume dependence on parents for financial support and care (Valentine, 1978). This aptly describes Danny's situation. Because he had no medical insurance and could not work, he chooses to live with his mother and stepfather and be dependent on them. Part of forming a healthy adult self-concept is finding a satisfying occupation. Danny seems to want to pursue this goal but has several obstacles in his path—the limitations imposed by his illness and the inability to complete high school. These have curtailed his occupational desires.

In the *intimacy versus isolation stage,* a person develops the ability to form a close, loving interpersonal relationship with another person, without losing his or her own identity (Valentine, 1978). Danny mentioned that it is difficult for him to develop a close relationship with a woman because of his illness. Even before his illness, he was having some difficulty in mastering the tasks in both of Erikson's stages just mentioned. He regrets now that he did not assume his full responsibilities in being a husband and father. He still seems to be experiencing conflict and remorse about his divorce. This analysis leads to the following nursing diagnosis for Danny: alterations in self-concept and disruption of interpersonal relationships related to illness.

Danny is aware that his disease may be fatal and apparently does have anxiety about his treatment and prognosis. He mentioned two ways in which he copes with his illness. He makes an effort to be cheerful, and he pretends that he doesn't have cancer. This seems to be a conscious denial of the reality of the situation. Denial is a normal protective means of adapting to the diagnosis of cancer, and some patients continue to use it throughout their entire cancer experience (Watson, 1978). Danny apparently receives acceptance and support from his family, physician, and friends. He may be coping adequately with his condition; however, the nursing diagnosis—anxiety related to life-threatening illness—is appropriate.

Interpersonal/Interfamily Stressors

From this first visit, little data support the perceived threat to family relationships, status, and goals. The only role change apparent at this time is Danny's change from husband and father to dependent son, which has a major impact on both Danny and the entire family. There is a data gap concerning the family's past experience with the same or similar situations and their response to the present situation.

Extrapersonal/Extrafamily Stressors

There are many data gaps regarding resources that are available to the family. How are the medical bills being paid? Is there financial strain on the family? Danny seems to receive spiritual support from the church that he attends. The spiritual resources of the other family members represent a data gap. Danny and his stepfather seem to have a closer relationship as a result of this illness, and Danny expresses a close relationship with his biological father.

NURSING DIAGNOSIS: Visit 1

Date	Diagnosis	Priority
10/22/93	1. Potential alterations in nutrition related to chemotherapy treatments	5
10/22/93	2. Alterations in comfort related to nausea and vomiting	1
10/22/93	3. Alterations in self-concept (body image) related to illness and treatment	2
10/22/93	4. Anxiety related to life-threatening illness	3
10/22/93	5. Potential alteration in family coping related to life-threatening illness of family member	6
10/22/93	6. Inadequate venous access related to repeated chemotherapy treatments	7
10/22/93	7. Alterations in interpersonal relationships related to life-threatening illness	4

Setting: Talked with Danny in living room of his family's home in a middle-class, suburban neighborhood. House is brick, three-bedroom, split-level with wood siding, 10 years old, and well kept. Client's house and lawn are neat, with motorboat and two cars in driveway. City bus line is one block away. Inside, home is orderly, clean, carpeted. Furniture appears new with two TV sets and a stereo system. Danny sleeps at the end of family room in an area set apart by room dividers. He has two posters and album covers decorating the wall, and his other personal items, bed, dresser, and shelves. Danny has a large collection of records and tapes. Mother keeps four poodles in the one-car garage. When nurse arrived for visit, Danny had just gotten home and said he forgot she was coming.

Subjective data	Objective data
Interactions	**Observations and measurements**

Biological data

I see my doctor Thursday. I may get more chemotherapy then, but my white blood count may still be too low.	
My pain medication was reduced to 1 mg every 4 hr from 4 mg every 4 hr. Now it does not relieve the pain in my back. It is a dull ache. I know my doctor is afraid I will become addicted to drugs, but I usually only need it in the evening when I am tired.	Indicated midlumbar back area as where pain was. Now takes Dilaudid 1 mg every 4 hr (previously 4 mg every 4 hr).
Mom gets *Prevention* magazine and has been trying to get me to eat green, leafy vegetables. She gets after me for eating junk food.	Pointed to end table where three or four *Prevention* magazines lay neatly stacked.
The doctor says it is okay for me to drink beer. It has helped me gain weight.	Talked with Danny in living room of home.
When I eat out with friends, I eat fast food. It's more convenient.	Danny sitting up in chair. Wearing plaid flannel shirt, corduroy pants, and slippers with heavy socks. Hair combed neatly. Alert and eyes bright.
What should I eat to increase my white blood count more rapidly?	
Mother and Jim both see a doctor in Englewood when they need medication; neither take any medication now except Ornade.	
Jim is a disabled vet—no physical disabilities now.	Danny smoked nine cigarettes throughout this interview.
The doctor says I am either in remission or entering remission.	
I have been exercising my arms with weights.	Danny extended arms and displayed his arm muscles.

Sociological data

Our family shops at the commissary once a month for food. We spend about $350. We have a freezer.	
Usually our family eats together in the evening. Mother fixes meals. One night a week everyone fixes their own dinner.	
Jim provides for the family. Mom contributes a little with money earned by grooming dogs or prize money from dog shows. I help buy food the last week of the month when food begins to run out.	
Mom cleans the house but everyone chips in a little. I keep my bedroom and family room straightened up. My sisters helps with the dogs.	
I went to Bowling Green Lanes last night with a friend. We drank beer, played pool, Tron, and other games.	
I lived with another family for 9 months while my mom and dad got their divorce. This family told me if I get my GED,* I would have a painting job with them. I don't know if I could physically handle the job yet.	
Jim told me that if I don't get my GED, I could stay in Florida with my real father.	
My mother and stepfather make the decisions in the family, but we do have family discussions.	
Jim, Jr., my stepbrother, is bused to high school.	
With five people living together in the house, sometimes things just blow up. (He mentioned disagreements between mom and stepfather, himself and stepfather, sister and stepfather. During one altercation, sister took mother's side against stepfather, who became angry, and threw coffee table, hit ceiling in family room; they had to have it repaired.)	Danny sat forward with an intense look in his eyes. He gestured with his hands as he described this incident. Then he frowned and shook his head from side to side.
I almost hit my stepfather with my crutch one time. He was angry because I wouldn't eat. We usually explode, then cool down, next day apologize, and forget all about it.	
I always lose in an argument with Jim.	
Every once in a while, when everyone is on edge, we all sit down together and just talk about things.	Sat back in his chair in a relaxed position with his arms at rest on the sides of chair and legs crossed.

Subjective data	Objective data
Interactions	**Observations and measurements**
My stepfather and mother have been involved in a group trying to get permission for a Vietnam veteran who is walking to Washington, D.C. to walk through Ohio. They finally took him to Kentucky, so he could walk from there.	Danny frowned, grimaced, and shook his head.
Jim is still talking about his Vietnam venture. When he does something, he wants to be sure everyone knows about it. I don't mean to belittle the man, but that is one thing I get tired of.	
I had a long talk with my girlfriend, and we ironed out our differences.	Smiled.
I have been getting General Relief ($67 a month). Now I will get $250 a month from Social Security.	
Jim's mom lives in Versailles. She sent cards when I was ill in the hospital	
I keep in touch with aunts, uncles, cousins on my real father's side; none live close. My mother is an only child, and all of her family are dead. She has one really close friend in Boston.	He sat back in chair and placed his hands behind his neck and cradled head in hands.
(When Danny was really sick, Jim handled things within the immediate family; the only outside help came from Cancer Control to help pay for medication.)	
My sister and I go places together. She has a car and I pay for the gas.	
Our family plays cards and watches TV together—programs like *Nova* and *Cosmos.* Jim insists that we watch these kinds of shows. I like the stereo especially.	Smiled. Got up and walked over to his stereo system.
Psychological data	
My real father is always on the run and likes to keep busy.	
I started going to vocational school to take classes for GED—two evenings a week for 2 hr each evening.	
After I get my GED, I would like to learn to play a synthesizer. I can take classes at the vocational school in reading music.	Eyes alert, bright; spoke animatedly.
I really enjoy music. I sang in the school choir for 6 yr. I could have made the best singing group in high school, but my grades weren't good enough. I was thought of as a "trouble maker."	
(Talked again about wife.) I called her parents to get her address, so I could have Social Security sent to my son. They told me their daughter was getting along fine without my money.	
When I was married I never saw my friends; now my friends are very important to me.	Thoughtful expression on face.
I really appreciate being able to stay at home and not have to pay for room and board.	
My mom is very particular about the house. I often have to wait for her when we're ready to go somewhere while she empties the ashtrays. If there is one piece of silverware in the sink, she washes it.	Rolled his eyes, then smiled.

*GED = Graduate equivalency diploma.

Analysis/Synthesis:
Visit 2—November 1, 1993
Intrapersonal/Intrafamily Stressors

Most of the previous analysis of October 22 continues to be appropriate. Using Neuman's model and considering the intrusion of this life-threatening illness on the basic lines of defense, the lines of resistance, and on the intrinsic core of energy, Danny continues to demonstrate acute symptoms. He is still experiencing back pain and also has pain in his left leg, especially in the evening when he is tired. The pain medication he is now receiving does not relieve the pain. He has some degree of leukopenia with his chemotherapy, which could put him at risk for infection (Brunner and Suddarth, 1992). He expressed an interest in what to do about this. A positive aspect of his illness is that his physician has told him that he is going into remission.

In considering energy conservation, a nutritional analysis is planned. On the positive side, his mother prepares meals for the family on most days and is apparently aware that good nutrition is important, but there is a data gap about what she prepares (tertiary and primary levels of prevention). Danny eats junk food and eats at fast food places when he is with friends, but it is not known how often this occurs. Danny seems to smoke regularly, which is detrimental to his energy level (Ardell, 1986). It might, however, be very difficult for him to quit smoking while having to cope with his illness. In conclusion, the nursing diagnoses are (1) alterations in comfort related to lower back pain, and (2) potential for infection related to leukopenia.

The basic core of the family appears intact, albeit somewhat stressed. It is normal that life-threatening illness challenges family stability, adaptability, resources, and, most intensely, beliefs and assumptions.

Interpersonal/Interfamily Stressors

Regarding Danny's personal response to shifting roles, new data support the diagnosis of alterations in self-concept. He is undecided about what kind of occupation he might like to pursue, but he has started working toward a high school diploma. It is unknown whether he is sufficiently motivated to do the required work or whether he has enrolled in the program only because other people have encouraged him to do so. Because of his ex-wife's and in-laws' attitudes, he is unable to fulfill his financial obligation to his son. Although he feels affection for his son, he is unable to be in touch with him. He does try to contribute what he can to his own immediate family.

In considering the perceived threat to family relationships, status, and goals, a data gap still exists because Danny is the only member of the family who has talked with me. The roles in the family seem to be mostly traditional, with the wife taking care of the home and cooking, and the husband providing most of the income. Their communication patterns seem somewhat dysfunctional, especially between the father and his stepchildren, and some members of the family have difficulty dealing with their anger in a functional manner. Some of the anger seems to be related to family tensions due to Danny's illness. Danny still seems to feel animosity toward his stepfather, and one gets the feeling from talking with Danny that he has little power in the family. The stepfather seems to be authoritarian in his approach to his grown children. Possible diagnoses could be family tensions related to Danny's illness and dysfunctional family communication.

Extrapersonal/Extrafamily Stressors

Some of the resources available to the family were identified in this visit. They live in a clean, well-kept home in a residential neighborhood, with adequate transportation available. Each member of the family has adequate money for food and other necessities. There is affection between Danny and his sister, and in spite of their difficulties, Danny's stepfather is concerned about him. The family spends time together at meals and watching TV or playing cards. Danny gets some support from his friends and the family he lived with while his parents were getting a divorce. The extended family has not responded to this crisis. According to Danny, his immediate family handled his hospitalization and initial illness, except for some help from the cancer control agency.

The next family visit will include Danny and his mother, to gather data about the effect of Danny's illness on the family, about communication and decision-making patterns, and about coping strategies used by the family. A review of Danny's systems will be done to see whether he is experiencing any other symptoms of Hodgkin's disease or any effects of chemotherapy. Also, the family support and communication patterns will be examined, which seems to have a great impact on the family functioning.

NURSING DIAGNOSIS: Visit 2

Date	Diagnosis	Priority
10/22/93	1. Potential alterations in nutrition related to chemotherapy treatment	6
10/22/93	2. Alterations in comfort related to nausea and vomiting	1
10/22/93	3. Alterations in self-concept related to life-threatening illness	7
10/22/93	4. Anxiety related to life-threatening illness	3
10/22/93	5. Potential alterations in family coping related to life-threatening illness of family member	8
10/22/93	6. Inadequate venous access related to repeated chemotherapy treatment	10
10/22/93	7. Alterations in intrapersonal relationships related to illness	4
11/1/93	8. Alterations in comfort related to lower back pain	2
11/1/93	9. Potential for infection related to leukopenia	5
11/1/93	10. Potential for dysfunctional family communication related to blending of two families	9

DATA COLLECTION: Visit 3—November 15, 1993

Setting: Meeting took place in living room of home. Mother wore new jeans, a bulky pink sweater, and loafers. Her hair is dark brown, shiny, and combed neatly off her shoulders. Eyes alert and facial expressions attentive. Danny wore a red T-shirt and jeans with Reebok running shoes. Danny and mother sat on opposite ends of couch, and nurse sat in chair facing them. The room is neat and orderly as in previous visit. (Jim came in later.)

Subjective data	Objective data
Interactions	**Observations and measurements**

Biological data (from client)

I weighed 140 lb before my illness, then lost and gained about 30 lb. Now I weigh 139 lb, and I'm 5'7" tall.

I had shingles on my left leg about 3 months ago. I wasn't able to walk on the leg for 6 weeks. That leg is still weak. Sometimes it buckles under me.

I still have pain in the tail bone area of my back. It aches worse when I lie down.

My doctor has taken me off Dilaudid. Now I can take Zomax but haven't tried this medication yet.

My doctor is concerned about the back pain. I was to have a bone scan Friday, November 12.

I received chemotherapy as an outpatient about a week ago (Adriamycin, bleomycin, and one other drug). I was very nauseated about 6 hr after treatment. The nausea lasted about 24 hr. I used THC and smoked marijuana at home to relieve nausea and vomiting.

(Review of systems revealed no other symptoms of Hodgkin's disease or side effects of chemotherapy at this time.)

Here is my 3-day diet diary. I was careful to keep track of almost everything I ate. I took 3 days that I wasn't nauseated.

Objective data (right column):

Good eye contact with nurse while talking.

Jim, Sr., walked into the room wearing a blue plaid shirt and corduroy trousers. Hair is shiny and combed back. He greets us, smiles, and sits next to Mary on the sofa.

Biological data from other members of family

Mary: My husband Jim has back and leg pain. He cannot sit or stand still for very long periods of time. Uses TNS* unit for pain relief. It goes back to Vietnam days.

I have no medical problems, except that my allergies kick up once in a while.

We all smoke except Jim, Jr. My husband and I each smoke about 3 packs a day. We seem to smoke more since Danny's been so sick.

Jim, Jr., is picky in his food habits, too. It's difficult to get him to eat his vegetables and salad greens.

Jim and I eat fairly healthy foods. Diane goes out a lot and eats at fast food places with Danny

3-Day diet diary

Day 1

1 egg	9 AM alone at home
1 pc toast w/butter	
1 glass milk	
1 quarter pounder	1 PM w/sister
1 reg french fry	
1 milk	
6–8 oz liver	5:30 PM at home w/ family
1 cup mashed potatoes (w/blue cheese, sour cream, garlic, onion, and butter)	
1 pc bread and butter	
2 glasses milk	
½ cup each of broccoli and brussel sprouts	
2 cookies	
6 beers	8–11 PM w/friends

Day 2

2 eggs	morning, alone
2 pc toast w/butter	
3 cup coffee	
2 big slices Godfather Pizza	6 PM at home w/family
1 glass milk	
single lg bag potato chips (4 oz)	in PM

Continued

Subjective data	Objective data
Interactions	**Observations and measurements**

	Day 3
	3 cups coffee — morning, alone
	2 Big Macs — 2 PM w/friends
	Small coke (8 oz)
	2 TV dinners, w/shrimp, fish, — 6 PM at home
	scallops, potato, peas
	2 glasses (8 oz) milk
	single bag potato chips (½ oz) — evening

Sociological data

Mary: When Danny first became so ill, we all got together and helped each other out in our chores and helped Danny, too. Even Jim, Jr., helped out.

Outside of our immediate family the only person to help out was Jim's mother, especially when Danny was hospitalized. She lives in Versailles. She prepared and brought food and provided emotional support to the entire family.

When Danny is feeling well, as he has been lately, he forgets how important a good diet is for him and stops eating well. This causes friction because Jim and I are concerned about him and realize how important diet is.

Jim: During the first part of Danny's illness, he was very weak and dependent (he couldn't walk 6 ft without becoming short of breath). Mary tried to let him do as much for himself as possible, but this was very difficult for her to do, I mean, stand by and watch heroic effort.

Roles in any family change during a crisis period. Diane, Jim, Jr., and I took over some of Mary's chores at home because she spent so much time at the hospital. I got up at 3:00 AM to study before going to school. That helps, but is exhausting after a while.

Psychological data

Mary: During the crisis period, Jim, Jr., did things to irritate me (left messes in the kitchen, etc). I knew this was for attention, but I just could not deal with it at that time. I tried to ignore his behavior—not easy.

Jim, Jr., is a loner; he has only one friend. He can talk with his father, but he really doesn't have much to do with other members of the family.

I get along well with Jim, Diane, and Danny. With Jim, Jr., our positive relationship is sporadic.

It was such a shock when Danny was so ill. We have always been very health conscious and wanted to know why this was happening. Jim and I read Jim's psychology and sociology books and got books from the library. We read about diseases being caused by stress.

I had feelings of helplessness. We wanted to help Danny as much as we could, but there didn't seem to be much we could do.

I read the book *Focusing* by Gendlin and encouraged Danny to use this technique to combat nausea and vomiting with chemotherapy.

I am not assertive (always afraid of hurting someone's feelings), so when I get upset with Danny, Jim, Jr., or Diane, I just keep it inside until I finally blow up and tell Jim about it. When he sees that I am upset, he lays down the law to the others.

Right column observations:

Mary leaned forward and gestured with her hands—eyes intense and focused on nurse.

Jim shifted position on couch and crossed legs to get more comfortable.

Look of concern on Mary's face. Jim's face also concerned as he looked at Mary.

Jim nodded his head in affirmation. Somber expression on his face.

Subjective data	Objective data
Interactions	**Observations and measurements**
My husband and I have the final say with most of the decisions in the family. My decisions mostly concern the running of the house and those concerning the children.	
Danny: I am worried that I will never again be as muscular and strong as I was before this illness.	Sad expression in Danny's eyes. He leaned forward and extended his right arm, which is very thin.
I missed my appointment last Friday for the bone scan because I forgot. I feel that Dr. Shelly was put out with me.	
Jim: The father of one of Danny's friends told Danny that he was worthless because he wasn't working—some friend!	
Danny: I was upset and angry because of this remark. Then I realized he just doesn't understand.	Danny's eyes alert at first; some expression of anger in voice and eyes. Then he settled back in chair and looked resigned.
Spiritual data	
Mary: Danny is the only one in the family who attends church right now. It's difficult for me to go to church and pray. Why would a good God let something like this happen to us? What have we done?	Eyes sad, intense. Jim reached over and took Mary's hand.

*TNS = Transcutaneous nerve stimulation.

Analysis/Synthesis:
Visit 3—November 15, 1993

Intrapersonal/Intrafamily Stressors

Previous analyses remain appropriate. Considering Danny's physical stamina and defense system, he still experiences back pain (lumbosacral area). His physician may suspect bone metastasis because he has ordered a bone scan. The left leg weakness that he is experiencing could be related to an episode of shingles, which he had about 3 months ago. Shingles or herpes zoster is an acute viral infection of the nervous system, characterized by a vesicular skin eruption, pain, and sometimes segmental motor and sensory loss along the course of a nerve or group of nerves, usually on only one side of the body (Patrick et al, 1991).

Considering energy and basic core structure, Danny is back to his pre-illness weight which is normal for his height (Williams, 1992). A comparison of Danny's 3-day diet diary with RDA standards reveals deficiencies in fruits, vegetables, and vitamin C. Vitamin A was adequate only because of one large serving of liver. Protein and calcium are adequate. He is eating more than twice as much meat and milk products as are recommended for an adult. He eats more than enough carbohydrates and fats and consumes adequate amounts of grains (Williams, 1992). An environmental condition that may be a family stressor is that four members of the family smoke, which is a potential for a multitude of problems. Smoking may be a coping mechanism used by individual family members to relieve stress in the family environment.

Interpersonal/Interfamily Stressors

Regarding Danny's other intrapersonal stressors, this interview revealed other ways in which his illness threatens his self-concept. It bothers him that others may think he is lazy because he doesn't have a job. He is also concerned about his physical appearance and stamina. New data from this interview support the previous cue that the mother and stepfather are concerned about his welfare and want to help him as much as they can.

New data were gathered about past experience with stressful situations. During the period when Danny was very ill and hospitalized, the family coped by doing some role changing and by learning more about the causes of his illness and how they might be able to help. Mary mentioned difficulty coping with Jim, Jr., at this time. This may be related to the fact that he seems to be an "outsider" in the family.

Mary seems to act as hub for most of the communication in the family. Everyone except Jim, Jr., seems to communicate well with her. New data support previous diagnosis of dysfunctional family communication. Jim, Jr., has difficulty talking with anyone but his father. Mary does not express her feelings until she really becomes upset and then she tells her husband, who speaks to the others. As other data indicate, Jim seems to use an authoritarian manner, which may be the reason that Danny and his sister have difficulty communicating with him.

Extrapersonal/Extrafamily Stressors

The family has expressed in many different ways that they get very little support from outside sources in times of crisis or stress.

Summary

Data gaps still exist concerning the spiritual resources of the family, their coping behaviors, and communication patterns. Information on these gaps will be completed in later interviews with as many family members as possible.

NURSING DIAGNOSIS: Visit 3

Date	Diagnosis	Priority
10/22/93	1. Alterations in nutrition related to chemotherapy treatment and lifestyle	2
10/22/93	2. Alterations in comfort related to nausea and vomiting	9
10/22/93	3. Alterations in self-concept (body image) related to life-threatening illness	5
10/22/93	4. Anxiety related to life-threatening illness	3
10/22/93	5. Dysfunctional communication related to blending of two families and illness in family	4
10/22/93	6. Potential inadequate venous access related to repeated chemotherapy treatment	10
10/22/93	7. Alterations in family coping related to illness of family member	6
11/1/93	8. Alterations in comfort related to low back pain	1
11/1/93	9. Potential for infection related to leukopenia	7
11/1/93	10. Social isolation related to life-threatening illness	8

DATA COLLECTION: Visit 4—December 1, 1993

Setting: Mary sat on couch dressed in jeans and yellow blouse. Hair shiny and arranged neatly off shoulders. Danny is dressed in plaid flannel shirt and faded blue jeans, wearing house slippers. He is sitting in a recliner chair tilted back.

Subjective data	Objective data
Interactions	**Observations and measurements**

Biological data

Danny: I still have back pain. Zomax does not relieve it.	Has redness and dryness at corner of right eye and corner of mouth. No sore areas or lesions within mouth.
I haven't had the bone scan yet, because I had the flu on the day of my appointment.	
I go to the hospital tomorrow for chemotherapy. I hope they find veins for the treatment.	Worried look on Danny's face.
I had flu last week. I vomited for about 8 hours, then I developed chest pain, could not breathe, and was very frightened. I went to emergency room at Sycamore Hospital. They took an x-ray and said maybe I had pulled a chest muscle, that it was an anxiety attack. They gave me Vistaril and sent me home. I felt better the next day.	Danny's face appeared more pale than usual.

Continued to sit contentedly in chair without much movement. |
I have a lot of numbness and weakness in my left leg.	
I have been urinating a lot and have needed more sleep lately, 10–11 hours per night.	
I drink about 12 beers a week.	
We have a lot of vegetables and greens but not much fruit. I don't like vegetables that much.	
Mary: Yes, Danny seems to be having some trouble with his leg—numbness and weakness too. Sometimes it buckles under him.	
I buy both fruits and vegetables, but the fruit gets eaten more quickly, especially by Diane and Jim Jr. Fruit in the winter is also more expensive, so we run out of it faster.	

DATA COLLECTION: Visit 4—December 1, 1993—cont'd

Subjective data	Objective data
Interactions	**Observations and measurements**

Sociological data

Danny: I did well in school. I plan to help mom with her math. She is considering getting her GED and starting her own business.

Mary: Yes, we've been talking about my getting my high school diploma. Jim thinks it's a good idea too. Danny has promised to help me with the math. He is good at that! I really can't go further, career-wise, if I don't have the basic diploma. I would like to operate my own business in dog grooming on a full-time scale. It's exciting!

Danny smiled and looked at his mom.

Mary's eyes lit up with enthusiasm, and her body posture became more alert and focused.

Psychological data

Danny: I dread going to the hospital tomorrow because the chemotherapy makes me feel so bad.

I am also concerned about the effects of the chemotherapy on my future children. I have one son who is perfect, but I will probably never see him again.

I am concerned about weakness in my left leg because this is the foot I used to support myself when riding my cycle.

You can call Dr. Shell. I told him you would be calling. Otherwise he probably won't tell you anything.

I am not interested in learning any other relaxation techniques to help me cope with nausea and pain.

I am also worried about whether they will have difficulty finding veins for my treatment.

Mary: I am aware that I need to be more assertive in some situations, especially within the family. (Mary expressed interest in reading *Stand Up, Speak Out, Talk Back.*)

Danny stared into space with a concerned look on his face.

Danny pointed to his left leg.

Spiritual data

Danny: Yes, I still go to church when I feel well enough to go. I always pray though, whether I go to church or not. It gives me a lot of strength, especially now when I have to deal with this illness and pain.

Mary: Jim and I used to go to church. None of us goes at this point. We've just gotten away from it.

Sometimes I wonder if there is a God when I see people with these terrible diseases and the suffering with it.

It doesn't make sense.

Looking thoughtful. Staring out of the window, speaking in a low voice almost to herself.

Analysis/Synthesis:
Visit 4—December 1, 1993
Intrapersonal/Intrafamily Stressors

The previous analyses are still relevant. Considering Danny's diminished physical stamina and penetration of lines of resistance, new symptoms are present that may be related to side effects of his chemotherapy.

Numbness and weakness of his left leg could be from neurotoxicity. Redness and dryness at corners of the eye and mouth are symptoms of skin and mucosal effects of bleomycin and Adriamycin. Drug effects are on the basal layers of mucosa, preventing replication and replacement of most superficial cell structures (Fredetta and Glorian, 1981). He has no lesions or sore areas within his mouth, however. Frequency of urination and increased need for sleep could be signs of a urinary tract infection. This and Danny's harsh bout of intestinal flu could be associated with leukopenia. Adriamycin suppresses bone marrow functions, especially granulocytes and neutrophils (Fredette and Gloriant, 1981). He seems to be having an increased problem with nausea during chemotherapy, so the diagnosis of discomfort related to nausea due to chemotherapy seems appropriate.

In considering diet and nutrition, there seem to be incongruencies about Mary's knowledge of good nutrition and concern about Danny's diet. In earlier interviews, Danny mentioned his parents' concern for his diet and his mother's knowledge in this area. But his food diary showing the meals eaten at home, along with Danny saying that there is not much fruit available at home, indicates the possibility that Mary does not actually have much knowledge about what is necessary for good nutrition. Although it is true that Mary spoke about greens, vegetables, and the family eating the fruits (and not liking vegetables), there is still a possible deficit in this area.

Interpersonal/Interfamily Stressors

Regarding interpersonal stressors, Danny is doing well in his schoolwork and also has offered to help his mother with her math classes when she goes back to school for a high school diploma. The bonding relationship between mother and son is being enhanced by their sharing of interests, talents, and time. This is definitely helping his self-concept. On the other hand, Danny's self-image is compromised because of the weakness in his legs and its effect on his ability and mobility in the future as well as now.

The diagnosis of anxiety related to diagnosis, treatment, and prognosis is still relevant. He dreads his chemotherapy because of the discomfort associated with the treatments and is concerned about iatrogenic effects of the drugs he is being given.

Few events in life provide deeper and more poignant emotions than a life-threatening illness of a young family member. It frequently shakes the very foundation, organization, and equilibrium of family life. Feelings of injustice, anger, hopelessness, and spiritual confusion are engendered among family members as they care for the endangered child (McFarland, Wasli, and Gerety, 1992). From the spiritual data obtained in this most recent visit, it seems that despite all of Danny's emotional fears, he is coming to peace with himself and with his God, for in this relationship he feels secure and loved. This assists him in coping with the illness. Conversely, it would seem that his parents are facing a sense of helplessness, powerlessness, and an overall anger directed toward God because of this illness, which has threatened the family's equilibrium. A diagnosis of the family's spiritual distress related to life-threatening illness seems appropriate at this time.

In summation, although Danny is exhibiting more symptoms and side effects from chemotherapy, he also is integrating his spiritual needs into his life in a wholesome manner. The family members continue to meet their physical needs but are having problems dealing with the group's spiritual integrity. Data gaps are in the areas of specific nutritional knowledge and knowledge of, and planning for, the eventuality of Danny's prognosis.

NURSING DIAGNOSIS: Visit 4

Date	Diagnosis	Priority
10/22/93	1. Alterations in nutrition related to chemotherapy treatments and possible lack of knowledge	2
10/22/93	2. Alterations in comfort related to effects of treatments	1
10/22/93	3. Alterations in self-concept (body image) related to effects of chemotherapy	3
10/22/93	4. Anxiety related to life-threatening illness	6
10/22/93	5. Dysfunctional family communication related to family member's illness	5
10/22/93	6. Inadequate venous access related to repeated chemotherapy treatment	8
11/1/93	7. Potential for infection related to leukopenia	4
12/1/93	8. Spiritual distress of family related to severe illness in family member	7

Interim—December 1 to January 25

Two appointments to visit with the family were canceled because one or more family members could not be there. Finally, on January 25 the nurse visited with Danny and his mother again; Diane was working and could not be there, and Jim declined to participate in any more visits.

Setting: Living room of home with Danny and his mother, Mary. Danny is dressed in corduroy pants, plaid shirt, socks, and slippers. He is sitting in a recliner. His hair is dry and lusterless. Mary is dressed in a green shirtdress with hose and black flat shoes. She had just returned from shopping. She is sitting on the couch. She looks tired (rings under eyes).

Subjective data	Objective data
Interactions	**Observations and measurements**

Biological data

Physician interview: Dan has recently been in the hospital for chemotherapy and various tests (EKG, chest x-ray, body scan). He is still in remission, and I am quite pleased with Danny's progress.	EKG, chest x-ray, body scan carried out. Results: he's still in remission. Physical exam revealed inguinal hernia.
Danny: I still have periods when all my muscles ache, and I feel very tired.	
I have been having less pain in my back.	
I have a right inguinal hernia, but my physician does not want me to have surgery at this time.	Danny pointed to his lower abdomen and rubbed that area gently.
I want to have my hernia repaired as soon as possible because it causes me some discomfort.	
The doctor says my leukocyte count is very good at this time.	
Mary: Danny will have just two more rounds of chemotherapy, and then he will be examined periodically.	
When receiving chemotherapy treatments, Danny eats very little—a light diet. He is usually able to eat more the day after the treatment.	
He has been out with his friends a lot and when not home for meals, he doesn't eat as well. I always check on this.	Mary's face showed concern—eyes intent, alert, and focused on both nurse and Danny.
He tends to forget that he is ill and that a good diet is important for him.	Mary's diet assessment shows she eats a well-balanced nutritious diet.
Danny: I am bothered that my hair is becoming dry and unruly.	
I try to prevent tension on my hair. I wash it only when necessary and let it air dry. I very seldom use a hair dryer.	
I realize that this is a side effect of my chemotherapy treatment.	

Psychological data/sociological data

Danny: My doctor has told me that I need to have another lymphography. I am really dreading the procedure because it was so painful when I had one last January.	Frowned—concerned look on face.
I will be relieved when chemotherapy is over. I am able to cope fairly well with nausea by sleeping or directing my thoughts on something else (focusing).	
I have been feeling bored and fed up with not being able to work and be as active as I would like. If I stay out late, I am tired for several days.	Voice indicated an irritable tone. He gestured widely with hands.
No, I don't think I would be interested in attending a support group.	
I cope well by having a positive attitude and not dwelling on the thought that I have cancer.	Voice had an emphatic tone.
It depresses me when I become acquainted with other cancer patients in the hospital who seem to be getting along fine, and then I find out later that they have died!	Voice sounded somewhat upset, almost an angry tone.
In a support group I wouldn't be able to tell people that because they hadn't experienced it. They couldn't understand what I've been through.	
I am still attending evening school, working toward GED.	
Mary: Dan is looking forward to visiting his real father in Florida for a few weeks, whenever it is possible.	Mary looked hopefully at Danny.
Although we had some difficulty coping with Danny's illness when he was first diagnosed, we have been able to cope well by maintaining a positive attitude, trying to accept things as they are, and doing what we can to help. We try to treat Danny as normally as possible—not like an invalid.	Mary smiled and glanced at Danny.
I have read most of *Stand Up, Speak Out, Talk Back* and find it helpful.	
I have decided I do not want to role play assertive behavior. I would rather just practice in specific situations where I want to be more assertive. Like with my own family at home, especially with Jim and the children. We have started to discuss things openly. It's a start but sometimes painful.	Facial expression alert, pleased with herself.
Yes, I know about the daily food guide and what should be eaten every day.	Mary repeated the elements of the food guide pyramid.

Spiritual data

Danny: I don't worry much about dying. I feel I can accept death if it happens. Just so they let me listen to my music.	Mary's eyes filled with tears. Danny appeared calm and assured.

Analysis/Synthesis:
Visit 5—January 25, 1994

Most of the previous analysis is still appropriate, with the following additional considerations. The reactions to the *interpersonal/interfamily stressors* during this visit indicate that Danny's energy integrity is still not in proper balance. Although he is having less back pain, he still complains of fatigue. Even though he understands what he should eat, Danny is apparently not motivated to eat fruits and vegetables, so his diet is still deficient in this area. His basic core structure and lines of resistance are penetrated by Hodgkin's disease. Now, however, he is in remission. His physician is evidently still assessing the extent of this remission because he feels it is necessary for Danny to have another lymphography. Danny also has recently developed a hernia, which is causing him concern. Although the family's values and belief systems have been challenged, role adjustments and interdependence have been maintained throughout. The basic core of the family is felt to be intact.

Intrapersonal/intrafamily stressors are those that impinge on a client's sense of identity and self-worth. Danny is still having problems working through the developmental tasks in the state defined by Erikson as identity versus role confusion (Eshleman, 1988). He says he is bored and "fed up" with not being able to work and be as active as he would like.

Danny still has anxieties about his treatment, especially in relation to the lymphography. Although he will be relieved when his chemotherapy is over, he is coping fairly well with the nausea. There are some incongruencies in what he says concerning the possibility that Hodgkin's disease may be fatal. He states he will be able to accept death if it happens, and he doesn't worry much about dying. It does bother him that other cancer patients seem to be getting along fine and then die. However, he is coming to terms with the possibility of his own death through a strong personal commitment to God. The family members, on the other hand, may be in spiritual distress, because they have not dealt with this problem and still express anger and powerlessness toward God.

The response of significant others in the family toward Danny's disease is still one of concern and support while, as Mary says, they try not to treat Danny as if he were an invalid. At this time, there still are a few perceived threats to family relationships, status, and goals due to Danny's illness, and his role change from independence to being again dependent on his parents. This role change began a year ago when he first became ill. Mary feels that learning some assertiveness skills may be helpful to their family communication, especially in some situations.

In regard to other *interpersonal/interfamily stressors*, the family is coping fairly well with Danny's illness at this time. Coping strategies include maintaining a positive attitude, trying to accept things they cannot change, and being as supportive of Danny as possible. Danny apparently still copes by denying his illness to a certain extent and does not think he would be interested in attending a support group. He feels that he is coping well at this time, and he thought that the people in a support group would not understand what he has been through.

No further information was obtained about the family's past experience with similar illness situations, so there is still a data gap in this area. All the previous diagnoses are still essentially correct.

NURSING DIAGNOSIS: Visit 5

Date	Diagnosis	Priority
Intrafamily (Intrapersonal)		
10/22/93	1. Alteration in nutrition—less than body requirements related to anorexia, nausea/vomiting, and malabsorption	2
12/1/93	2. Activity intolerance, fatigue	3
10/22/93	*3. Alteration in comfort: pain and discomfort related to illness and treatment	1
12/1/93	4. Alteration in tissue integrity (alopecia) related to chemotherapy treatments	6
10/22/93	*5. Altered body image and self-esteem related to changes in appearance, functions, and roles	5
10/22/93	6. Anxiety related to life threatening illness	4
Interfamily (Interpersonal)		
11/1/93	*1. Alterations in family process related to dysfunctional communication	9
10/22/93	2. Disrupted interpersonal relations related to illness	7
11/15/93	3. Difficulty with role changes related to family member's illness	8
12/15/93	*4. Grieving related to anticipatory loss	10
12/1/93	5. Spiritual distress related to search for meaning in family member's illness	11

NURSING DIAGNOSIS: Visit 5—cont'd

Date	Diagnosis	Priority
Extrafamily (Extrapersonal)		
12/1/93	1. Inadequate resources related to impact of catastrophic illness in family	13
11/15/93	2. Inadequate support group related to Danny's diminished self-concept and life-threatening illness	12
12/1/93	3. Potential for financial crises related to illness and required therapy	14

*Plans for nursing implementation for these diagnoses are shown on p. 262.

Summary

In using Neuman's systems model to assess the stressors that impinge on Danny and his family, it is felt that although Danny's inner structure of defense is not in proper balance yet, the disease is in remission and Danny is on a trajectory toward reconstitution. Other intrapersonal stressors that relate to Danny's in-

ability to work and anxieties about his treatment are still present. Although he is not interested in a support group, information about such a group was given to him in the event he would reconsider this option.

Whereas the family in general is coping, it is felt that some education in assertiveness skills may assist them in improving family communication, thereby helping them to reach a higher level of functioning.

PLANS FOR IMPLEMENTATION

Nursing diagnosis 1: Alteration in comfort: Pain and discomfort related to illness and treatment (10/22/93).
Long-term expected outcome: The client will use various methods to relieve pain and discomfort by 12/15/93.

Short-term expected outcomes	Nursing orders	Scientific rationale	Evaluation
1. Danny will have less intense pain and discomfort by 12/15/93.	1a. Nurse will assess pain and discomfort characteristics: location, quality, frequency, duration, timing, disruption of activities, etc. 1b. Danny will verbalize the specific characteristics of his discomfort (same as above). 1c. Nurse will assure Danny that she knows pain and discomfort are real and will facilitate some measures to reduce them: • Pain medication to be taken before pain peaks • Use of humor and distraction • Adequate rest periods	*Content:* Pain. *Strategy:* Principles of nursing practice. 1a. Baseline data provides information for assessing changes in pain level and evaluation of intervention (Brunner and Suddarth, 1992). 1c. A client's fear that pain will not be considered real increases anxiety and reduces pain tolerance (Brunner and Suddarth, 1992).	**Ongoing** Danny reported that level of pain and discomfort has decreased with use of measures such as humor, music, analgesics, relaxation, and rest. Analgesic therapy was modified to adjust to the level of pain and to prevent narcotic addiction.
2. Danny will verbalize awareness of those factors that contribute to pain in order to prevent them by 12/1/93.	2a. Nurse will explain and list the many factors that can contribute to pain, such as fear, fatigue, anger, etc. 2b. Client will identify those factors in his life that contribute to his pain (i.e., lack of rest)	2a. Holistic assessment provides a basis for dealing with other factors that decrease a client's ability to tolerate pain and increase pain level (Brunner and Suddarth, 1992).	Danny reported less disruption from pain and discomfort. He verbalized that fatigue and fear contributed to the severity of pain and discomfort. He used pain medication as prescribed and reports an increased level of relief after adjustment.

Continued

PLANS FOR IMPLEMENTATION—cont'd

Nursing diagnosis 1: Alteration in comfort: Pain and discomfort related to illness and treatment (10/22/93).
Long-term expected outcomes: The client will use various methods to relieve pain and discomfort by 12/15/93.

Short-term expected outcomes	Nursing orders	Scientific rationale	Evaluation
3. Danny will use 3 or 4 new strategies to deal with pain by 12/15/93.	3a. Client will verbalize how he responds and deals with pain (i.e., tenses up muscles, goes to bed, takes too many analgesics, tires easily, etc.). 3b. Nurse will explain and teach new and different strategies in dealing with pain: • Use of humor • Relaxation techniques • Imagery, distraction • Cutaneous stimulation • Use of analgesics before peak in cycle • Music 3c. Client will select and use appropriate measure to deal with pain and discomfort: • Analgesics within prescribed regimen • Relaxation techniques • Diversion, humor, and music	3a. To fully relieve pain, a total assessment is necessary, and all additional information provides basis for appropriate intervention. 3b. The use of humor in relieving pain and discomfort has a therapeutic effect in relieving the accompanying depression and one overpowering aspect of stress (Prerost, 1988). 3c. Analgesics tend to be more effective when administered early in pain cycle (Brunner and Suddarth, 1992); McCaffery, 1979). Client's participation in his own self-care improves self-esteem and gives more control over his illness (Pohl, 1981).	Danny verbalized the ways he responded to pain: weary, tired, fatigued, irritable, and grimacing. He identified additional effective pain relief strategies He reported the effective use of new pain relief strategies and the decrease in pain intensity: • Imagery, music • Humor • Diversion
4. Danny will identify measures that maintain a pain management regimen by 12/15/93.	4a. Danny will cooperate and collaborate with nurses, physician, other health care team members, as well as family, when changes in pain management are necessary (i.e., when medication does not appear to relieve pain, the dosage is too small, side effects are present, relief of stress is needed, etc).	4a. New methods of administration of analgesics must be acceptable to patient, physician, health care team members, and family to be effective: the patient's participation decreases his sense of powerlessness (Brunner and Suddarth, 1992).	Danny exhibits decreased physical and behavioral responses to pain: • Interest in surroundings • Interest in school Danny takes responsibility for taking analgesics at appropriate times. **Concluding** Danny achieved more relief from pain and discomfort through use of new coping strategies and adjustment in medications.

*Nursing diagnosis 2: Altered body image and self-esteem related to change in appearance, function, and roles (10/22/93).
Long-term expected outcomes: The client will develop an improved body image and self-esteem by 12/15/93.

Short-term expected outcomes	Nursing orders	Scientific rationale	Evaluation
1. Danny will identify concerns related to body image and self-esteem by 11/5/93.	1a. Nurse will assess client's feelings about body image and level of self-esteem: • Dependence on family • Inability to provide for his son (infant) • Changes in appearance.	*Content:* Body image. *Strategy:* Principles of nursing practice; therapeutic use of self; and stress management. 1a. Provides baseline assessment for evaluation of changes and assessing effectiveness of interventions (Brunner and Suddarth, 1992).	**Ongoing** Danny identified areas of importance: • Loss of strength • Loss of hair • Loss of role as father • Dependence on family by not being able to work

PLANS FOR IMPLEMENTATION—cont'd

*__Nursing diagnosis 2:__ Altered body image and self-esteem related to change in appearance, function, and roles (10/22/93).
Long-term expected outcome: The client will develop an improved body image and self-esteem by 12/15/93.

Short-term expected outcomes	Nursing orders	Scientific rationale	Evaluation
	1b. Nurse will identify potential threats to self-esteem (altered appearance, decreased sexual function, hair loss, energy, role changes). Danny will validate with nurse his specific concerns.	1b. Anticipation of changes permits client to identify the importance of these areas to self. Effective learning requires active participation (Redman, 1993).	
2. Danny will continue an active role in activities and decision-making by 11/15/93.	2a. Nurse will encourage continued participation and decision-making in personal and family life.	2a. Active participation of client in his own self-care is critical to reconstruction and upward trajectory (Neuman, 1990).	He continued to take an active role in both personal and family decision-making.
	2b. Danny will be active in choices of social life, family decision-making, and responsibilities in household.	2b. Active role in ramily living reduces depersonalization and emphasizes patient's self-worth (McFarland et al., 1992).	He verbalized his feelings and reactions to impending losses (fatherhood, sexuality, loss of muscle tone and activity, loss of body image: hair, muscles).
	2c. Nurse will encourage Danny to voice concerns regarding self-care.	2c. Identifying concerns is an important step in coping with them (Brunner and Suddarth, 1992).	
	2d. Danny will voice concerns to himself, family, and nurse.		
3. Danny will participate in self-care when side effects compromise his independence by 12/1/93.	3a. Family (or other caregivers) will assist Danny when fatigue, lethargy, nausea, vomiting, and other symptoms alter his independence (appropriate foods for a nutritious diet; adequate rest periods provided, etc).	3a. Physical well-being improves self-esteem (Brunner and Suddarth, 1992).	Danny allowed nurses and family to assist him when in distress from chemotherapy (diet; passive exercise [ROM], walking, etc).
	3b. Client will maintain self-care yet accept assistance in times of severe distress (choosing eating times and types of food that are less aggravating to his system; taking appropriate rest periods).	3b. Accepting assistance with appropriate self-care measures when possible assists in maintaining self-esteem and helps with upward trajectory in rehabilitation (reconstruction) (Neuman, 1983; Hill and Smith, 1990).	
4. Danny will select activities that will increase his general well-being in dealing with his illness by 12/1/93.	4a. Nurse will provide information about methods of problem solving with hair loss, loss of muscle tone, general body image, and self-esteem (use of hairpiece; care of hair and skin; preservation of muscle tone).	4a. Providing current information to client regarding prostheses, and activities that maintain an improved body image are necessary and preliminary to self-care measures (Hill and Smith, 1990).	Danny exhibited interest in appearance and was anxious to participate in self-care. He does not use a hairpiece yet but is very cautious in taking care of his hair (washes with gentle shampoo; uses no hair dryer).
	4b. Danny will choose alternatives and ways to work with these impending losses: • Hair care • Weight lifting • Extended rest periods	4b. Client participation in improving body image will increase self-esteem (Brunner and Suddarth, 1992). Alternating rest periods with passive exercise will maintain and improve physical well-being (Brunner and Suddarth, 1992).	

Continued

***Nursing diagnosis 2:** Altered body image and self-esteem related to change in appearance, function, and roles (10/22/93).
Long-term expected outcome: The client will develop an improved body image and self-esteem by 12/15/93.

Short-term expected outcomes	Nursing orders	Scientific rationale	Evaluation
5. Danny will share concerns about possible altered sexual functions and social relationships with partner by 12/15/93.	5a. Nurse and client will explore and verbalize concerns about socializing with girlfriend (sexual relationships; effects of illness on time commitment; knowledge about illness). 5b. Danny will share these concerns with girlfriend. 5c. Danny and girlfriend will explore alternatives and various ways to express affection. 5d. Nurse and Danny will provide knowledge and encourage girlfriend to verbalize her concerns regarding his illness.	5a. The client's participation in selecting options and in decision-making regarding the socialization process is paramount to preserving self-esteem (Hill and Smith, 1990). 5b. The provision of both knowledge and opportunity for expression of concern, affection, and acceptance is basic to maintenance of self-esteem (Stuart and Sundeen, 1991; Brunner and Suddarth, 1992).	Danny participated with others in conversations, social events, and activities (he and his sister go to parties, or go "cruising"). He verbalized concern about his girlfriend's reluctance to get involved after he told her of his illness. Danny is willing to explore better ways to communicate with girlfriend and to explore alternate ways of expressing concern and affection. **Concluding** Danny fulfilled the short-term outcomes and verbalized that he was coping and feeling good about himself.

Nursing diagnosis 3: Grieving related to anticipatory loss (altered role functioning) (11/15/93).
Long-term expected outcome: The client and family will progress within the grieving process by 1/22/94.

Short-term expected outcomes	Nursing orders	Scientific rationale	Evaluation
1. The family and ill client will verbalize expressions of grief by 12/1/93.	1a. Nurse will encourage and explore verbalization of fears, concerns, and questions regarding disease, treatment, and future implications: • Chemotherapy and side effects • Role changes • Prognosis/remission	*Content:* Grief/loss. *Strategy:* Therapeutic use of self and stress management. 1a. An increased and accurate knowledge base will decrease family anxiety and dispel misconception.	**Ongoing** Mother just beginning to express grief (crying), and also expressed spiritual distress. Danny describes feelings openly.
2. The family will identify internal and external resources available to aid coping strategies during grieving by 12/15/93.	2a. The nurse will encourage active participation of both ill client and family, in care and treatment decisions: • Medications • Pain relief • Decisions about work 2b. Nurse will visit family frequently to maintain interpersonal relationship and physical closeness. 2c. Nurse will inform Danny of support groups for those with cancer. 2d. Danny and family will speak with clergy or counselors as needed. 2e. The nurse will offer other aids such as the book *When Bad Things Happen to Good People* by Rabbi Harold Kushner (nurse and family can read and discuss this book together).	2a. Active participation from ill client along with family helps with client independence and control. 2b. Frequent contacts promote trust and security and reduce feelings of fear and isolation. 2c. Support from others who are experiencing same problems reduces isolation, and the added knowledge releases anxiety. 2d. Professional support can aid the grieving process.	The family included Danny in household chores and in financial support and management of the home. A schedule was set up for visits from nurse as needed. Danny refused to go to support groups because of fear of members dying. This was a way to preserve his own use of denial. Mary expressed an interest in this resource (book).

Nursing diagnosis 3: Grieving related to anticipatory loss (altered role functioning) (11/15/93).
Long-term expected outcome: The client and family will progress within the grieving process by 1/22/94.

Short-term expected outcomes	Nursing orders	Scientific rationale	Evaluation
3. The family will openly express grief as they need to by 1/10/94.	3a. The nurse will encourage the ventilation of feelings including projected anger and hostility within acceptable limits: • Oppositional behavior • Verbalize anger at nurse • Verbalize anger at God	3a. Ventilation of feelings allows for emotional expression without destruction of self-esteem. It also reverses the denial mechanism when use of this defense technique becomes destructive and dysfunctional (Rawlins and Heacock, 1993).	*Short-term outcomes not met:* Anger was expressed somewhat openly in Danny's refusal to use a support group. Jim, Sr., not coming to these meetings was an expression of negative behavior. Anger was expressed indirectly.
	3b. The nurse will support and give permission for periods of crying and expression of sadness: • Support client through touch • Verbal affirmation • Cry with client • Offer spiritual support and reinforcement	3b. The expression of emotional grief (crying and sadness) are necessary to progress through the grief process (McFarland et al., 1992). The meeting of spiritual needs is basic to integrating the human spirit (Carson, 1989).	Only mother directly expressed sadness and crying (other members still in denial?).
4. The family will relieve their spiritual distress by 1/22/94.	4a. The nurse will assess the spiritual needs of ill client and family as they relate to grieving in life-threatening illness: • Search for meaning • Sense of forgiveness • Hope • Love 4b. Danny and family will become aware of these needs as nurse explores these concepts with them.	4a–b. Providing spiritual care is a requirement of holistic nursing. (1) As people approach finitude, they want to view their lives as having *purpose and meaning*. They need to integrate dying with personal goals and values. (2) When people review their lives, guilt is experienced if their self-expectations are unfulfilled. They must have a sense of *forgiveness*. (3) *Hope* is a feature of human existence critically ill patients need, with concrete and abstract hope to carry them through the dying process. (4) One of the spiritual needs of the dying is to experience love. This can be demonstrated through words and acts of kindness (Conrad, 1985).	Danny seemed to be at peace with himself and his God. The family continues to struggle and is displacing their anger at God.

	4c. The nurse will provide spiritual care support for this family:
	(1) Use of communication skills:
	  a. Openness
	  b. Listen for cues; respond appropriately
	  c. Willing to be involved with family
	(2) Other intervention such as
	  a. Prayer
	  b. Meditation
	  c. Guided meditation or imagery
	  d. Reading
	  e. Music and art
		4c. Prayer is powerful and effective when used cautiously. Music has tremendous power for meeting the emotional and spiritual needs of a dying person. It can produce laughter and tears. It can sedate or stimulate (Conrad, 1985).	Danny verbalized his peace with God. The family has not yet done this.
			Danny used music as his own support system.
			
			Concluding
			Long-term expected outcome partially met.

Continued

PLANS FOR IMPLEMENTATION—cont'd

Nursing diagnosis 4: Alteration in family process related to dysfunctional communication (11/1/93).
Long-term expected outcome: Family will improve communication among its members by 1/15/94.

Short-term expected outcomes	Nursing orders	Scientific rationale	Evaluation
1. Mary (mother) will verbalize her knowledge of assertiveness skills by 12/15/93.	1a. Nurse will assess Mary's knowledge and "feelings" concerning assertiveness, that is: • Meaning of word *assertive* • When she is or isn't assertive • When she would like to be assertive • How she feels about it (guilt, etc) 1b. Nurse will explain: • Difference between *passive, assertive,* and *aggressive* behavior • That the key concept in learning assertiveness is choice 1c. Mary will read the book *Stand Up, Speak Out, Talk Back* by Alberti and Emmons (1990) before next visit and relate this to her own situation, giving specific examples. 1d. Nurse and client will discuss important points in above book and clarify together any parts of book about which client has questions.	*Content:* Communication *Strategy:* Teaching and learning. 1a. Assertiveness training is a type of behavior therapy in which the client learns to communicate both positive and negative feelings in an open, honest, direct, and appropriate way (McFarland et al, 1992). 1b. It is important to differentiate passive, assertive, and aggressive behavior so that client can make an informed choice about appropriate action to take (McFarland et al, 1992). 1c. Clients cannot change others, but they can change their own behaviors so that self-esteem and self-respect are enhanced (Rawlins and Heacock, 1993).	**Ongoing (primary prevention)** Mary and nurse explored what her concept of assertiveness was: • How she felt about it • The discomfort • Fear of antagonism • Fear of confrontation Mary read *Stand Up, Speak Out, Talk Back.* She felt she understood it and had no particular problems with it. She gave examples in her own family situations where it applied (i.e., with children and husband; taking care of situation when it occurs).
2. Client (Mary) will use assertive techniques to improve family communication by 12/30/93.	2a. Nurse will teach client the techniques and steps in assertiveness training using Alberti and Emmon's book as a guide. 2b. Client will practice these steps using "I" message and role playing with nurse in practice situations. 2c. *Nurse* will *serve* as a *role model* in seeking clarification, showing respect, listening to expression of feelings, giving suggestions, expressing opinions, setting limits, and making clear statements. 2d. The nurse will give support by: • Clarifying "I" and "we" messages • Supporting trials of new behaviors	2a. Each person should choose for himself how he or she will act (Alberti and Emmons, 1990). 2b. Effective learning requires active participation of the learner (Redman, 1993). 2c. Teaching requires effective communication (Rorden, 1987). 2d. Changed behavior leads to changed attitudes about oneself and one's impact on people and situations (Alberti and Emmons, 1990)	Mary practiced the steps and techniques of assertiveness as outlined in book. She felt the book was helpful to her. She only role played one situation and then decided against this method of learning. She said she would rather practice on her own. Mary practiced new behaviors with her family and felt rather awkward the first week. The family gave positive feedback at end of first week.

PLANS FOR IMPLEMENTATION—cont'd

Nursing diagnosis 4: Alteration in family process related to dysfunctional communication (11/1/93).
Long-term expected outcome: Family will improve communication among its members by 1/15/94.

Short-term expected outcomes	Nursing orders	Scientific rationale	Evaluation
	• Listening to expressions of fear of change • Giving feedback after role play • Helping client learn positive self-reinforcement 2e. Client will try out new behaviors with the family and ask for feedback for 1 week and then discuss these interactions with nurse. 2f. Client will continue for 3 more weeks and meet with nurse to discuss progress.	Positive reinforcement of behavior increases its occurrence (Bower and Bevis, 1984). 2e. Client has the right to make a request, and others have a right to refuse the request. Rights have accompanying responsibilities (Rawlins and Heacock, 1993).	Mary states that she still feels uncomfortable in being assertive. **Concluding** Long-term expected outcome partially met.

REFERENCES AND READINGS

Alberti R and Emmons M: *Stand up, speak out, talk back,* New York, 1990, Pocket Books.

Ardell D: *High level wellness,* New York, 1986, Bantam Books.

Backanan BF: Human environment interaction: a modification of the Neuman systems model for aggregates, families, and the community, *Public Health Nurs* 4:1, 1987.

Bower F and Bevis E: *Fundamentals of nursing practice,* St Louis, 1984, Mosby–Year Book.

Brunner LS and Suddarth DS: *Textbook of medical surgical nursing,* ed 7, Philadelphia, 1992, JB Lippincott.

Carson VB: *Spiritual dimensions of nursing practice,* Philadelphia, 1989, WB Saunders.

Conrad NL: Spiritual support for the dying, *Nurs Clin North Am* 20(2):415, 1985.

Cross J: Betty Neuman. In George J, editor: *Nursing theories: the base for professional nursing practice,* ed 2, Englewood Cliffs, NJ, 1985, Prentice-Hall.

Eshleman JR: *The family: an introduction,* ed 5, Boston, 1988, Allyn Bacon.

Fredette S and Gloriant F: Nursing diagnoses in cancer chemotherapy, *Am J Nurs* 11:2013, Nov 1981.

Gerald MC: *Pharmacology: an introduction to drugs,* Englewood Cliffs, NJ, 1981, Prentice-Hall.

Hill L and Smith N: *Self-care nursing,* ed 2, Norwalk, Conn, 1990, Appleton & Lange.

Kushner H: *When bad things happen to good people,* New York, 1983, Avon Books.

Lauer P et al: Learning needs of cancer patients: a comparison of nurse and patient perceptions, *Nurs Res* 31(1):11, 1982.

Leahey M and Wright LM: *Families and life threatening illness,* Springhouse, Pa, 1987, Springhouse.

LeBlanc D: People with Hodgkin disease: the nursing challenge, *Nurs Clin North Am,* 13(2):281, 1978.

Levitt DZ: Cancer chemotherapy, *RN* Dec.:33, 1980.

Mahan K: *Krause's food, nutrition and diet therapy,* ed 2, Philadelphia, 1992, WB Saunders.

Mayer MG and Watson AB: Nursing care plans and the Neuman systems model: I. In Neuman B, editor: *The Neuman systems model,* East Norwalk, Conn, 1982, Appleton-Century-Crofts.

McCaffery M: *Nursing management of the patient with pain,* Philadelphia, 1979, JB Lippincott.

McFarland G, Wasli E, and Gerety EK: *Nursing diagnosis and process in psychiatric mental health nursing,* ed 2, Philadelphia, 1992, JB Lippincott.

Miller S and Winstead-Fry P: *Family systems theory in nursing practice,* Englewood Cliffs, NJ, 1982, Reston Publishing.

Neuman B: The Neuman systems model: a theory for practice. In Parker ME, editor: *Nursing theories in practice,* New York, 1990, National League for Nursing.

Neuman B: Family interventions using the Betty Neuman Health Care Systems Model. In Clements I and Roberts B, editors: *Family health: a theoretical approach to nursing care,* New York, 1983, John Wiley & Sons.

Patrick ML et al: *Medical surgical nursing: pathophysiological concepts,* ed 2, Philadelphia, 1991, JB Lippincott.

Pohl M: *The teaching function of the nursing practitioner,* ed 4, Dubuque, Iowa, 1981, Wm C Brown.

Porth CM: *Pathophysiology: concepts of altered health states,* ed 3, Philadelphia, 1990, JB Lippincott.

Prerost FJ: Use of humor and guided imagery in therapy to alleviate stress, *Ment Health Counsel* 10(1):16, 1988.

Rawlins RP and Heacock PE: *Clinical manual of psychiatric nursing,* ed 2, St. Louis, 1993, Mosby–Year Book.

Spiegel D et al: Group support for patients with metastatic cancer, *Arch Gen Psychiatry* 38:527, May 1981.

Story EL and Ross MM: Family centered community health nursing and the Betty Neuman systems model, *Nursing Papers: Perspectives in Nursing,* 18:2, Summer 1986.

Stuart GW and Sundeen SJ: *Principles and practice of psychiatric nursing,* ed 4, St Louis, 1991, Mosby–Year Book.

Suddarth DS: *The Lippincott manual of nursing practice* ed 5, Philadelphia, 1991, JB Lippincott.

Valentine AS: Caring for the young adult with cancer, *Cancer Nurs* 12:385, 1978.

Veninga K: An easy recipe for assessing your patient's nutrition, *Nursing 82* 12(11):57, 1982.

Watson P: Psychosocial aspects of the cancer experience, *Can Nurse* 14:45, 1978.

Williams SR: *Nutrition and diet therapy,* ed 9, St Louis, 1992, Mosby–Year Book.

Wright LM and Leahey M: *Nurses and families: a guide to family assessment and intervention,* 1994, Philadelphia, FA Davis.

CHAPTER 16

NURSING PROCESS OF THE FAMILY CLIENT
Application of Friedman's and Roy's Models

Cynthia Makielski Martz, RN, MS

The client in this chapter is a young family: husband, wife, and 2-year-old son, who are facing the birth of a new baby in the next 6 weeks. The community health nurse received a routine referral from the clinic physician for a home visit. No specific health concerns were identified in the referral other than the pregnancy and the changing family unit.

During the initial home visit, the nurse chose Friedman's (1992) Structural-Functional Model as the guide for the family nursing process. This model was chosen because it facilitates analysis of the interactions among family members and the family's interactions with the community, such as the educational and health care systems. Roy's (1991) Adaptation Model is also applied in this chapter for an appropriate focus on individual family members. Roy's model is congruent with Friedman's model in examining role function and interdependence. However, Roy's model also addresses the physiological and self-concept areas that the nurse believes are very important aspects of individual health.

The Structural-Functional Model by Marilyn Friedman (1992) describes the structure of the family as the manner in which it is organized. Four basic dimensions or subconcepts are considered: (1) role structure, (2) value systems, (3) communication patterns, and (4) power structure. Family functions, according to Friedman, are those outcomes of the family structure that meet the needs of the family members. Five family functions are considered: (1) affective functioning, (2) socialization and social placement, (3) reproduction, (4) economic function, and (5) health care function. Both structure and function need to be addressed in a family nursing process.

In Roy's Adaptation Model, the individual is viewed as a whole being in interaction with the environment, who adapts to changes through four adaptive modes: physiological needs, self-concept, role function, and interdependence. Friedman's Structural-Functional Model and Roy's Adaptation Model are more fully described in Chapter 2.

In this chapter, the nursing process begins with an overview of the demographic data. Subjective and objective assessment data follow and are presented in three columns. The left-hand column shows interaction data; the middle column is the observations; and the right-hand column indicates the measurements. The nursing process is organized as follows: first, the assessment and analysis/synthesis for the first visit are presented, followed by the list of nursing diagnoses. Next, the second and third assessment visits and analysis/synthesis are included, along with an updated list of nursing diagnoses. The nursing plans, which include expected outcomes, strategies, nursing orders, scientific rationale, and evaluation, are presented last. The plans are last because they are ongoing and subject to revision, and because they demonstrate the continuity of the entire nursing process. However, they are initiated, implemented, and evaluated concurrently with the assessment visits.

Biographical data and initial contact

Biographical data

Father	David Smith	Age 24	Full-time student, first-semester college senior
Mother	Carla (Jones) Smith	Age 23	High school graduate
Son	Gabe	Age 2 years, 4 months	

Race: Caucasian

Ethnicity: Mother, German and English; father, English and Swiss

Religion: Mother, Methodist; father does not attend religious services

Occupation: Father, full-time sales clerk, Guaranteed Auto Store; mother not employed outside the home

Language spoken: English

Marital status: Parents married to each other; neither married previously

Carla and Dave have been married 4½ years. They both grew up in Kokomo, Indiana, but did not meet until they were out of high school. They dated 6 months before getting married. They moved to Bloomington 3½ years ago so Dave could go to Indiana University and pursue a degree in political science.

Carla's mother, father, and sister (4 years younger) still live in Kokomo. Dave's mother, stepfather, brother (3 years younger), and sister (4 years younger) also live in Kokomo. Dave's mother and father were divorced when Dave was 5 years old. Dave does not know where his father lives and has not seen him since the divorce.

Source of referral

Physician at clinic where Carla was seeking prenatal care

Initial contact

Initial contact was with Carla by telephone on Tuesday, Oct. 25, 1994. At that time the nurse explained that all clinic patients received a home visit by the community health nurse to discuss concerns of pregnancy or any other health concerns of the family. Carla was very pleasant and seemed eager to cooperate. After discussion with Dave, a date was set for the first visit.

Time: Monday, November 7, 1994, 2 PM

Place: The Smith home. Carla and 2-year-old Gabe were present. Dave had planned to be present but was called to work to cover for someone who was sick. Carla had been watching television but turned it off. Gabe had just awakened from a nap. Carla offered the nurse something to drink. The visit lasted 1½ hours.

Nursing goals: (1) to establish rapport with the family members, (2) collect a health history on each family member, (3) begin to assess family life patterns, and (4) initiate at least one plan of intervention based on nursing diagnosis made during this visit.

Subjective data		Objective data	
Interactions		**Observations**	**Measurements**

Carla provided Gabe's health history

Gabe was born July 7, 1992, after 18 hours of labor. Low forceps were used. I had epidural anesthesia, and I received one pain shot during labor. I don't know what kind of medicine it was.		
No allergies that I know of.		
No childhood diseases.		
Immunications are up-to-date; at least that's what the pediatricians have told me.	Carla went to desk and immediately found Gabe's immunization record booklet with the pediatricians' names on front of booklet.	
Not on any medications.		
No chronic illnesses, only two or three colds, and he had a really bad ear infection about a year ago.		Diptheria, pertussis and tetanus (DPT) given: 9-4-92; 11-6-92; 1-15-93; 1-13-94
No surgeries or hospitalizations.		Oral polio vaccine (OPV) given: 9-4-92; 11-6-92; 1-15-93; 1-13-94
We have a car seat for him, and we always strap him in it.		Measles, mumps, and rubella (MMR) given: 10-14-93
		Haemophilus influenzae type b (Hib vaccine) given: 9-4-92; 11-6-92; 1-15-93; 10-14-93
		Hepatitis B vaccine given: 7-7-92; 8-7-92; 1-15-93

Continued

DATA COLLECTION: Visit 1—cont'd

Subjective data	Objective data	
Interactions	**Observations**	**Measurements**

Gabe's current health status provided by Carla

I give Gabe a bath every night before bedtime, and I usually wash his hair about twice a week. We're in the process of potty training, and he does pretty well, but he usually has one or two accidents a day. Of course, that means my laundry builds up quickly. Thank God I have that washer and dryer. They were gifts from my mom and dad.

Well, I guess you could call me a health food nut when it comes to diet. I never bought any baby food that had salt or sugar in it. And Gabe never gets candy. He doesn't each much, but I always make him eat a little bit of protein and some fruits and vegetables. He loves milk, and I make my own cookies with whole wheat flour and honey, which he loves. He usually has two or three snacks a day besides his three small meals. Gabe weighs 27 lb and is 35" tall.

Gabe is such an active boy. We go for a walk every day, and I have to walk fast to keep up with him. He loves to do puzzles, and he loves it when Dave roughhouses with him.

I usually put Gabe to bed at 8 or 9 o'clock, and he sleeps till 6 or 7 in the morning. But sometimes I do keep him up later if he hasn't seen Dave. You know, with classes and work, some days Dave isn't home at all. Anyway, then Gabe usually takes a 2- or 3-hour nap during the day.

I get awfully tired being the only one here with Gabe all day. But I understand that Dave doesn't have a choice right now. Besides, if Dave didn't work full time, I'd have to work. And with the new baby coming, that isn't very feasible. I guess it won't last forever.

Gabe really is a mama's boy. And I know I let him get away with more than he should. But it takes so much more energy to fight with him than to let him have his way. I'm a little concerned how he will react when we bring the new baby home.

Observations:

Gabe is dressed in shirt and overalls that fit neatly, navy blue tennis shoes with white shoe laces. Hair is straight, brown, combed, and cut neatly.

Carla helped Gabe wash hands before snacktime and washed his face and hands after snack. Carla also helped Gabe wash hands after urinating in the potty chair. Carla washed her own hands before giving Gabe his snack and after emptying the potty chair receptacle. Washer and dryer are in the small bathroom off the kitchen.

Gabe is a 2-year-old with dark-brown eyes and fair complexion. Skin soft, well hydrated.

Gabe half runs whenever he goes somewhere. Gabe did a four-piece puzzle quickly and easily. When Carla turned the TV on to "Sesame Street," Gabe became very excited and then settled in front of TV, sucking his thumb and holding a blanket. There are a few toys scattered over the living room floor: a small round ball, two puzzles, a large plastic truck, three books, and a See 'n Say talking toy about farm animals. Gabe played with all the toys during the visit but seemed to prefer the puzzles. He smiled, clapped his hands, and looked at Carla at the completion of the puzzles.

Gabe speaks several words clearly: Mommy, milk, no, potty, ball, Ernie, Bert, blanky, go, baby, tummy, and a few others. He speaks in three- to four-word sentences. Gabe said no to many of Carla's requests and demands, and Carla did not insist that he comply. Most of the time Carla would ignore Gabe's no's and

Measurements:

Gabe had a snack of about 4 oz 2% milk and 25 raisins.
Gabe has 16 teeth, missing only his second molars.

Gabe was on and off Carla's lap seven times in 5 minutes. Gabe sat still for 10 minutes while watching TV show (the only quiet period of any length during the 1½-hour visit).

DATA COLLECTION: Visit 1—cont'd

Subjective data		Objective data	
Interactions		**Observations**	**Measurements**

Interactions	Observations	Measurements
	let him do as he pleased. However, besides the negative behavior, Gabe was also openly affectionate with Carla, hugging and kissing her many times during the visit. Carla was also physically and verbally affectionate with Gabe, stroking his head and back, hugging and kissing, and saying, "Mommy loves you." At one point, Gabe said, "Gabe a good boy."	
Well, we've talked about the new baby. He knows the baby is in my belly, and we encourage him to love the baby.	Gabe pats Carla's abdomen and says, "baby."	
We're going to move Gabe into a youth bed that my mother has in her attic, and then the new baby will sleep in Gabe's crib.		
My mother said she could come to take care of Gabe while I'm in the hospital, but we haven't made anything definite yet. I know Dave won't be able to stay home; he'll be getting ready for final exams.		
I'm willing to do anything that will make this easier for Gabe and for Dave and me. The little girl next door started wetting her pants all the time after her baby sister was born. How can I deal with that if it happens with Gabe?		
So should I have a special time with Gabe every day while the baby's sleeping and have Gabe help care for the baby in simple ways?		
Well, it will be easy to keep telling Gabe how good and special he is and how much we love him. Dave and I have always been very demonstrative with Gabe.		
Getting Gabe in the youth bed as soon as possible makes sense, too. I'm sure my mother would bring the bed this weekend if I asked her. I'd kind of enjoy a visit with her anyway. And then we could finalize the plans for her coming when the baby is born. I know, that's when we could talk to Gabe about grandma staying with him when mommy is gone. Don't you think that's a good idea?	Carla becomes more animated. She speaks faster, and the pitch of her voice gets higher.	
I have another good idea! Since you say Gabe won't understand 1 or 2 days, do you suppose it will help if Dave and I go out for awhile when my mom is here? Gabe really does love my mom.		
You know, all of this seems vaguely familiar. When Dave and I took prenatal classes before Gabe was born, it seems the instructor talked a little bit about preparing the older children for the new baby. But of course, Dave and I didn't pay much attention, since Gabe was our first. We didn't take the classes this time because of Dave's hectic schedule.		
I'm going to call my mom tonight and try to set it up for her to come and bring the bed this weekend. I can let you know how it all goes the next time you come. At least this way, if Gabe reacts badly to the new baby, I'll know we did everything we could to prepare him.		

Continued

DATA COLLECTION: Visit 1—cont'd

Subjective data		Objective data	
Interactions		**Observations**	**Measurements**

Carla's health history

No allergies

I know I had the chickenpox. And I must have had rubella vaccine because my obstetrician took a test for that and he said I don't have to worry about getting it because my titer is high.

No chronic illnesses, and no medications. I really am very healthy. Oh, I do take prenatal vitamins.

Carla smiled and said this in a very prideful tone of voice.

My mother's father died of a heart attack, but everyone else in my family is okay.

I had a tonsillectomy when I was 10, and I had a D and C last summer after I had my miscarriage.

Started my period at age 12, had a period every month, and had no problems with periods except occasional bad cramps.

I've been pregnant a total of three times. A year ago August when I had my miscarriage, I was only about 2 months along.

No problems with Gabe's pregnancy, except I had a lot of problems holding water near the end of my pregnancy. The doctor kept a close watch on my blood pressure. He said it was okay.

I always wear my seat belt.

Carla's current health status

No problems with this pregnancy either, but I do get awfully tired chasing after Gabe all day.

Carla has a gravid uterus, apparently near term. She appears to have edema of the hands and feet and has dark circles around her eyes.

Carla is wearing an attractive maternity top and blue jeans. Her hair is shiny brown, curly, and neatly styled. She is wearing makeup. Her fingernails are nicely shaped, medium length, and painted with a light pink polish. Carla's loafers are polished.

The drinks Carla offered the nurse were orange juice and herbal tea.

LMP: 2-24-94; EDC: 12-1-94
Blood type A, Rh pos.
Uterus measures 35 cm from symphysis pubis to fundus.

As I said, I'm a health food nut. I loved home ec in high school. Then I worked in a nursing home in the kitchen after Dave and I were married. So I understand about the basic foods and vitamins and all. Luckily, Dave will eat anything I fix. I like to try new recipes, and I make great salads. It's a good thing, too. I lost all my baby weight after Gabe was born by eating mostly salads.

No, I don't smoke or drink coffee or pop. Dave and I have an occasional glass of wine, but I haven't had any while I've been pregnant.

My recreation consists mostly of socializing with the other mothers in the apartment complex. A lot of them have husbands in school, too, and we sort of get together and bolster one another. About once a week this one girl and I trade babysitting, so I get out during the day to run errands or go shopping. I really enjoy that. Dave and I try to get out about once a month to one of the free things on campus. We trade babysitting for that, too. Oh, I almost forgot: I love to take care of my plants. And I do a little needlepoint while I'm watching TV.

There are many healthy and exotic-looking plants throughout the living room and kitchen. There are also two or three needlepoint pictures hanging on the wall. A large stack of women's and home decorating magazines sits by the living room couch.

I'm tired all the time. I'm sure it's the pregnancy and running after Gabe. I wasn't this tired before I got pregnant. Anyway, I try to sleep whenever Gabe takes a nap, and I always get at least 8 hours at night.

Subjective data	Objective data	
Interactions	**Observations**	**Measurements**

Like I said, I take a walk every day. That's nice. And I do a few of the exercises that I remember from prenatal classes. The pelvic rock really helps the low back pain.

I certainly intend when Dave is through school to take my turn. I've heard too many stories about wives who put their husbands through school and end up divorced. I know I'll have to go part-time because of the kids, but I think it would be a lot more fun taking only one class at a time. Not so much pressure, like Dave has. I'd like to study interior decorating or home design.

Carla is an articulate woman who uses grammar correctly.

I feel pretty good about myself. I truly enjoy being a mother, even though someday I want to be an interior decorator. I feel sorry for some of the other mothers in the complex. They're always complaining about their boring lives. Well, sure, some days are rough, but Gabe and this new baby won't be little forever. I'm not going to be one of those mothers who complains when they're around and then complains when they're gone.

Carla walks with head and shoulders erect and speaks with confidence when talking about her role as a mother and about her plans to go to school and become an interior decorator.

I come from an emotional family. We love family get-togethers, and we're always hugging and kissing one another. Dave's family isn't that way, and I think it really took some getting used to on his part. But now I think he really enjoys all the affection.

Carla laughs and smiles appropriately. She also frowns and shows concern appropriately. No evidence of anger during this visit.

I weigh 142 lb, and I'm 5'4" tall. I've gained 22 lb so far in the pregnancy. I guess you've noticed the water in my hands and feet. It's the same problem I had before. The doctor says my blood pressure is okay, though.

Family life patterns

Boy, making ends meet is tough, especially with only a sales clerk's income and a full-time college student. Luckily, our parents have been great. I don't know what we'd do without them. Dave's folks pay for all his tuition. They're just so happy he's finally getting a degree. And every time my mom and dad come down for a visit, they're always bringing several sacks of groceries and clothes for Gabe and me. Then, of course, we have our student loans, which we'll probably be paying back 50 years from now. And Dave's employee health benefits plus the student health insurance policy we took out cover most of the medical bills.

We've been in this apartment about 3 years. We had a one-bed-room apartment down by the College Mall when we first moved here. Then when I got pregnant with Gabe, we needed a bigger place. It's not a bad place. As I said, a lot of the families in the complex are going to school. I think most of the others work at Otis or Cook's or RCA. This place is sort of like college: we know we won't have to be here forever, and it's okay for now.

Upstairs there are two bedrooms, a bathroom, and a linen closet.

Smiths live in a two-bedroom town-house apartment in a large complex on Bloomington's west side. Several large factories are located on the west side, and the Smiths are within a mile of several grocery stores (supermarkets), fast-food places, and discount stores (e.g., K-Mart). The apartment has an 11' × 15' living room furnished with a couch and chair, a Boston-type rocking chair, a bookshelf made of bricks and planks, a stereo tape and CD player with two small speakers, and an antique-looking desk. The dining room is an area between the living room and kitchen. It has a card table with two placemats, napkins and napkin rings, and a small vase with a few

Continued

Subjective data		Objective data	
Interactions		**Observations**	**Measurements**

Observations

silk flowers in it. There is also Gabe's high chair next to the card table. The kitchen has a window over the sink, overlooking an approximately 6′ × 8′ fenced-in patio area. Off the kitchen is a half-bath, where the washer and dryer and Gabe's potty chair are located. The nurse did not go upstairs. Everything looked orderly except the few toys scattered on the floor. The furnishing were few, but the plants made the apartment look very unique and well decorated. A small TV rests on the bookshelves. There is also a coat closet inside the front door and a closet under the stairway that is used for storing Gabe's toys. (See floor plan on this page.)

Interactions

I belong to the first Methodist Church, you know, the one downtown. But I don't go very often. Sunday morning is one of the few times Dave and Gabe and I all have together, and frankly, I don't want to give up our time together to go to church. Does that sound awful?

I don't belong to any other organizations and neither does Dave. We do have friends, though. I still see some of the girls I used to work with at Sears and, of course, the girls here in the complex. Dave has his college friends and some friends from Guaranteed Auto. I guess our best friends are the Gibsons. They live almost directly across the parking lot from us. They have a 6-month-old girl, and Gary goes to IU, too. Sharon and I probably talk on the phone or in person almost every day. The four of us sometimes get together on weekends and play Trivial Pursuit or cards, and eat popcorn. They're the ones we trade babysitting with so Dave and I can get out alone. They really are fun.

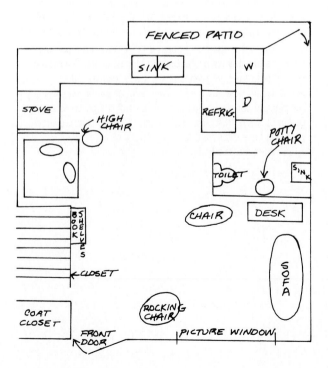

Subjective data		Objective data	
Interactions		**Observations**	**Measurements**
Well, I've already said our folks have been great. My mom and dad are terrific, and even though Laura [sister] is 4 years younger, we're good friends besides being sisters. I love Dave's dad. We get along great. Dave's mom is okay. I guess we are typical mother-in-law and daughter-in-law. Luckily, Dave usually agrees with me that his mom is being a little too nosy and pushy. But she has her good side, too. She sure loves Gabe. I'd say either my folks or Dave's come down or we go to Kokomo at least once every 2 months. It's easier for us to go there because we don't really have any room for them to stay here. We'll go up for Thanksgiving. The nice thing about Kokomo is that it's only 2 hours away, so if we want to go up for just a day's visit, it's not too bad a trip. I hope my mother can come this weekend. It's been awhile since we visited.		On the top of the desk are Carla and Dave's wedding pictures taken with each of their separate families (along with several pictures of Gabe).	
Sure, we can set up a time for you to come again. How about next week on Dave's day off? That's next Wednesday. Same time? I'll check with Dave and call you at the clinic, if it's not okay.		Carla goes to the desk and looks at a calendar.	
I enjoyed your visit. Thanks for the information. We'll work on the bed thing, hopefully this weekend. Bye.		Gabe waves bye-bye at Carla's suggestion.	

Analysis/Synthesis of Data: Visit 1

Analysis/Synthesis of Individuals

An analysis/synthesis of the individuals according to Roy's (1991) adaptation model is presented first.

Physiological Mode

Gabe is very active most of the time and takes a walk with his mom nearly every day. He gets 12 to 13 hours of sleep in a 24-hour period, which according to Mott, James, and Sperhac (1990) is normal. Gabe eats small amounts of food, but Carla claims he eats from the food guide pyramid. Gabe is in the process of being toilet trained, but no information was obtained on elimination patterns, which is a data gap. Gabe's skin is soft, intact, and well hydrated, which indicates adequate intake of fluids and electrolytes. Gabe's height of 35 inches and weight of 27 pounds put him in the 25th percentile for his age, according to Mott et al (1990). A total of 16 teeth is normal for his age. All this information, plus the fact that Gabe's health history reflects current immunizations and no disease, indicates that Gabe is adapting physiologically. Data gaps exist in the areas of oxygenation, elimination, the senses, and neurological and endocrine functions.

Carla gets adequate exercise and rest. Her diet includes foods from all groups in the food pyramid, and weight gain of 22 lb in 8 months of this pregnancy is adequate (Bobak and Jensen, 1993). No elimination information was obtained. Although edema of the hands and feet is a common phenomenon of pregnancy and Carla's blood pressure is "okay" according to her doctor, further assessment of Carla's edema is needed before ruling it out as a physiological threat. Carla's complaint of constant fatigue may also be a phenomenon of pregnancy; however, other causes, such as anemia, have not been ruled out. Therefore a data gap exists. Carla's health history is negative for disease, and Carla considers herself a healthy person. From the evidence gathered, physiologically she is adapting, which is a strength.

Self-Concept Mode

Gabe appears to be adapting in the self-concept mode, as evidenced by his stating, "Gabe a good boy," and by his obvious pleasure and pride after completing a puzzle.

Carla's self-concept can also be described as adaptive. She is attractively dressed and wears makeup. She states, "I feel pretty good about myself." She has a plan to get further education when Dave is through college.

Strengths are good self-concepts for both Gabe and Carla.

Role Function Mode

Data relating to Gabe's role as a 2-year-old first-born son show that he is complying with toilet training, eating, and hygienic habits expected of him. He appears to be in Erikson's (1963) stage of development: autonomy versus shame and doubt, which is appropriate for his age. He is developing autonomy as he learns to control himself and his environment.

Regarding Carla's role as mother, she states, "I truly enjoy being a mother," and feels it is important for her to be home with the children. She is conscientious in her mothering role, as evidenced by her attention to eating and hygienic habits, as well as her concern for Gabe's emotional well-being. Data gap: Carla's role as wife. It can be concluded that Gabe and Carla are both adapting to their respective roles identified during this visit.

Interdependence Mode

Gabe appears to be still in the working stages of achieving independence from his mother. Getting on and off her lap frequently may represent his working through needing her in close proximity and exploring the environment. He gives and gets verbal and nonverbal affection openly. Data gaps: separation anxiety/behaviors when Carla leaves the house without him, behaviors at bedtime, and interdependence with Dave.

Carla obviously enjoys giving to and getting from Gabe verbal and nonverbal affection. She recognizes Gabe's dependence on her (calls him a mama's boy), yet recognizes the need to, and actually does, get out of the house without Gabe. Carla's interdependence with her family and Dave's shows that she can depend on them and is grateful for their help and support. Yet, independence also exists in that a family visit every 2 months seems reasonable. Data gap: Carla's interdependence with Dave.

Strengths from the evidence gathered: Gabe is at an appropriate level of interdependence adaptation for his age. Carla is adapting in the interdependence mode with Gabe and the extended families.

Analysis/Synthesis of Family

An analysis/synthesis of family data is presented according to the structural-functional approach. The four concepts of structure are addressed first, followed by the six concepts of family functions.

Family Structure

1. *Role*. The roles of Gabe as a 2-year-old firstborn son and Carla as mother have been addressed under Roy's model. However, the coming birth of the new baby will bring new roles for Gabe and Carla. Gabe will become a brother and for the first time have to share his parents' attention on an everyday basis. Carla is concerned about Gabe's adjustment to the new role, which is a strength. However, she has done very little (only talks about the new baby to Gabe and has him pat her belly as a way of loving the baby) to prepare Gabe or help him accept the new role. This is a potential concern.

Carla's role as mother of one 2-year-old will change to mother of two children, including a newborn baby. More information is needed regarding Carla's new role. Another data gap is Dave's roles in the family.

2. *Values*. Carla's apparent values are health (good nutrition, good hygiene, exercise, prenatal care), education, and time together as a nuclear family, as well as an extended family. The data gap is values that Dave and Carla hold together as a nuclear family.

3. *Communication*. Communication patterns between Carla and Gabe reflect much use of touch, stroking, and sitting on the lap. When Gabe and Carla speak, they look at one another, and Carla encourages the expression of feelings, which Reidy and Thibedeau (1984) say is a characteristic of a healthy family. Data gap: Dave's communication with the rest of the family, and theirs with him.

4. *Power*. Carla makes the decisions about nutrition and food, but that is the only definite data collected related to power structure. It is possible that Gabe's many "no" responses have become manipulative, and in that way Gabe may exert some power over Carla. However, more assessment is necessary, because the "no" could simply be a result of his age and stage of development. Data gaps: who makes what decisions and how; power hierarchy.

Family Functions

1. *Affective*. The open affection between Carla and Gabe has been mentioned and can be considered a strength. Data gaps: Dave's part in the family's affective function; his psychological response to members' needs.

2. *Socialization*. Initial assessment shows that child-rearing practices in the Smith family are permissive, inasmuch as Carla does not insist that Gabe do what she asks. But a data gap exists because Dave's input on child-rearing practices is not known, and child-rearing practices were not actually discussed. Also, the environment was somewhat artificial because of the nurse's presence. Carla may have let Gabe go to avoid any hassles during the visit. According to Piaget, Gabe should be in the preconceptual period of the preoperational phase of cognitive development. In this period the emergence of the symbolic function is shown in the rapid development of language (Mott, James, and Sperhac, 1990). Data related to cognitive development show that Gabe is at the proper period, which is a strength.

Dave is in college, and Carla intends to get further education in the future. This will influence Gabe's attitude toward education.

In the area of community contacts, Dave is involved with an educational organization and with his work organization. Carla belongs to church but goes infrequently. So their contacts with actual organizations are somewhat limited. However, they do have contact with the community in terms of their friends and family, which is a strength.

3. *Reproduction.* Carla and Dave are participating in the reproductive function of the family. Data gaps: Were any of the three pregnancies planned? Are more children wanted? Sexual history; family planning.

4. *Economics.* The family income is apparently meager, but the Smiths are able to provide for their food, clothing, shelter, and health care by using a variety of resources, such as help from family, loans, medical insurance, and even trading babysitting and attending free functions at the university for entertainment. The apartment is modest but satisfactory to Carla until something nicer can be afforded. The Smiths' economic function, according to Carla, is a strength. Data gaps: provision of transportation; Dave's attitude toward economic function.

5. *Health Care.* The physical functions of food, clothing, shelter, and protection against danger are provided by Carla and Dave. Gabe's immunizations are current, he eats an appropriate diet and gets adequate sleep, and Carla always belts him in his car seat. Carla seeks regular prenatal care, eats an appropriate diet and gets adequate sleep and rest, does not smoke or drink, and always wears her seat belt. These data indicate positive health care and health practices, which

are a strength. Data gaps exist in the areas of Dave's health care and health practices, and dental health for the whole family.

The Smith family strengths are as follows:

1. Adequate activity and rest, nutrition, fluids, protection, and physiological adaptation for Gabe
2. Adequate activity and rest, nutrition, fluids, and physiological adaptation for Carla
3. Gabe and Carla have good self-concepts
4. Role adaptation of Gabe, and of Carla in her mothering role
5. Appropriate level of interdependence adaptation of Gabe for his age
6. Adaptation in the interdependence mode of Carla with Gabe and with the extended families
7. Carla's concern for Gabe's adjustment to his future new role as brother
8. Open expression of feelings between Carla and Gabe, with much verbal and nonverbal affection shown
9. Good contact with friends in the community and family for Carla
10. Adequate economic provisions
11. Positive health care and health practices for Gabe and Carla

NURSING DIAGNOSES: Visit 1

Date	Diagnoses	Priority
11/7/94	1. Potential role conflict for Gabe related to inadequate preparation for new baby	1
11/7/94	2. Incomplete database, especially in areas related to Dave	2

DATA COLLECTION: Visit 2

Time: Wednesday, November 16, 1994, 2:00 PM
Place: The Smith home. Dave opened the door, introduced himself, and immediately apologized for not having been present at the last visit. Carla greeted the nurse and told her that Gabe was still napping. The visit lasted 1 hour.
Nursing goals: To (1) establish rapport with Dave, (2) fill in the identified data gaps related to Dave and family life patterns, (3) evaluate previous nursing interventions, and (4) initiate at least one plan of intervention based on nursing diagnosis made during the previous visit.

Subjective data		Objective data	
Interactions		Observations	Measurements

Dave's health history (provided by Dave)

I'm not really sure about my childhood diseases. My mom would know. She kept records just like Carla does for Gabe.
I don't have any chronic illnesses, and I don't take any medications. I do take Alka-Seltzer Plus when I have a cold.

Dave is dressed in a flannel shirt and blue jeans. He is clean-shaven with shiny, dark-brown straight hair that is cut just cov-

Continued

DATA COLLECTION: Visit 2—cont'd

Subjective data	Objective data	
Interactions	**Observations**	**Measurements**

Interactions	Observations	Measurements
I couldn't really tell you whether or not my dad has any illnesses. I guess Carla told you I haven't seen him or talked to him in almost 20 years. I hardly remember what he looks like. But my family is all healthy. No surgeries, but I did have to go to the hospital in high school when I broke my arm playing touch football, of all things. I wear my seat belt most of the time.	ering the top of the ears. His nails are clean, and his oral hygiene is good. Dave is a trim-looking man with a muscular physique who does not have dark circles around his eyes.	
Dave's current health status (provided by Dave) Carla's a great cook. I'll eat anything she fixes. No, I don't smoke. But I do drink wine and an occasional beer. My greatest recreation right now is sleeping. I know that sounds terrible, but with my schedule and all the studying I have to do, it's such a luxury to get a good night's sleep. When I'm not in the midst of a semester, I like sports of all kinds, to watch and play. I used to run 3 miles every day, but I've even given that up, too. Now my only real exercise is walking on campus between classes.		
School is going great, in spite of the pressure it creates. My grades are good, and if everything goes according to schedule, I'll graduate next May. We'll both be glad.	Carla is smiling.	
You know, I feel good about myself, but I also feel a little selfish and guilty. I know my being gone all the time is hard for Carla. It will be worse when the new baby comes. I also know how much Carla wants to go to college. I guess I am grateful that I get to be the first one to go. I'll support her all the way when it's her turn.	Dave is an articulate man, uses correct grammar.	
Well, having Gabe has been great, although as I've said, I don't get to spend as much time with the family as I'd like. I think because my own father ran out, I want to do a good job as a father. Speaking of Gabe, there's the little guy now.	Gabe comes walking down the stairs carrying a blanket in one hand and a stuffed Snoopy dog in the other hand. Dave smiles as Gabe enters the room. Gabe goes immediately to Carla and climbs on her lap.	
Dave: Carla told me that Gabe may wet his pants more and throw more temper tantrums and maybe even hit the new baby. I guess it's gonna be rough on him, huh?		
Carla: Well, maybe not. We did all the things to prepare him, and I'm sure I can spend a little time with just him every day, and I know I'll be careful about him getting rough with the baby. So maybe it won't be so bad.	Carla and Dave are now sitting on the couch about a foot apart. They look at each other when they talk.	
My mom did come this past weekend and brought the youth bed. Gabe is really proud of his new bed now, but the first couple nights were pretty hairy. I think he was out of bed 50 times at least.		
Dave: Gabe, come to daddy.	Gabe crawls into his dad's lap.	
What's going to happen when mommy goes to the hospital to have our new baby?		
Gabe: Mommy go bye-bye. Gabe stay with Gram.	Dave looks at Carla, smiles, and then gives Gabe a hug.	
Dave: Good boy, Gabe. Mommy and daddy love you.		
Carla, if you tell me what you want Gabe to have for a snack, I'll get it.	Dave helps Gabe use his potty chair and washes his hands; then Dave washes his own hands and gets Gabe's snack.	Gabe ate half a banana and 4 oz 2% milk.

DATA COLLECTION: Visit 2—cont'd

Subjective data	Objective data	
Interactions	**Observations**	**Measurements**

Carla: You know, something has been on my mind. I know it would be best if I nursed this baby, and I want to, but I'm afraid to try. I breastfed Gabe for about 2 weeks and had to quit. I don't want to feel like such a failure again.		
I think I received bad advice and conflicting advice from the nurses in the hospital and the clinic.		
Gabe was really sleepy at first, and my nipples are kind of flat. So a nurse gave me a nipple shield to use. Things were going fine until another nurse told me to get rid of the shield. Then came the sore nipples! After we went home, I used the bottles of formula they sent home with us to give my sore nipples an occasional break. Well, by the end of a week it seemed like I didn't have enough milk. Poor Gabe wanted to eat every hour. And of all things, the nurse at the clinic told me to let him cry and not to nurse that often. I couldn't just let him cry, so I'd give him a bottle. By the end of 2 weeks I hardly had any milk at all, so I gave up and switched completely to formula.	After Gabe's snack and during the discussion on breastfeeding, Dave and Gabe are on the floor stacking and knocking down building blocks. Gabe is giggling loudly.	
Carla: I didn't decide for sure to breastfeed until about 3 weeks before Gabe was born. I don't think I really listened to the pre-natal instructor when she was talking about breastfeeding because I didn't think I would be doing it. My mom didn't breast-feed either of us, and Dave didn't really care one way or the other. So I didn't make that much effort to learn about it. I figured if I decided to do it, it was just a natural thing.		
I just wasn't prepared for those awful sore nipples. They said in prenatal classes to rub the nipples with a towel in the last months of pregnancy to prepare them. And I did that. But my nipples got sore anyway.		
My neighbor always looks so at ease breastfeeding. I think I need to know more about it. It was never easy for me.		
Oh, I love to read, and I'm certainly interested in the subject. I read the little booklet the obstetrician gave me in the clinic, but I didn't get that much information from it.	Carla goes to the bookshelf and pulls out the booklet. It is a 10-page booklet on feeding your baby published by a formula company.	
I've heard of LaLèche League, and I know its a bunch of breast-feeding mothers getting together, but that's about all I know.		
I could go to at least one meeting and see what it's like. It's good to know they allow toddlers to come along. I'll be happy to have you bring the books about breastfeeding over, too. As for the nipples, I'll try to start preparing them. But if they're going to get sore anyway, I'm not sure it's worth the bother.		
Dave: I'll sure support Carla if she decides to breastfeed. But I really feel the decision is up to her.	Dave resumes his position next to Carla on the couch. Gabe promptly squeezes between Dave and Carla, then hops down and begins playing with some plastic trucks.	
Carla: We're really pretty flexible about decision-making, don't you think, Dave?		
Dave: Uh, huh.		
Carla: I make most of the household decisions. It's what I know best. I also make most of the decisions about Gabe because I'm with him the most. But Dave and I always talk it over first.		
Dave: I make the decisions about the car, and we make joint decisions about how to spend our money and what to do when we go out.		

Continued

Subjective data		Objective data	
Interactions		**Observations**	**Measurements**
Dave: How do I feel about family? You mean my mom and dad and brother and sister? The great thing about Mom and Dad is that they're giving us the money for my tuition, with no strings attached. It seems to me that after forking over that kind of dough, they'd think they would have a right to tell us how to live our lives. But they don't. I always thought my parents were terrible dictators when I was in high school. I certainly have a different opinion of them now. I'm not sure how we'll ever repay them, even though I know they don't expect it.		Gabe continues to go from toys to the couch, climbing on Dave and Carla and chattering constantly. Carla looks at Gabe and several times says, "shh" to Gabe and puts her finger over her mouth.	
I'll have to say that Carla is my best friend. Oh, I have buddies at work and at school, but I'm not real close to any of them. Gary and Sharon across the way are a fun couple, and we get together fairly often.		Dave puts his hand on Carla's shoulder. Carla smiles.	
Carla: Of course you may come again. I'd especially like to discuss breastfeeding with you after I've had a chance to do some reading. But next time, let's make it in the evening when Gabe will already be in bed.			
A week from today will be fine.		Dave nods his assent.	

Analysis/Synthesis of Data: Visit 2

Analysis/Synthesis of Individuals

The previous analysis of Carla and Gabe is still appropriate. To be consistent, the data will be analyzed according to Roy's model first, followed by the structural-functional approach to family life patterns. Only new pieces of data are addressed.

Physiological Mode

Dave gets adequate exercise at least some of the time and has been able to maintain a trim, muscular physique. He does not always get adequate rest but does not appear tired. Carla is nutrition-conscious, and Dave says that he enjoys her cooking. However, there is insufficient data to indicate adequate activity, rest, or nutrition. Data gaps exist in the area of elimination, fluids and electrolytes, oxygenation, and protection, as well as endocrine function. Strengths are Dave's overall good health, determined from his health history and current health status.

Self-Concept Mode

Dave's self-concept is a strength. He feels pretty good about himself, enjoys being a father and student, and takes care of his physical appearance.

Role Function Mode

Data relating to Dave's role as a husband indicate that he considers his wife to be his best friend, is grateful for her support of his education, and wishes

he could spend more time with the family. Dave's feelings about his roles as father and student are enjoyment. His positive attitudes toward his role show adaptation, which is a strength. Data gaps: Dave's role as a worker, Carla's role as a wife.

Interdependence Mode

Dave, like the other members of the Smith family, openly gives and takes affection. He and Carla are adapting in the interdependence mode in that they can function and make decisions independently and yet confer with and support one another. Dave also appears to have appropriate interdependence with his extended family, accepting their help, yet "living his own life." These are strengths.

Analysis/Synthesis of Family

Family Structure

1. *Role.* Carla fears failure, as she experienced it with Gabe, at breastfeeding the new infant, yet expresses a desire to breastfeed. Data indicate that Carla has done little reading about breastfeeding and received misinformation or no information at all from health professionals. There is a potential concern for repeated failure in Carla's role as a new nurturing mother.

2. *Values.* Data gathered during the second visit show that Dave's values are the same as Carla's, which were identified as health, education, and time together as a nuclear family, as well as an extended

family. The fact that Dave and Carla have no value conflicts is a strength.

3. *Communication.* Dave is openly affectionate verbally and nonverbally with Gabe and Carla. Dave and Carla look at one another when speaking, they sit close to one another on the couch, they take turns speaking, and their communication appears to be open and honest with freedom to express feelings. According to Reidy and Thibedeau (1984), these are effective means of communication and a strength for the family.

4. *Power.* Carla and Dave have separate areas of decision-making responsibility, but admit to flexibility, some joint decision-making, and some conferring before decisions are made. This can be considered a strength. More information is needed before a power hierarchy can be identified. The data gap of Gabe's power over his parents still exists.

Family Functions

1. *Affective.* A major strength of the Smith family is the open and free expression of verbal and nonverbal affection. A data gap still exists in the area of a response to members' needs.

2. *Socialization.* Child-rearing practices were not discussed. However, data indicate that Dave takes an active role in Gabe's care. He readily helped Gabe use the toilet, gave him a snack, and seemed to enjoy playing with him. There is still no information on discipline and whether Carla and Dave agree on how Gabe should be raised.

3. *Health Care.* Dave is a nonsmoker and occasional drinker. He wears his seat belt most of the time. He considers himself healthy, but the data are insufficient to say that health care and health practices are appropriate and positive. There is no new data related to reproduction and economics.

The Smith family's strengths determined from this visit are as follows:

1. Dave's physiological adaptation
2. Dave's positive self-concept
3. Dave's adaptation toward his role as husband, father, and student
4. Dave's appropriate interdependence with Carla and extended family
5. No conflict of values between Carla and Dave
6. Open communication patterns
7. Flexibility in decision-making
8. Mutual expression of affection

NURSING DIAGNOSES: Visit 2

Date	Diagnoses	Priority
11/7/94	1. Potential role conflict for Gabe related to inadequate preparation for new baby	2
11/16/94	2. Potential role failure for Carla related to lack of knowledge about breastfeeding	1
11/16/94	3. Incomplete database	3

DATA COLLECTION: Visit 3

Time: Wednesday, November 23, 1994, 7:30 PM
Place: The Smith home. Dave answered the door. Gabe was playing on the floor, dressed in his pajamas. Carla was not on the first floor, and Dave called her down from upstairs. Carla greeted the nurse with tears in her eyes and stated that she found out at the clinic today that she will have to have a cesarean section. The visit lasted 45 minutes.
Nursing goals: To (1) fill in identified data gaps related to family life patterns, (2) evaluate previous nursing interventions, and (3) initiate at least one plan of intervention based on nursing diagnosis made during this visit.

Subjective data		Objective data	
Interactions		Observations	Measurements
Carla: I do need to talk, but I'd rather talk about this thing after Gabe goes to bed. Dave: I have some concerns, too.		Carla is fighting back tears, voice is quivering. Gabe is playing with a puzzle with one hand while sucking his thumb on the other hand. He sits still, not moving about as during the last two visits.	

Continued

DATA COLLECTION: Visit 3—cont'd

Subjective data	Objective data	
Interactions	**Observations**	**Measurements**

Subjective data	Objective data
Carla: Yes, I've read one of the books on breastfeeding, and I've started a second.	
The LaLèche League women were very nice and helpful, but some of them seem kind of fanatic. I'm not sure I'll go back to the meetings.	
I am feeling more confident, but I'm still not sure about nipple preparation. I haven't really done anything about that.	Gabe begins to whine, but Dave picks him up and gives him a piggy-back ride upstairs after goodnight hugs and kisses to mommy. Gabe is giggling during the ride upstairs.
I'd like to keep the books until after the baby's born, if you don't mind—especially now that I have to have a cesarean section.	Dave came downstairs, offered the nurse a drink of juice, got himself and Carla a drink of juice, then resumed his position next to Carla on the couch. Gabe came downstairs, and Dave immediately took Gabe back upstairs to bed.
I'm down to 1-week visits now because my due date is so close. I went in for my regular visit this morning and the doctor said, "The baby's in frank breech position, and your pelvis is only borderline. You know, we had to use forceps to get Gabe out, and he weighed only 6½ pounds. This baby weighs much more than that. You're going to have to have a cesarean section." That's about all I remember. I was so shook up I couldn't even think of any questions to ask. But now I have a million. I'm so scared.	Carla takes a deep breath before beginning.
I guess I'm mostly afraid of the pain. You hear so many gruesome stories. But I'm also afraid of not getting off to a good start with the new baby and not being able to take care of Gabe when I get home. I don't even know what frank breech position is.	Dave puts his arm around Carla's shoulder. She begins to cry again.
(The nurse explained what breech position is and encouraged further exploration with the obstetrician.)	
Dave: You mean talk to the doctor (in response to nurse asking what could be done to relieve the anxiety). I think he owes her a much better explanation of what's going to happen. I think I'll find some time and go to talk to him with you, Carla. Maybe he'll be more apt to give you the information you deserve.	
Carla: I'm sorry! I was so shook up.	
Dave: I'm not blaming you, honey. I just hate to see you so upset. And we're not dumb. We have a right to know.	
Carla: Well, I need some time to think about what I'd like to ask him. I have an appointment next Wednesday. Do you think that would be soon enough? (in response to nurse asking when they would talk with the doctor).	
Dave: Let's not take a chance of you going into labor. Let's call tomorrow and make an appointment for this week. Want to?	
Carla: You're probably right. We'll call tomorrow. Maybe we should make a list of questions tonight.	Carla goes to the desk and gets a pad of paper and pen.
Dave: Well, I want to know if I can still be in the delivery room and how long Carla will have to stay in the hospital.	
Carla: As I said before, I'm afraid of the pain, so I want to know how much pain I'll have—both during the surgery and after—and what kind of scar I'll have. Will breastfeeding be harder?	

DATA COLLECTION: Visit 3—cont'd

Subjective data		Objective data	
Interactions		Observations	Measurements
It's good to know the different positions (in response to nurse showing her ways of positioning a baby for breastfeeding after a cesarean section). I hope the nurses in the hospital will help me.			
Dave: Yes, I've read about the cesarean birth support group in the paper.			
Carla: I guess we could call them. But I hope they're not as fanatic as LaLèche League.			
I feel better now that we have a plan.		Carla smiled for the first time during this visit.	
Dave: All I want from the doctor and the hospital personnel and any other health person is the knowledge to make informed decisions and a healthy outcome for my wife and new baby.			
Carla: I'll second that!			
Dave: I'd have to say that I'm stricter with Gabe than Carla is.			
Carla: But that's because you're with him less time. If you were with him as much as I am, he'd wear you down, too.		Carla raises her voice, sounds defensive.	
Dave: Oh, I agree with you, Carla, but you know how often we've talked about the importance of consistency.			
Carla: I know you're right. It just doesn't always work out that way.			
Dave: We do discuss how to deal with Gabe a lot. We'll probably do that even more when the new baby comes.			
Carla: We agree on most things, too. We both think manners are important, and teaching Gabe responsibility. We're trying hard to get him to pick up his toys and take care of them.			
Dave: We're not opposed to an occasional spanking, but it's not the only method of punishment we use, and we try hard not to do it when we're very angry. Right now, making him sit on a chair seems to work the best.			
Carla: I'm always questioning if how we're raising Gabe is right. I fight the "guilts" a lot.			
Dave: And I keep telling her that we're better parents than most.			
Carla: Of course, we'll be glad and grateful to have you visit after the baby is born (in response to nurse's inquiry about a postpartum visit).			
Dave: If you could visit in the hospital, that would be good too.			

Analysis/Synthesis of Data: Visit 3
Analysis/Synthesis

The previous analyses are still appropriate. No new information was obtained relating to Roy's adaptation model used to analyze the individuals. Only the categories from the structural-functional approach pertinent to new data are included at this analysis/synthesis.

Family Structures

Previous analyses remain relevant.

Family Functions

1. *Affective.* The open and free expression of verbal and nonverbal affection continues to be evident during this visit as a major strength of the Smith family. With regard to the previous data gap of members' needs, it was shown that Dave provided comfort, support, and help in developing a plan during Carla's time of need. Dave also admits to bolstering Carla's confidence when she has doubts about being a good parent. It is still not known if Carla provides the same for Dave during his times of need.

2. *Socialization.* Carla and Dave perceive themselves as agreeing on "most things" in relation to child-rearing practices. They use a variety of disciplining methods, and value manners and teach Gabe responsibility. Dave and Carla feel that Dave is stricter with Gabe than Carla, but both understand the reason for this, and they try to be consistent. Overall, the childrearing area of socialization in the Smith family is functional. This is a strength.

3. *Reproduction.* Carla's reproductive function has been altered because of the need for a cesarean section. Carla fears pain and the loss of control, and is also stressed by her lack of knowledge. Dave is also stressed and is concerned about a healthy outcome for his wife and baby. This is a concern.

Data gaps previously identified that still exist are Carla's role as wife, Dave's role as worker, Gabe's separation anxiety, power hierarchy, sexual history, family planning, family dental health, Dave's health care and health practices, and provision of transportation.

The Smith family strengths determined from this visit are as follows:

1. Functional affectional response by Dave for Carla
2. Functional child-rearing practices.

NURSING DIAGNOSES: Visit 3

Date	Diagnoses	Priority
11/7/94	1. Potential role conflict for Gabe related to inadequate preparation for new baby	3
11/16/94	2. Potential role failure for Carla related to lack of knowledge about breastfeeding	2
11/23/94	3. Stress related to need for cesarean section and lack of knowledge about cesarean delivery	1
11/23/94	4. Incomplete database	4

PLANS FOR IMPLEMENTATION

Nursing diagnosis 1: Potential role conflict for Gabe related to inadequate preparation for new baby (11/7/94).
Long-term expected outcome: Gabe will be prepared for new baby to decrease potential role conflict by 11/16/94.

Short-term expected outcomes	Nursing orders	Scientific rationale	Evaluation
1. Client will list behaviors indicative of role conflict and possible strategies for dealing with conflict by 11/16/94.	1a. Client will verbalize behavior expected of Gabe after baby is born by 11/7/94.	*Content:* Sibling rivalry. *Strategy:* Teaching and learning. 1a. New learning must be based on previous knowledge and experience (Redman, 1993).	**Criteria statement** Client will cite the following behaviors: Reversal of bowel and bladder control. Attention-getting behaviors such as temper tantrums. Physical violence aimed at new baby (e.g., hitting the baby, throwing things at the baby). Negative verbalization about the baby (e.g., "Baby bad").
	1b. Nurse will provide additional information to family about possible behaviors expected by Gabe after baby is born by 11/7/94. 1c. Client will verbalize possible strategies to use in dealing with above behaviors by 11/7/94. 1d. Nurse will provide additional information about possible strategies to use in dealing with behaviors by 11/6/89.	1b. Cognitive learning is the acquiring and development of concepts (Johnson, 1986). 1c. Effective learning requires active participation (Redman, 1993). 1d. Knowledge of what to expect increases the client's sense of control and powerfulness (Haggard, 1989).	**Criteria statement** Client will cite the following strategies: Put Gabe in new youth bed and take down crib. Discuss with Gabe Carla's absence when baby is born and who will stay with him. Spend time each day with Gabe when baby is not around. Include Gabe in care of baby (e.g., getting a diaper, rubbing lotion on baby). Reinforce verbally to Gabe how good and special he is.

Nursing diagnosis 1: Potential role conflict for Gabe related to inadequate preparation for new baby (11/7/94).
Long-term expected outcome: Gabe will be prepared for new baby to decrease potential role conflict by 11/16/94.

Short-term expected outcomes	Nursing orders	Scientific rationale	Evaluation
			Ongoing Nurse implemented orders 1b and 1d on 11/7/94. Client implemented orders 1a and 1c on 11/7/94. Carla mentioned all four behaviors and five strategies on 11/16/94. She had discussed them with Dave. Short-term outcome met.
2. Client will take steps to prepare Gabe for coming of new baby by 11/16/94.	2a. Client will decide which steps to take to prepare Gabe by 11/8/94. 2b. Client will obtain a youth bed, put Gabe in the youth bed at night, and take the crib down by 11/13/94. (Taking Gabe out of crib and putting new baby in crib will be two separate events.)	2a. An individual must be motivated to learn (Pohl, 1981). 2b. Effective learning requires active participation (Pohl, 1981). Concept of centricism causes child to think all events revolve around him or her (Mott, James, and Sperhac, 1990)	**Ongoing** Carla and Dave discussed and decided which preparatory steps to take with Gabe on 11/9/94. Carla's mom did bring the youth bed down on 11/12/94, and the crib was taken down and Gabe put in the youth bed on 11/12/94. Gabe's apparent reaction to the bed was pride, but he had trouble staying in bed the first few nights.
	2c. Client will discuss Carla's absence with Gabe repeatedly, stressing her assured return by 11/16/94	2c. Repetition strengthens learning (Pohl, 1981).	Carla and Dave discussed Carla's absence with Gabe many times since 11/7/94. Gabe says "Mommy go bye-bye, Gabe stay with Gram."
	2d. Client will confirm that Carla's mom will stay with Gabe during Carla's hospitalization by 11/13/94. 2e. Client will leave Gabe with Carla's mom and then discuss with Gabe how that will be like when mommy goes to have the new baby by 11/13/94	2d. Separation anxiety is high for the toddler (Mott, James, and Sperhac, 1990). 2e. Separation anxiety is high for the toddler (Mott, James, and Sperhac, 1990).	It was confirmed on 11/8/94 that Carla's mom would stay with Gabe at time of birth. Carla and Dave left Gabe with Carla's mom 11/14/94, and then discussed it with Gabe. **Concluding** Carla and Dave have taken steps to prepare Gabe. Actual effectiveness of steps will be evaluated after baby is born.

Nursing diagnosis 2: Potential role failure for Carla related to lack of knowledge about breastfeeding (11/16/94).
Long-term expected outcome: Carla will use her increased knowledge about breastfeeding to decrease her potential for role failure by 11/30/94.

Short-term expected outcomes	Nursing orders	Scientific rationale	Evaluation
1. Client will discuss at least five new things learned about breastfeeding on 11/16/94.	1a. Client will verbalize at least five points already known about breastfeeding by 11/16/94.	*Content:* Breastfeeding. *Strategy:* Teaching and learning. 1a. New learning must be based on previous knowledge and experience (Redman, 1993).	**Criteria statement** Client will verbalize understanding five of the following: Supply and demand principle Importance of adequate fluid intake; importance of adequate rest
	1b. Nurse will provide several books about breastfeeding and phone number of LaLèche League leader by 11/17/94.	1b. Cognitive learning is the acquisition and development of concepts (Johnson, 1986).	Need for alternating breasts to begin feeding

Continued

Nursing diagnosis 2: Potential role failure for Carla related to lack of knowledge about breastfeeding (11/16/94).
Long-term expected outcome: Carla will use her increased knowledge about breastfeeding to decrease her potential for role failure by 11/30/94.

Short-term expected outcome	Nursing orders	Scientific rationale	Evaluation
	1c. Client will select two breastfeeding books to read by 11/23/94. 1d. Client will try to attend at least one meeting of LaLèche League by 11/23/94.	1d. Effective learning requires active participation (Pohl, 1981). Learning may occur through imitation (Pohl, 1981). Provision of support group enhances learning.	Importance of avoiding emotional upset Positions of mom and baby Engorgement Let-down reflex Breast/nipple care Amount of time to nurse Quality/content of breast milk Avoidance of drugs during lactation Importance of support person
2. Client will implement techniques to promote breastfeeding by 11/26/94.	2a. Client will decide whether to breast-feed or bottle feed by 11/23/94. 2b. Nurse will support the client's decision on infant feeding by 11/23/94. 2c. Client, if she decides to breast feed, will identify techniques to facilitate successful breastfeeding by 11/25/94. 2d. Client will begin prenatal nipple preparation (if breast-feeding) to reduce nipple soreness during nursing by 11/26/94.	2a. The choice of infant feeding method is up to the mother (Bobak and Jensen, 1993). 2b. Support and encouragement may facilitate client's action on a decision. Therapeutic use of self (Wilson and Kneisl, 1992). 2c. Effective learning requires active participation (Pohl, 1981). 2d. Nipple preparation may reduce soreness when breastfeeding (Bobak and Jensen, 1993).	**Ongoing** Nurse implemented plan 1b. On 11/23/94, Carla stated she had read all of *The Womanly Art of Breastfeeding* and had started *Breastfeeding Today: A Mother's Companion* by Woessner, Lauwers, and Bernard. She stated she enjoyed reading them and sounded enthusiastic. On 11/21/94, Carla attended a LaLèche League meeting. She was impressed with the knowledge and skill of the mothers, but was concerned about what she called "fanaticism." Carla decided to try breast-feeding again and stated that nipple rolling, a rough towel massage, and expression of colostrum prenatally may help with breastfeeding. Carla sheepishly admitted that she had not done anything about nipple preparation. This was probably because she was not convinced of its value. **Concluding:** Carla discussed five things she learned about breastfeeding on 11/23/94. She stated she felt more confident about trying it again, but was especially concerned about the effects of the cesarean section on her efforts to breastfeed. Carla has increased her knowledge, and the potential for role failure is reduced, although more support and evaluation should take place after the baby is born.

PLANS FOR IMPLEMENTATION—cont'd

Nursing diagnosis 3: Stress related to need for cesarean section and lack of knowledge about impending cesarean delivery (11/23/94).
Long-term expected outcome: Carla and Dave will report decreased stress regarding the cesarean delivery by 11/30/94.

Short-term expected outcomes	Nursing orders	Scientific rationale	Evaluation
1. Clients will identify their specific stressors regarding cesarean delivery by 11/23/94.	1a. Nurse will encourage Carla and Dave to express their feelings and concerns regarding cesarean delivery by 11/23/94. 1b. Clients will identify their major concerns regarding cesarean delivery by 11/23/94.	*Content:* Stress/anxiety. *Strategy:* Therapeutic use of self (Wilson and Kneisl, 1992). 1b. Areas of stress must be identified before handling them.	Nurse implemented 1a on 11/23/94. Carla and Dave stated their main concerns were the need for a cesarean delivery because of breech presentation; the effects of this delivery on the baby and on Carla; type of anesthesia; and duration of physical recovery for Carla.
2. Clients will discuss at least five concerns about cesarean section during next visit with doctor by 11/28/94.	2a. Clients will make a list of questions and concerns about cesarean section by 11/23/94. 2b. Nurse will provide information about cesarean section by 11/23/94. 2c. Clients will visit the doctor and discuss questions and concerns by 11/29/94. 2d. Clients will contact the cesarean birth support group in Bloomington before the birth of the baby, if possible.	*Strategy:* Teaching and learning. 2a. Learning needs of the client must be determined (Pohl, 1981). 2b. Cognitive learning is the acquisition and development of concepts (Johnson, 1986). Information reduces anxiety and fear. 2c. Information reduces anxiety and fear. 2d. Learning may occur through imitation (Pohl, 1981). Provision of a support group is one way of coping with stress.	**Criteria statement** Client will verbalize understanding of five of the following: Frank breech position Borderline pelvis Turn, cough, deep breathe Type of incision Type of anesthesia Length of hospital stay Pain medication available Consequences of cesarean birth to baby Consequences of cesarean birth to father Positions for breastfeeding after cesarean delivery **Ongoing** Client implemented orders 1b and 2a on 11/23/94. Nurse implemented plans 1a and 2b on 11/23/94. Orders 2c and 2d not implemented because dates had not occurred yet. Short-term outcome not met. **Concluding** Long-term expected outcome is not met. Evaluation will take place after next visit to doctor.

REFERENCES AND READINGS

Bobak IM and Jensen MD: *Maternity and gynecologic care: the nurse and the family*, ed 5, St Louis, 1993, Mosby–Year Book.

Duvall EM and Miller BL: *Marriage and family development*, ed 6, New York, 1985, Harper and Row.

Erikson E: *Childhood and society*, ed 2, New York, 1963, WW Norton.

Friedman MM: *Family nursing: theory and assessment*, ed 3, New York, 1992, Appleton-Lange.

Haggard A: *Handbook of patient education*, Rockville, Md, 1989, Aspen.

Johnson SH: *High risk parenting: nursing assessment and strategies for the family at risk*, ed 2, Philadelphia, 1986, JB Lippincott.

LaLèche League: The womanly art of breastfeeding, Franklin Park, Ill, 1991, LaLèche League International.

Mott SR, James SR, and Sperhac AM: *Nursing care of children and families*, ed 2, Redwood City, Calif, 1990, Addison-Wesley.

Pohl ML: *The teaching function of the nurse practitioner*, ed 4, Dubuque, Iowa, 1981, Wm C Brown.

Redman BK: The process of patient education, ed 7, St Louis, 1993, Mosby–Year Book.

Reidy M and Thibedeau M: Evaluation of family functioning: development of a scale which measures family competence in matters of health, *Nurs Papers* 16:42, 1984.

Roy Sr C and Andrews HA: *The Roy adaptation model: the definitive statement*, ed 2, Norwalk, Conn, 1991, Appleton-Lange.

Wilson HS and Kneisl CR: *Psychiatric nursing*, ed 4, Redwood City, Calif, 1992, Addison-Wesley.

Woessner C, Kauwers J, and Bernard B: *Breastfeeding today: a mothers' companion*, Garden City Park, NY, 1991, Avery.

CHAPTER 17

NURSING PROCESS OF THE COMMUNITY CLIENT

Karen Saucier Lundy

his chapter examines a hypothetical aggregate in the community of Rosetown, a small rural community with black and white mixed ethnic groups. The population has a low median income, high unemployment, and a high rate of teenage pregnancies. The aggregate is made up of pregnant teens enrolled in Rosetown High School.

The nursing care plan is presented using the Community-as-Client Assessment Framework as the organizing model (Stanhope and Lancaster, 1992).[31] This framework was selected to guide the assessment and analysis of this specific aggregate because of its emphasis on systems within a community and how each is related to the goal of health. The Community-as-Client Assessment Framework is useful in the examination of a community or aggregate located in a geopolitical community. Structure and process both are assessed with emphasis on structural components of an aggregate or community. Because the aggregate of pregnant teens resides in a geopolitical community, this nursing framework is an appropriate application. For a more complete explanation of the Community-as-Client Framework, see Chapter 6.

Most of the references for this hypothetical aggregate and community are fictitious but provide the reader with a sample format for documentation.

Data collection. Data have been collected using the methods of observation, interaction, and measurement, and categorized into structure and interacting subsystems. The data were all collected before the analysis and implementation of plans.

Data analysis and diagnosis. During the analysis, models and principles are used. Data are compared with standards, and judgments are made as to strengths and concerns of a community's functioning. Health resources are analyzed by examining the direct services provided according to the three categories of services recommended in *Healthy People 2000: National Health Promotion and Disease Prevention Objectives.* These categories are *preventive health services*—services that can be delivered to individuals by health providers; *health promotion services*—activities that individuals and communities can use to promote healthy lifestyles; and *health protection services*—measures that can be used by governmental and other agencies to protect people from harm.[34]

Planning and implementation. Knowledge regarding functioning of the community directs the appropriate change strategies to be used. The process of change according to Lewin is used, and involves three steps: unfreezing, moving to the new level, and refreezing at the new level.[30]

Evaluation. Evaluation data are not collected because this is a hypothetical situation. Questions that indicate appropriate data are provided, and criteria standards are established.

Text continued on p. 303

DATA COLLECTION*

Subjective data	Objective data
Interactions	**Measurements**

Core structures

Self-concept

"People in school looked down on me when I was pregnant, like I had done something shameful or something."[1]

"I like being in a special class for pregnant girls 'cause they understand how I feel and the problems I am having."[1]

History

"When I became pregnant, I read all about the problems of having a baby when you're a teenager."[1]

"The nurse at school told me about the things that have happened to pregnant girls in my school, like divorce and getting sick and dropping out of school and welfare."[1]

Statistics

Observations

Adolescent pregnancy has been identified as a risk factor in this century as societal changes resulted in such trends as increased age at first marriage, increased need for advanced education, and increased life span resulting in changes in acceptable sexual experiences for teens.[3,4]

Pregnant teens are not actively involved in school activities, such as clubs, sports, or recreational activities. Aggregate members are often observed in school with each other.

Live births to women younger than 20 years by race and ethnic group, in county of aggregate[36]

	Total under 20	Under 15	15-17	18-19	% All births
All races	292	7	135	150	20.1
White	59	1	15	45	17.4
Black	233	6	120	105	31.4

Age distribution of community[36]

18 and younger	48.2%
18-45	20.2%
45-62	18.6%
62 and older	13.0%

Total population of town and county of aggregate[18,36]

Year	Rosetown	County	State
1980	2793	42,500	2,520,638
1990	2791	45,034	2,598,000

Population of Rosetown High School[13]

Year	Rosetown High
1980	442
1989	450

Birth rate = $\dfrac{\text{No. live births per year} \times 1{,}000}{\text{average (midyear) population}}$ [14,35,36]

(See refs. 17, 35, 36.)

Rosetown High		County of aggregate	
No.	Rate	No.	Rate
15	33.3	832	18.5

State of aggregate		U.S.	
No.	Rate	No.	Rate
43,432	16.7	3,749,000	16.3

Mortality rates = $\dfrac{\text{No. deaths per year} \times 1{,}000}{\text{Average midyear population}}$ [35,36]

	Rosetown		State		U.S.	
Type of mortality	No.	Rate	No.	Rate	No.	Rate
Neonatal deaths						
White	0	0.0	127	5.5		
Nonwhite	12	21.1	241	11.8		
Totals	12	16.9	368	8.5		
Infant deaths						
White	0	0.0	213	9.3		
Nonwhite	14	24.6	383	18.7		
Totals	14	19.7	596	13.7	39,500	10.5

Infant mortality rates by age of mother, 1981, 1985, 1994 (state)[36]

Age of mother	1981	1985	1994
10-19	21.9	21.2	18.1
20-29	13.2	14.0	13.1
All ages	15.2	15.1	14.1

Continued

*See reference list for sources of data indicated by superscript numbers.

Subjective data

Interactions

Objective data

Observations

Measurements

Percentage of female-headed households, 1994[15,36]

Rosetown	County	State	U.S.
61%	47%	34%	25%

Gender distribution[13,18]

	Rosetown High	Rosetown
Males	49.7%	47.1%
Females	50.3%	52.9%

Income of families[18,36]

	Rosetown	State
Under $3,000	4.2%	3.8%
3,000-5,999	17.3%	12.7%
6,000-9,999	26.9%	17.3%
10,000-14,999	21.8%	22.7%
15,000-24,999	18.4%	24.3%
25,000 +	11.4%	19.4%
Median	$11,216.00	$14,500.00

Education of persons 25 years and older[26]

	Rosetown	State
No schooling	0.9%	0.7%
H.S. graduate	42.4%	54.8%
Attended college	16.4%	19.4%
Median school yr completed	10.6	12.2

Unemployment rate, 1994[18,36]

Rosetown	State	U.S.
12.4%	10.2%	8.1%

Leading causes of death in county of aggregate

Cause	White	Nonwhite	Total
Diseases of heart	69	78	147
Malignant neoplasms	44	52	96

Cerebrovascular disease	14	40	54
Accidents (all causes)	9	16	25
Atherosclerosis	7	8	15

High school completion rate by age at first birth for women age 20-26 (U.S.)[35]

Age at first birth	Percentage of Women who complete high school (%)
15	45
16	49
17	53
18	62
19	77
20	90

Birth outcome/prenatal care by age in the United States[35]

	Under 15	15-19	20-24
Babies born at low birth-weight (5.5 lb or less) (%)	14.5	9.0	5.6
Babies born at very low birth weight (3.5 lb or less) (%)	7.0	3.4	2.1
Babies born to mothers who received early prenatal care (%)	33.0	53.0	71.1

Percentage of sexually active U.S. females who use contraception[35]

Age	Percentage
10-15	4
16-19	21
20-25	65

"We have a real problem getting these girls in before the second trimester. They try to deny the pregnancy, pretend it doesn't exist. We don't have statistics on Rosetown, but a significant number of these girls' babies are small."[3]

Culture

"Pregnant girls are usually interested in childbirth, and most are interested in baby care. They are aware that they are different than other girls their age."[3]

"I really want to finish high school even though I am pregnant. Some of the girls in my class have dropped out and gotten married and all they think about is being with a guy and having his baby. I want to be able to make sure my baby has what he needs, so I need to get a job that pays money."[1]

The pregnant teens are easily identifiable as the pregnancy advances.

Continued

DATA COLLECTION—cont'd

Subjective data	Objective data
Interactions	**Measurements**

Interactions

"I don't understand a lot of what is going on inside of me, but I know that my baby is going to be perfect and it will be all I want it to be (childbirth)."[1]

"The older people in our community are very religious, and most of their lives center around church meetings. The young are not as interested in church but still value religion. Whites value family, career, education, and good health. The black culture places much more emphasis on the rearing of children and recreation."[6]

"Rosetown is predominantly Southern Baptist. Values and customs vary among age and social groups."[6]

"We are seeing girls engage in sexual intercourse at a much younger age here in Rosetown. They talk about it more openly now, and they still believe that it (pregnancy) won't happen to me."[4]

Social network/support

"I am really scared about having a baby; I mean I can't believe all of this is happening. My mother is not really thrilled, but I know she is there for me anyway."[1]

"We have this special class at school for pregnant girls, and they help us with doctor appointments and food stamps and things like that."[1]

"I don't know where I will put the baby if I come back to school. My mother works, and I don't know anybody who can keep it."[1]

"We all kind of stick together like we all understand what this is all about cause we have the same problems."[1]

"We really don't have much help for these girls in Rosetown. The health department has the prenatal clinic and baby clinic and WIC, and we have a welfare office. I meet in a support group for girls out of school. There is really no baby care and very little follow-up if the girls drop out of school."[4]

"My boyfriend isn't too good about this whole thing. When I'm scared or need something, I call my teacher or my mother, not him. He don't know what to say or do."[1]

Observations

Measurements

There are five Southern Baptist churches and one Episcopal church in Rosetown.

Percentage of adolescents aged 15-19 who have had sexual intercourse (US)[25]

	1970	1980	1990
White	23.2	33.6	42.3
Black	52.4	64.8	71.4
Total	27.6	46.0	53.4

Continued

Rosetown—4.52 square miles with an estimated population of 2793.[5]

Topography—flat terrain at an average of 150 inches above sea level.[5]

Nearest neighboring towns—25 miles to the east and 20 miles to the north.[5]

822 housing units in Rosetown; 316 tenants occupied.[8]

Value of houses in Rosetown—from $8500 to $150,000; average—$21,400 ($90,000 median for the US).[9]

Average temperature	64.2° F
Maximum temperature	85.5° F
Minimum temperature	48.3° F
Average rainfall	26.2"
Average relative humidity	57.7%

Interacting subsystems
Physical environment

Appearance

Rural farming community bordered by Strong River on western boundary and surrounded by farmland, artificial boundaries on east, north, and south. State routes 61 and 8 divide the area. Area is combination of residential and farmland.

Many houses in need of repair; houses very close together, particularly in black segregated areas. One neighborhood observed with larger lots and houses in good condition, lawns well maintained with shrubbery and flower gardens. New housing projects provide low-cost housing for lower income families. Animals roaming free in streets. Farm houses older than housing in town; many houses do not have adequate plumbing or protection from weather. Roofs in bad condition. Yards littered with old cars and farm equipment. Streets in need of repair. Speed limit is 35 mph in rural areas, 15 mph in town. No center line markings on streets other than highway. Children seen riding bikes on streets. People observed "hanging around" bars and stores all during day and night.

High school built in 1921 and in need of repair. Inadequate lighting, no air conditioning, gas heat, crowded classrooms. Students seen laughing and talking quietly outside building. Class change quiet and orderly.

Parenting class for pregnant teens held in spacious home economics classroom with fetal models, growth charts, and pelvic models present. Audiovisual equipment observed and used. Students in class actively participating in activities with obvious interest.

"Some of our houses are in real bad shape. We have a federal grant which will help us remodel for some of these folks."[6]

"We are real proud of our housing projects in town. They help out our poor a great deal."[6]

"We have the richest soil in the world here in the Rosetown area. We can grow anything."[2]

"The unemployment situation is very serious in our town. Folks just stand around with nothing to do."[2]

"We desperately need more room in our high school, and our buildings need repair."[3]

"We have a very friendly school with well-behaved students. We don't have the problems that a lot of the city high schools do, with drugs and guns."[14]

"We can walk to our doctor's appointments from school, which helps a lot. The welfare office is only 10 minutes from school, too."[1]

Subjective data	Observations	Objective data
		Measurements

Interactions

Interacting subsystems—cont'd

Physical environment—cont'd

"I have been trying to get a neighborhood watch up for 2 years without success; no one seems concerned or interested."[10]

"We have a real friendly, quiet little town."[11]

"We fry everything around here, and we tend to use salt pork in all of our vegetables. We really eat a lot of salty foods."[12]

"My favorite foods are hamburgers and pizza, and my doctor won't let me eat them while I'm pregnant 'cause of my blood pressure. I can't wait until I can have my mother's french fries again."[1]

Health and welfare services

The city has applied for a federally funded physician and clinic.[6]

"Most of our patients in Rosetown do not pay fees because of their income."[3]

"The girls from the high school use the prenatal and well-child health dept. services and are encouraged to do so by their teachers. They rarely miss appointments. The problem as I see it is that they don't come to family planning. They just don't seem to want to prevent pregnancy. We just aren't getting to them."[3]

Observations

No neighborhood watch. Business district located in center of town.

Sounds

No heavy industry present in town; loud cars without mufflers evident.

Tastes

Southern style cooking preferences: fried chicken, fried vegetables, steak, and tamales. Fast-food hamburgers and pizza establishments frequented by teens. People very friendly in local restaurants, eager to share recipes and ingredients.

Smells

Pleasant smell of flowers. Noxious odors noted in rural areas from aerial spraying of pesticides on crops. No pollution index available. Gas fumes noted around highways.

Health department and physician's office within walking distance of school. Welfare office—3 blocks away.

No hospitals in Rosetown. A 135-bed regional hospital is 21 miles away in neighboring city.

Physician's office within five blocks of high school.

No emergency center services in Rosetown.

Medical/health services, including dental and eye clinics, are provided free by the Levee Clinic, which is federally funded. There are two physicians, one nurse, two dentists, and a part-time optometrist. There are two pharmacists in two different drug stores. Ambulance service is available within a 25-mile radius of Rosetown, 24 hours a day, housed in the fire department and staffed with four

Continued

The health dept. offers comprehensive services 5 days a week:
- Immunizations
- Midwife and physician services 2 days a week at prenatal clinic (Tue and Thurs)
- TB screening at schools once a year and three times a week at clinic
- Well-child clinic, 2 days a week (nurse practitioner, pediatrician)

Large number of persons in waiting room of health department and welfare office.

There is one school nurse, but her services are limited to the elementary and junior high schools.

Home health care services available on referral from physician.[8]

Occupational safety services are provided in various industries. There is no occupational health service in Rosetown.

For developmentally disabled children and adults: services available on referral from State Mental Health and through local school system.[8]

For ages 5 years to 21 years: developmental classes, physical and speech therapist services, psychological services.[8]

No health profession training available within 50-mile radius; nearest nursing school (A.D. and B.S.N.)—62 miles; nearest medical school in state medical center—150 miles away.

Rosetown Connection bus with full load.

By calling federally funded bus line (Rosetown Connection) 1 day in advance, any resident may be picked up at home and transported free of charge to any health or social service location.

Services for mentally handicapped in school and through mental health center in town 21 miles away.[14]

"We could really use one more bus. The people in Rosetown depend on us since most all services are in Cleveton."[17]

No utilization statistics readily available.

One private day care center accepts children over the age of 9 months.[16]

No low-cost child care services are available for children under the age of 4. Headstart available at 4 years free to all residents.[16]

Health promotion activities:
- Physical education classes in junior and senior high schools.
- Stress management taught in home economics
- Smoking and drug education offered twice per year at high school
- Recreational activities primarily organized by individuals
- Nutrition classes offered in home economics and through home demonstration office[13]

All health and social services are available on a sliding scale with most residents classified as "A," which means they are below poverty level and do not pay fees.[16]

Mental health services are available free in the county seat 21 miles away. Includes all counseling: drug abuse, teens, children, and psychiatric referral.[8]

No counseling available in Rosetown except through local ministers.[16]

No parenting classes for community at large.[3]

"Sometimes I think that Rosetown is in the middle of nowhere. I have problems with my blood pressure and sugar diabetes, so I have to go to the medical center 100 miles away once a month. I have to miss school for a day, and my mother or aunt has to miss work to take me. I wish we had these special doctors closer."[1]

No crisis intervention, except in neighboring town's mental health center and hospital emergency room.[16]

No telephone hot line services within 100 miles.[16]

Meals on Wheels by the Commission on Aging for the town's elderly residents.[16]

Audiologist and speech pathologist 20 miles away. Available through referral from health dept. and school system.[3]

Subjective data		Objective data
Interactions	**Observations**	**Measurements**

Welfare services:
Welfare department has a branch office located in Rosetown, which is open 5 days a week and dispenses food stamps and welfare payments.[16]

"I worry that too many of our residents, particularly our young girls, get dependent on the welfare system. I like to see this as temporary assistance only until girls can get an education and get a job. The office really needs to encourage education for pregnant girls more than they do."[6]

Observations: High degree of usage, as indicated by full waiting room in welfare office each day.

Economics

"We need more jobs for our young men and women. They have to move away to get off welfare."[2]

Observations: Farming is the leading occupation, and industry is second. Leading crops are soybeans, rice, cotton, and catfish.[5]

Measurements:
County unemployment rate (1994): 11.6%[18], state unemployment rate: 10.2% (1994).[36]
Unemployment rate 18 and under: 72% (1994).[18]
Unemployment rate for aggregate: 100% (1994).
No pregnant high school girls are employed.[4]
Median family income: $11,216.00[18], state median family income: $14,500.00.[36]
50.2% of families are below poverty level (1994).[18]
Shopping facilities:
Four grocery stores, four appliance/hardware supply stores, three gas stations, two banks with combined assets of $32,828,000.00, two drug stores, three attorneys, one CPA, and one insurance agent.[6]
Three major industries are located in Rosetown: Apco Metal Products employing 260 persons: 175 females and 85 males; Riverco, a marine construction company employing 139 persons: 135 males and 4 females; Searight, a grain-processing company employing 100 persons: 85 males and 15 females.[6]

Safety and transportation

"Sometimes I feel unsafe in the crowded halls of school, like I could fall or something and hurt my baby."[1]
The crime rate is low in Rosetown, with no murders or homicides recorded in the past 6 years.[19]
"We have a quiet, safe little town. No one really bothers anyone else here. Our biggest crime problem is with petty theft and breaking and entering."[19]
An airport and a Greyhound bus station are 25 miles away; train services 30 miles away.[17]
Handicapped services not readily available except through welfare services in town 21 miles away. Rosetown Connection is accessible for wheelchairs.[17]

Observations: Transportation is primarily through private car or on foot.
Bus service is available free to surrounding towns for needed services.

Measurements:
Police protection: five full-time and two part-time police officers; three police cars with two-way radio contact with county police department.[19]
Fire protection: 35 man volunteer fire dept. two 500 gpm (gallons per minute) pumper trucks, one utility truck available in town; ambulance housed in fire department building.[20]
Flouridated water via three wells. Water is treated at waste water treatment plant. Plant has 1,663,200 gpd (gallons per day) and peak capacity of 420,000 gpd. Plans are to overhaul complete system to update equipment.[21]

Continued

Informal leaders: two ministers and a local café owner.

Formal communication
School paper produced monthly.
Two radio stations accessible to community.
Three television stations accessible to residents.
75% of residents have telephones.
90% of residents have televisions.[5]

The average number of years of education in the US for an adolescent who has a child prior to age 20 is 10.8.[28] This information was unavailable from Rosetown.
One public library in Rosetown, open 9-12 AM Mon–Fri.[25]
There are two elementary schools, two junior high schools, and one high school.

Compact treatment plant with a 0.4 million gpd capacity.[21]

No political activism observed.

Aggregate leadership not formally identified. Teacher of class for pregnant teens holds formal leadership position.

Aggregate members communicate through parenting class experiences and through common experiences at clinic.

Informal communication
Billboard advertisements frequently are of liquor and restaurants.
The newspaper contained no stories about available contraception services or risks of teen pregnancy.
National media observed focusing on teen pregnancy.
No members of aggregate visible at community meetings.

"Our treatment plant is quite adequate since we are using it at 50% capacity."[21]
Entire community has access to sewage disposal.[22]
Garbage disposal is done with city trash collection. Sanitary landfill 5 miles outside city limits.[21]
Mosquitos are continuous vectors: problem is due to the rice fields. Spraying to control mosquitos is done in city limits weekly during peak season of summer.[21]

Politics and government
Weekly town meetings open for the first hour.[6]
Mayor and four council members from the Rosetown city government structure. Current issues: attract a clinic from federal government and decrease unemployment.[6]
"We are pretty much conservative Southern Baptists here in Rosetown."[2]
"If you want to get anything started or finished, talk to Reverend Taylor; everybody respects and listens to him."[23]
"We listen to our teacher when she directs us; she knows better what we need than any of us. She's looking out for us."[1]

Communication
"Sometimes the only people I can talk to are the girls in my parenting class—they understand what I'm going through better than anybody."[1]
"If you want to know something about our town, hang out at Hank's Barber Shop—you'll soon find out."[2]
Barber shop is center of information dissemination for residents of Rosetown.[24]
Bulletin boards in local supermarkets and businesses advertise parenting class at high school for girls who have dropped out of school.[4]
Rosetown News published weekly, carries pictures and announcements of local events.[24]
About ¾ of community residents receive local newspaper.[24]

Education
One class per day at Rosetown High offered to pregnant girls and to girls with infants up to 1 year of age. A night parenting class has been available for girls who have dropped out of school for 6 months. The teacher reported that at least three students from the night class have started back to school. Number of students varies from 6-9 per class.[4]

Subjective data	Objective data	
Interactions	Observations	Measurements

Interacting subsystems—cont'd

Education—cont'd

Special services available for physically and mentally handicapped students. Bus services provided free to students living within the district.[13]

"I like having classes with all of the students, but I also like having a special class for pregnant girls. I look forward to hearing from the other girls about how they're getting along."[1]

Recreation

"I usually don't feel much like getting out in shorts anymore and going out for gym. I would rather walk after school."[1]

"I get enough exercise out in the fields—I just want to rest when I'm off."[26]

Rosetown has no physical fitness center.

No organized recreational program in Rosetown. Physical education is available as an option to all high school students.

Recreational facilities are widely observed to be used at a high rate.

All pregnant teens at Rosetown High are or have been enrolled in physical education classes.

Public recreational facilities:
- three ball fields
- one swimming pool
- four tennis courts
- two local parks

There is one private country club available to members only with the following facilities: one golf course, one tennis court, and one swimming pool.[27]

Analysis/Synthesis of Data

Core Structure

The aggregate of pregnant teens of Rosetown High School participates in very few community activities and appears to be marginal to the community structure. The *self-concept* of these pregnant teens varies from feeling special to feeling ashamed. *Historically,* adolescent pregnancy has been demonstrated by national and state statistics to be a risk factor in terms of low birth weight infants, infant mortality, unemployment, poverty, and low educational achievement. Nationally, the number of teens who engage in sexual intercourse has steadily increased to an estimated 53%. *Culturally,* Rosetown is an ethnically mixed community with a large percentage of the population younger than 45 years. The total population has remained essentially unchanged at 2791 persons. The population of the high school has remained consistent. The infant mortality for the county of the aggregate is high, the percentage of teens who gives birth is high, and the state infant mortality rate of the aggregate is high.

Rosetown teens seek prenatal care later than adults and are much less likely to use any type of birth control before or after the first pregnancy, according to the local public health nurse. The birth rate for the aggregate based on number of *known* pregnancies is more than twice that of state and U.S. rates and significantly higher than the county rate. The median number of years of school completed by the aggregate is 10.6 compared with 12.2 for the state.

Statistics show that the greatest number of residents is between 18 and 45 years of age. Almost half (48.2%) of the population is younger than 18 years; the gender ratio is about equal. The aggregate has a birth rate twice that of the national and county birth rate average. The percentage of female-headed households in Rosetown is over twice the U.S. average, and the median income is $11,216, well below the state average of $14,500 and the national average of $23,300. The unemployment rate is 12.4%, higher than the state average of 10.2% and the national average of 8.1%. The aggregate of pregnant teens has a 100% unemployment rate of those in high school.

Teen pregnancy exposes the young female to economic, social, and biological risks based on research and statistics from national and state sources. Consequently, teenage pregnancy is considered a stressor that has the potential for causing disequilibrium in the system. Pregnant teens are much less likely to complete high school, more likely to deliver a low birth weight infant, and less likely to seek prenatal care during the first trimester.[28] Pregnancy affects the teenager's future and, according to Neuman's system model, would cause a significant degree of reaction.[29] *Degree of reaction* is the amount of disequilibrium or disruption that results from stressors affecting an aggregate's lines of defense.[29]

Social support is provided to pregnant teens through special classes, the prenatal clinic, their family, and WIC. However, no child care is available for teens who want to complete high school after giving birth.

These statistics reveal that Rosetown is *economically* and socially depressed, and that the aggregate is at specific risk. The age distribution and birth rates for the area provide documentation of the need for specific health care facilities and services for females of childbearing age.

The leading causes of death in Rosetown are in the same rank and order as that for the nation, as indicated in the Surgeon General's Report on Health Prevention.[34]

Interacting Subsystems

Rosetown is a rural community interspersed with farmland, housing developments, and business. The *physical environment* is adequate and in a temperate climate. Community residents have an adequate supply of clean water for drinking, bathing, and recreational needs. The area is adequately supplied with telephone service and energy sources. The pollutants were identified as pesticides and gasoline odors. The positive environmental aspects of pure water and clean air is congruent with Nightingale's environmental standards.

There is adequate police and fire protection. *Safety* is a major community strength.

The rural isolation of Rosetown affects the members of the community and members of the aggregate, specifically regarding health care services for specific needs. The primary mode of *transportation* is the private car, with the Rosetown Connection free bus service available for transport to social and health services in nearby cities.

The community of Rosetown is *governed* by a mayor and elected aldermen. Council meetings are poorly attended, and *political* interest appears low. Decision-making power is concentrated in the leadership of the community, formal and informal, with little involvement of the community residents. The aggregate of pregnant teens has very little power within the school and the community. Their needs are represented through a spokesperson, a teacher in the high school.

Communication exists through both formal and informal channels. The aggregate members communicate with each other in a class specifically designed for their special needs. A variety of modes are used to transmit information to the community residents. Citizens and aggregate members appear to be informed about social and health services available to them. Community meetings are not well attended; no aggregate involvement was observed. A school newspaper and community newspaper are published for school and community residents, respectively.

Educational services are delivered through a total of two elementary schools, two junior high schools, and one high school. Special services are available for mentally and physically handicapped students. Free bus service is provided to all students living in the school district.

Recreational facilities are limited, primarily restricted to public parks. Protective services are provided by fire and police departments. Services appear to be adequate to cover Rosetown's needs. Housing varies in quality, with much of the population living in substandard living conditions. The average value of a house in Rosetown is $21,400 compared with $90,000 nationally.

Health and welfare services for pregnant teens are described under preventive health services, health promotion, and health protection.

Preventive health services. Childbearing during teenage years is a high-risk experience for both mother and child; it also presents social risks for the community. A major concern that urgently needs addressing is underutilization of contraceptive counseling and services available free 5 days a week at the health department. These services serve as *lines of resistance,* which, according to Neuman's model, are internal mechanisms that act to defend against stressors. They represent a community strength. Special needs of the adolescent mother, as a result of biological risks and child care services needed, are not available in the local community.

Comprehensive prenatal care services are available in Rosetown through the health department and private clinics. Clinics are within walking distance of the high school. Infant care is available after the age of 9 months through a private day care center. Child care for low income persons is not available until the child reaches 4 years of age. Well-child care is available through the health department. Special health care services are available in neighboring towns, with transportation provided free. The residents and members of the aggregate were aware of the availability of services.

Health promotion services. Health promotion activities for the aggregate are primarily offered at the high school, including nutrition classes, physical education classes, and stress management. Health promotion activities are sporadic in Rosetown. The high school offers special programs twice a year on tobacco and drug use. Sports are organized by residents, with no planned recreational program. Facilities for recreation are limited to public parks and the country club (members only). Benefits of these recreational activities are low costs, open participation, promotion of community cohesiveness, and family involvement. Constraints are the time and energy required for the organization and execution of the activities.

Residents of the community who are involved in farming engage in physical exertion activities. Other occupations do not require physical activity, and the aggregate members do not reflect an interest in the benefits of exercise. No community effort has been made to educate the public regarding these types of health promotion activities.

Health protection. Environmental protection services are provided by the health department, including sanitation and environmental inspection. Vector control is a significant problem in Rosetown, and mosquitoes are prevalent. Accident safety and education are offered in all grades of the schools. Occupational safety services are provided for workers in local industries.

Nursing Diagnosis

Two nursing diagnoses have been identified and arranged in order of priority. Plans have been formulated for only the first diagnosis.

1. Potential for increased incidence of teen pregnancy related to increased sexual activity and nonuse of contraceptive services
2. Potential for increased school dropout of teen mothers related to inaccessibility of child care services for children younger than 4 years

Nursing diagnosis: Potential for increased incidence of teen pregnancy related to increased sexual activity and nonuse of contraceptive services (3/12/94).

Long-term expected outcome: The Rosetown High School population will have a decreased pregnancy rate by June 1996.

Short-term expected outcomes	Nursing orders	Scientific rationale	Evaluation
1. Community will have access to information regarding the risks of teen pregnancy by October 1994.	1a. Interview health care providers regarding perception and incidence of problem.	*Content:* Teen pregnancy. *Strategy:* Change process and principles of community health nursing practice. **Unfreezing** 1a. Implies that for change to take place, community has to become dissatisfied with status quo.[30] Local health care providers often serve as community gatekeepers; community residents tend to respond to those with informal power.[33] Empirical rational mode of change implies that humans are rational and will make informed decisions after information is presented.[32]	**Outcome criteria** 1. Media will communicate informative news stories concerning incidence, risks and prevention of teen pregnancy. 2. Community residents will acknowledge and respond by discussion with each other about above information. 3. Specific community organizations and groups will request programs to inform the aggregate of teen pregnancy risks. **Ongoing:** Who was contacted and what was their response?
	1b. Contact local newspapers regarding incidence of teen pregnancy in community. Offer to write series of articles regarding Incidence and risks of teen pregnancy to teen and community Interviews with local leaders physicians, teachers, clergy, school board members, and public health officials regarding the problem	1b. Essential elements for reducing teen pregnancy include education of public to understand economic, biological, and social risks.[28]	Was newspaper contacted? Were articles printed?
	1c. Solicit several people to write to newspapers commenting on the problem and suggesting measures to decrease incidence of teen pregnancy.	1c. Quoting community residents and leaders promotes concern necessary for social action.[31]	Were letters to newspapers written and printed?
	1d. Encourage aggregate and community residents to call local talk radio station and comment on articles.	1d. Keep issue before public to raise consciousness of community residents.[31]	Were radio stations contacted? What was the response? Did health professionals participate in community talk shows?
2. Community will take action to inform the aggregate population of risks of teen pregnancy by April 1995.	2a. Encourage school board to form a task force to plan sex education, including contraceptive counseling, to be offered in junior and high school courses: Task force to be composed of parents, teachers, clergy, physician, nurse, and other health professionals and aggregate members	**Moving to the new level** 2a. Community involvement will influence whether change will be accepted.[30] Formal and informal community leaders, as well as aggregate members, need to be involved in decision-making.[33]	**Outcome criteria** 1. School board will have teen pregnancy as an agenda item at monthly meeting. 2. A task force will be formed with active participation by members. 3. The program will include information on incidence, risks, and prevention.

Continued

Nursing diagnosis: Potential for increased incidence of teen pregnancy related to increased sexual activity and nonuse of contraceptive services (3/12/94).

Long-term expected outcome: The Rosetown High School population will have a decreased pregnancy rate by June 1996.

Short-term expected outcomes	Nursing orders	Scientific rationale	Evaluation
	Task force to look at specific content and the options of program: Elective or required With parental permission During school or after school hours.	It is important to encourage collaboration between and among groups.[33]	4. A contraceptive counseling course will be implemented in junior and senior high schools. 5. A citizen's task force will be formed with active participation by members.
	2b. Support total community involvement and acceptance by supporting task force effort in local media. 2c. Contact health department, local health care providers, and service organizations regarding available services, cost, and community acceptance of this type of service.		**Ongoing** Was a task force formed? When? Who was on task force? Was there interest evident by task force members? What content will be taught? Where and when will course be taught? Who will teach it? Who will be required to attend? Was health department contacted? Was information shared with members of aggregate? What was the response?
	2d. Suggest to school board the formation of a citizen's task force to look further into the concern.	2d. Decisions regarding content and course planning by community facilitates community acceptance.[33]	Was a citizen's task force formed? Why or why not? Was there interest evident by task force members?
		Refreeze at new level	**Outcome criteria**
3. Community will provide contraceptive education in junior and high schools by August 1995.	3a. Act as resource for implementing contraceptive education, including class involvement and evaluation. 3b. Encourage school staff to share information about progress of contraceptive education with parents and community residents through the following: PTA meetings Media Written and oral correspondence	3a. Provided change has been brought about through community forces, it should continue.[30] 3b. Essential elements of controlling teen pregnancy are sex education, contraceptive counseling, and decision-making.[28] Rosetown has demonstrated active participation in community decisions; acceptability of services is more likely when community is involved in decision-making.[31]	1. There will be an increase in contraceptive services offered by the health department. 2. Everyone in community will have access to such services, regardless of ability to pay. 3. Confidentiality will be ensured. **Ongoing** Was program implemented as planned? If not, why not? What modifications were made in the original program?
	3c. Monitor contraceptive services of health department utilization by aggregate members and sexually active teens.	3c. Essential to successful program planning is determining what community residents perceive that they need and the motivation to achieve these needs.[31]	Who was contacted? By whom? When? What facilities available? What was cost? Community acceptance? Did meeting evaluation criteria lead to goal achievement? **Concluding** Were evaluation criteria met?

REFERENCES*

1 Aggregate members: Interviews.
2 Community residents: Interviews.
3 Rosetown Health Department nurse: Interview.
4 High school faculty member (teaches class for pregnant teens): interview.
5 Chamber of Commerce: This is Rosetown (pamphlet).
6 Mayor of Rosetown: Interview.
7 National Weather Service: National Weather Service Bulletin.
8 Rosetown Bureau of Social Service: Resource Directory.
9 President of Board of Realtors: Interview.
10 PTA president: Interview.
11 Rotary Club President: Interview.
12 County home economist: Interview.
13 Rosetown High School principal: Interview.
14 Rosetown High School guidance counselor: Interview.
15 United States Bureau of the Census, 1990.
16 Social worker, Rosetown Welfare Department: Interview.
17 Rosetown transportation manager: Interview.
18 Rosetown annual report.
19 Rosetown Police Chief: Interview.
20 Rosetown Fire Chief: Interview.
21 Health Department environmental engineer: Interview.
22 Rosetown City Manager: Interview.
23 Rosetown Town Council member: Interview.
24 Newspaper editor, *Rosetown Review:* Interview.
25 Rosetown Public Library Director: Interview.
26 Community resident, farmer: interview.
27 Rosetown Recreational Services Director: Interview.
28 Alan Guttmacher Institute: *Teenage pregnancy: the problem that hasn't gone away,* New York, 1981, The Institute.
29 Neuman B: *The Neuman systems model: applications in nursing education and practice,* ed 3, Norfolk, Conn, 1989, Appleton and Lange.
30 Lewin K: *Field theory in social science,* New York, 1951, Harper & Brothers.
31 Stanhope M and Lancaster J: *Community health nursing,* ed 3, St Louis, 1992, Mosby–Year Book.
32 Bennis WG et al: *The planning of change,* ed 3, New York, 1976, Holt, Rinehart, & Winston.
33 Klein DC: *Community dynamics and mental health,* New York, 1968, John Wiley & Sons.
34 US Department of Health, Education, and Welfare: *Healthy people 2000: national health promotion and disease prevention objectives,* Washington, DC, 1990, US Government Printing Office.
35 US Department of Health and Human Services: National Center for Health Statistics, Monthly Vital Statistics Report, 1988.
36 Research Development Center: *Handbook of selected data,* (state and US), 1990.

*References 1-27 are fictitious.

Glossary

accountability Ability to explain rationale for actions taken that is consistent with the responsibility for which the nurse contracted.

advocate One who acts in the interest of the health care consumer.

assessment Ongoing process of data collection and analysis/synthesis of data that results in conclusions about the client's health concerns and strengths.

autonomy The freedom to develop and control oneself.

biomedical domain Collaborative, interdependent nursing actions related to the client's pathological condition or medical treatment.

caring Concerned with or interested in another's well-being.

catalyst Person who promotes actions and reactions and enables them to proceed under optimum conditions.

client Individual, family, group, or community.

collaboration Joint effort for the purpose of creating change toward a mutually desired outcome.

colleague Peer functioning in a group in which each member openly shares knowledge and has equal opportunity to exercise power and authority.

communication techniques (facilitative) Methods used to promote open dialogue between people.

clarifying Asking the client what was meant by a particular statement or question.

consensual validation Asking client the meaning of a particular word that was used in the conversation.

focus Restrict discussion to obtain specific information.

open-ended statements and questions Statements and questions that cannot be answered with a "yes" or "no" answer.

reflect feelings or content Share with the client your (interviewer's) thoughts or feelings of the content spoken.

related questions Questions that are relevant to previous statements for the purpose of obtaining more information about the topic.

restate, repeat main idea Restate what the client said verbatim or pull together the main idea of what the client said and state it. This is used to promote elaboration on the topic or validation of what was said.

sharing perceptions Telling the client what your (interviewer's) impressions are of a given statement or situation.

summarize Share with the client succinct impressions or conclusions drawn from data.

verbalize the implied State what the client implied to validate the interviewer's impressions.

community Specific population living within a defined perimeter; or group that has common values, interests, or needs.

community process How the components of a community system function.

community structure Arrangement of animate or inanimate properties or parts of a community at a given moment.

comprehensive Reflecting the totality or wholeness of the client's life experiences.

concept Complex mental formulation of objects, events, or ideas that can be symbolized by a word.

conceptual model Matrix of concepts, theories, or ideas that are interrelated but in which the precise interrelationships among the concepts are not clearly defined.

concluding evaluation Description of whether and to what degree the long-term expected outcomes have been achieved.

concurrent evaluation Ongoing examination of activities as they occur.

consultation Invited communication with an expert who serves in an advisory capacity for the purpose of information exchange or analysis.

continuum Continuous whole whose fundamental common character is discernible amid a series of variations.

coordination Regulation and combination of effort for harmonious performance.

criteria statement Statement reflecting the expected qualities, attributes, or characteristics that measure a client's achievements toward expected outcomes.

data Units of subjective and objective information obtained through the use of the senses and the designated methods of observation, interaction, and measurement.

dependent Relying on or requiring the support of others for the authority to perform activities.

depleted health Alteration in the dynamic pattern of functioning whereby there is an inability to interact with internal and external forces as the result of a temporary or permanent loss of necessary resources.

developmental needs Any requirement arising from the natural process of situational concerns of growth and differentiation.

diagnosis Clear, concise, definitive statement of the client's health status and concerns that can be affected by nursing intervention.

empirical knowledge Knowledge obtained through the conscious use of the senses and grounded in scientific investigation; the science of nursing.

esthetic knowledge Knowledge or meaning gained by the creation or appreciation of subjective expression; the art of nursing.

ethical knowledge Knowledge that includes both goals and actions in an attempt to do what is good or right; the moral component in nursing.

evaluation Systematic, continuous process of comparing the client's response or observable behavior with the established expected outcomes.

family Dynamic system of two or more individuals who consider themselves a family and share a history, common goals, obligations, instrumental and affectional bonds and ties, and a high degree of intimacy.

family process Functions and group interactions by which the family operates; salient features that differentiate it from another collection of individuals.

family structure Names, ages, health states, and occupations of family members.

health Dynamic pattern of functioning whereby there is continued interaction with the internal and external forces that results in the optimal use of necessary resources that serve to minimize vulnerabilities.

health care system Organized distribution of services and personnel to meet the health needs of others.

health care team Organized group of health care workers who have common goals, cooperative relationships, and coordinated activities related to the health care needs of the client or group of clients.

health concern Actual or potential health problem, disability, deficit, or limitation.

health maintenance Act of protecting and preserving patterns of maximum potential for health.

health promotion Advancement of patterns of functioning that foster and encourage optimal health.

health restoration Advancement of patterns of functioning from depleted or impaired health to health maintenance.

health status State of health.

holistic View that an integrated whole has a reality independent of and greater than the sum of its parts.

impaired health Alteration in the dynamic pattern of functioning whereby there is a diminished ability to interact with internal and external forces as the result of a reduction in necessary resources.

implementation Nurse and client executing the plans.

independent Assuming autonomous authority to perform activities.

inference Judgment made from data obtained compared with health norms, concepts, principles, or standards.

interdependent Mutually collaborative effort in performing health care activities with other health care professionals and the client.

interpretation (personal) Individually biased perception of a given event that may be judgmental.

interviews Transitory relationships or exchanges of information that are goal directed.

　directive-interrogative Discussion between client and nurse for the purpose of obtaining information.

　open-ended Discussion between client and nurse for the purposes of obtaining information and building rapport.

　rapport-building Discussion between client and nurse for the purpose of establishing a relationship.

intuition Awareness of meanings, relationships, and possibilities by way of insight without conscious knowledge.

leader Person with foresight who is able to influence others in a positive direction, who is accountable for his or her own beliefs, who is willing and able to take risks, and who accepts power and uses it judiciously.

leadership Complex relationship between individuals whereby interpersonal influence is exercised through the process of communication toward the achievement of specific goals.

long-term expected outcome Broad or abstract statement of a client-expected observable behavior that is relatively long-term in nature.

maximum potential for health Client's ability to achieve or develop the highest pattern of functioning possible within his or her health perimeter.

measurable Able to be determined in terms of extent, dimension, rate, rhythm, quantity, or size; used for a given behavior, performance, or characteristic.

methods for data collection Means by which the nurse obtains data from the client.

　interaction Mutual or reciprocal exchange of verbal information.

　measurement Use of all the senses, as well as instruments, to allow quantitative value of observations.

　observation Use of all the senses to obtain information about a client.

multifocal View that clients are composed of multiple foci, such as biophysical, spiritual, psychological, developmental, and sociocultural.

nonjudgmental Free from personal interpretation and bias.

norm Generally accepted range of behavior, performance, or characteristics.

nursing domain Independent nursing actions related to health promotion, health maintenance, health restoration, and referral.

nursing orders/nursing prescription Actions chosen by the nurse and client to achieve the short- and long-term expected outcomes.

nursing process Deliberate intellectual activity whereby the practice of nursing is approached in an orderly, systematic manner. Components consist of assessment, diagnosis, planning, implementation, and evaluation.

ongoing evaluation Ongoing process for determining the completion of the short-term expected outcomes.

optimal health See maximum potential for health.

outcome domains Categories on which to base expected learning outcomes.

affective domain Reflects interests, attitudes, values, or feelings.

cognitive domain Reflects knowledge or intellectual abilities and skills.

psychomotor domain Reflects ability to perform a manipulative or motor skill.

pattern Composite sample of traits or behaviors that is characterized by rhythm, rate, intensity, duration, and amount.

perception Individual's idea of an event or situation that is based on the use of all senses and past experience.

performance Any behavior or outcome of a client that can be directly or indirectly assessed.

personal knowledge Knowledge gained through introspection, intuition, and the intentional development of self-awareness; the self in nursing.

philosophy Statement of a person's beliefs, values, and assumptions about a given phenomenon (e.g., nursing).

planning Determining how to assist the client in resolving concerns related to the restoration, maintenance, or promotion of health.

principles Guiding rules or laws that have been supported over time through research and/or practice.

process Interaction of the components of a given system.

process evaluation Examining the actions and interactions of the nurse.

reliable Stable, dependable, accurate, consistent, and relatively predictable.

research Systematic inquiry to discover facts or test theories to obtain valid answers to questions raised or solutions for concerns identified.

resource External or internal source of strength or assistance.

responsibility Obligation to fulfill the terms of implied or explicit contractual agreement in accord with professional and legal nursing standards.

retrospective evaluation Examining the nurse's actions for effectiveness after the client is discharged from care.

role Dyad that is an actual or expected behavior pattern determined by socialization, including the interaction and interpretation of given norms, status, or position.

short-term expected outcome Statement describing a specific client-expected observable behavior that is relatively short-term in nature.

spiritual Internal essence or quality that gives meaning to a client's existence.

standard Acceptable, expected level of performance that is established by authority, custom, or general consent.

strategy (nursing) Overall method or approach that serves as a guide for individual nursing orders.

structure Arrangement of animate or inanimate properties or parts of a given system at a given moment.

structure evaluation Examining physical facilities, types and availability of equipment, and organizational components.

synthesis Integration of theories and concepts into varied patterns.

systematic Organized and planned method of completing a given project.

theoretical framework Collection of concepts whose interrelationship describes or explains phenomena that have not been proven.

theory Internally consistent body of relational statements and concepts that describes, explains, controls, or predicts phenomena.

unique Way clients differ from each other by virtue of heredity, environment, particular experiences, perception of such experiences, and the manner in which they react to such experiences.

valid Quality of data or data collection method to accurately reflect what was intended to be reflected.

validation Process of determining accuracy of data.

verifiable Capable of having authenticity of data confirmed through a variety of sources.

vulnerability State of being at risk or susceptible.

APPENDIX B

Guidelines for the Nursing Process

A. Assessment
1. A systematic format is used for data collection.
2. The data are comprehensive and multifocal.
3. A variety of sources is used for data collection.
4. Appropriate methods are used for data collection.
5. The data are verifiable.
6. The data reflect updating of information.
7. The data are recorded and communicated appropriately.

B. Diagnosis
1. Analysis and synthesis of data
    a. Data are categorized.
    b. Data gaps and incongruencies are identified.
    c. Cues are clustered into patterns.
    d. Appropriate theories, models, concepts, norms, and standards are applied and compared with patterns.
    e. Health concerns and strengths are identified.
    f. Etiological relationships are proposed.
2. Diagnostic statements
    a. The nursing diagnosis is a statement of an actual, high-risk, or wellness health concern.
    b. The nursing diagnosis is written as a descriptive and etiological statement.
    c. The nursing diagnosis is concise and clear.
    d. The nursing diagnosis is client-centered, specific, and accurate.
    e. The nursing diagnosis provides direction for nursing intervention.
    f. The nursing diagnosis is the basis for independent and collaborative nursing actions/interventions.
    g. The nursing diagnoses are validated with the client.

C. Plans
1. Priorities
    a. Actual or imminent life-threatening concerns are considered before actual or potential health-threatening concerns.
    b. Temporal, human, and material resources are examined deliberately.
    c. The client is involved in determining the priority of concerns.
    d. Scientific and practice principles provide rationale for decisions.
2. Expected outcomes
    a. Expected outcomes are client-focused and reflect mutuality with the client.
    b. Long-term outcomes are appropriate to their respective diagnosis, and short-term outcomes are appropriate to their respective long-term outcome.
    c. Expected outcomes are realistic, reflecting the capabilities and limitations of the client.

d. Long-term expected outcomes include broad or abstract indicators of performance.

e. Short-term expected outcomes include specific indicators of performance.

f. Short-term outcomes are numbered in the appropriate sequence to achieve the long-term outcome.

g. Scientific and practice principles guide the establishment of long-term outcomes and development of short-term outcomes.

3. Strategies

a. Major strategies for implementation are identified.

b. Strategies are appropriate to their respective outcomes.

c. Strategies are based on scientific rationale.

d. Strategies are mutually determined with the client.

4. Nursing orders

a. Nursing orders are appropriate to their respective outcomes and strategy.

b. Scientific and practice principles provide rationale for orders.

c. Nursing orders incorporate the autonomy and individuality of the client.

d. Nursing orders indicate specific intended behaviors, giving direction to the nurse, client, and others.

e. Nursing orders reflect consideration of human, temporal, and material resources.

f. Nursing orders are numbered in sequence to achieve the short-term outcome.

g. Nursing orders are dated and include the signature of the responsible nurse.

h. Nursing orders are kept current and are revised as indicated.

i. Nursing orders include plans for termination of nursing services.

D. Implementation

1. The actions performed are consistent with the plan and occur after validation of the plan.

2. Interpersonal, intellectual, and technical skills are performed competently and efficiently in an appropriate environment.

3. The client's physical and psychological safety is protected.

4. Documentation of actions and client responses is evident in the health care record and care plan.

E. Evaluation

1. The nurse reviews the client's expected outcomes and identifies relevant indicators to monitor changes in the client's health status.

2. The nurse continuously monitors, appraises, and reassesses the client's response to nursing actions.

3. The client's response to nursing actions is compared with the client's short-term outcomes to determine the extent to which these outcomes have been achieved (*ongoing evaluation*).

4. The client's progress or lack of progress toward achievement of long-term expected outcomes is determined (*concluding evaluation*).

5. The nursing care plan is reviewed to determine which actions are effective or ineffective in assisting the client's progress.

6. The nursing care plan is revised to reflect changes in the client's condition, or when the short-term or long-term expected outcomes have not been adequately met.

Assessment Tools for the Individual Client

Example of a Nursing History Form Based on Marjory Gordon's Functional Health Patterns.*

ROCKFORD MEMORIAL HOSPITAL ADMISSION/ASSESSMENT RECORD

GENERAL INFORMATION

Date _____ Time _____ Mode of Entry _____ From _____ To Room _____

Accompanied by: Name _____ Phone _____

Person to Contact _____

Disposition of: Clothes _____ Money/Jewelry _____ Meds _____

Oriented to: Bed _____ Bathroom _____ Intercom _____ Call Light _____

Personal electrical equipment inspected: (list) _____

Vitals: Temp _____ P _____ R _____ BP _____ HT _____ WT _____

PROCEDURES/TREATMENTS/NOTES *Documentation for Same-Day admission surgical patients*

_____
_____
_____
_____
_____

Signature _____

HEALTH AND ILLNESS PERCEPTION

STRENGTH _____ CONCERN _____
Remainder of this page omitted due to completion of pre-admission history ☐

Reason for this admission as stated by patient: (Describe symptoms) _____

Patient's understanding of problem: ☐ Excellent ☐ Good ☐ More explanation needed

Describe previous general health: _____

HEALTH HISTORY

Medical:	Surgical	Allergies and Transfusions: (describe reaction)

HEALTH MAINTENANCE

Menstruation _____ Self Breast Exam _____ Pap Smear _____ Last Period _____

Contraceptives _____ Testicular check/Prostate _____

Smoking _____ Pack/Day Caffeine _____ Alcohol _____ Recreational Drugs _____

Last Meal _____

Strength _____ Concern _____

FAMILY HISTORY

Diabetes _____   Arthritis _____
Cancer _____   TB _____
Hypertension _____ Seizures _____
Cardiac _____   Anemia _____
Renal _____
Other _____

MED/DOSE	TIMES	LAST DOSE	MED/DOSE	TIMES	LAST DOSE

Have you had problems maintaining your medication schedule: _____

ACTIVITY-EXERCISE-SELF CARE
(Please circle any positive findings)

STRENGTH _____ CONCERN _____

Exercise/Work Pattern/Energy Level: _____

Self-Care Abilities:
Grade ADL by 0 = independent; 1 = Needs Equipment; 2 = Needs Person; 3 = Equipment & Person; 4 = **Dependent**
Personal Hygiene: _____ Dressing: _____ Feeding: _____ Ambulating/Transfers: _____
Disabilities: _____ Prosthesis: _____ Equipment: _____

CARDIAC
Apical/radial strong and regular, chest pain, neck vein distention, pacemaker, palpitations, fainting, orthopnea, vertigo _____

PULMONARY
Normal/Abnormal breath sounds, coughing, asthma, hemoptysis, sputum, dyspnea, cyanosis

PERIPHERAL VASCULAR
Peripheral pulses present, varicosities, claudication, vascular access: (Describe) _____

NEURO-MUSCULAR-ORTHO
Orientation: _____
Sensation: _____
Movement: _____
Gait: _____

*Used with permission from Rockford Memorial Hospital, Rockford, IL.

ROCKFORD MEMORIAL HOSPITAL ADMISSION/ASSESSMENT RECORD

NUTRITIONAL & METABOLIC — STRENGTH — CONCERN

Special diet/Weight loss diet
Supplements — Intolerance
Weight gain or loss within last six months
Appetite
Poor swallowing, nausea and vomiting, poor dentition, change of taste

INTEGUMENTARY — STRENGTH — CONCERN

Warm and dry, rash, lesions, petechiae, jaundice, discoloration
Number identified areas and describe:

MUCOUS MEMBRANES/MOUTH — STRENGTH — CONCERN

Pink and moist
Teeth: — Dentures — Upper — Lower — Partial Plate
Hair: Distribution, texture, loss
Nails: Changes in color, texture

ELIMINATION — STRENGTH — CONCERN

BOWEL: Pattern: — Last Bowel Movement: — Bowel Sounds:
Bowel Management
Constipation, diarrhea, hemorrhoids, bleeding, incontinence, ostomy:
Change in appearance of stools:
URINE: Clear, incontinence, dribbling, retention, dysuria, urgency, frequency, hesitancy, nocturia, discharge, urinary diversion
Changes in appearance of urine:
Urinary Devices:
ABDOMEN: Soft, tender, distended, rigid

COGNITIVE & PERCEPTUAL — STRENGTH — CONCERN

Vision: — Visual Aids:
Hearing: — Hearing Aids:
Communication Barriers:
Thought Process Disturbances: Describe changes in memory, learning abilities, decision making:

PAIN — STRENGTH — CONCERN

Location:
Description:
Intensity (0-10): — Precipitating Factors:
Relieving Factors:

SLEEP - REST

STRENGTH
CONCERN
Sleep Pattern:
Hrs/Night: — Times:
Naps: — Aids/Rituals:
Problems getting to sleep, waking early, dreams, nightmares, confusion at night:

HOME MAINTENANCE — STRENGTH — CONCERN

1. Prior to this admission lived: Alone, With Family or other person, in Long Term Care Facility (— Name of Facility).
2. Prior to this admission, required assistance for activities of daily living: — Never, — days/month.
3. If support services were used at home, who provided them:
4. Considering the current reason for admission and recent history, what level of service is likely to be needed at discharge: None — Home Services — Long-Term Care

VALUES - BELIEFS — STRENGTH — CONCERN

Spiritual Needs: — Referral to Pastoral Services:

GROWTH AND DEVELOPMENT-ROLE RELATIONSHIP-COPING — STRENGTH — CONCERN

Who lives with you:
Occupation: — Who or what helps you handle stress:

Have you had any major life changes?

SAFETY

LEVEL I
— No problems noted at this time
— Inability to understand/follow directions

LEVEL II
— Age over 70
— History of falls prior to this admission (within 6 months)
— Hypotension, including orthostatic
— Incontinence - bowel or bladder
— Uncompensated Sensory Impairment - visual, auditory, or tactile
— Dizziness/balance problems

LEVEL IV
— Disoriented and restless
— One occurrence of falling during hospitalization
— Triad of ambulation difficulty, bowel/bladder incontinence or urgency, and inability to follow directions.

LEVEL III
— Disorientation or history of intermittent confusion

Level Assignment — Safety brochure discussed
Level Reassignment
Primary Nurse:
Signature: — Date
Signature: — Date

Example of a Nursing History Form Based on Dorothea Orem's Model.*

DATE_____ TIME_____ ARRIVAL TO UNIT: CART ☐ W/C ☐ AMBULATE ☐ ID BAND APPLIED ☐

ADMITTED FROM: HOME ☐ ER ☐ ECF ☐ OPSC ☐ Other _____

VALUABLES: Policy Explained ☐ Valuables: None ☐ Sent Home ☐ To Hospital Safe ☐ Kept by Patient ☐ _____

ASSISTIVE DEVICES BROUGHT IN: Glasses ☐ Dentures ☐ U ☐ L ☐ Partial ☐ Contact Lens ☐ Hearing Aid ☐ Prosthesis ☐ Brace ☐ Splint ☐

Walker ☐ Cane ☐ Crutches ☐ W/C ☐ Biogard Mattress ☐ Equipment labeled? Yes ☐ No ☐ Other_____

HEIGHT_____ **WEIGHT**_____ **SCALE**_____ T_____ P_____ R_____ BP_____

ORIENTATION TO ROOM: Bed ☐ Phone ☐ Call System in Reach ☐ Visiting Hours ☐ Smoking Policy ☐ TV ☐ CCTV ☐

TIME OF LAST FOOD/DRINK_____ Side Rails: UR ☐ UL ☐ LR ☐ LL ☐

INFORMATION GIVEN BY: Family Member ☐ Friend ☐ Patient ☐

Unable to Take History - Patient Unresponsive/Not Accompanied by Friend/Family ☐

SIGNATURE/TITLE_____

HEALTH DEVIATION

ALLERGIES Medication Allergies Document Reaction/Sensitivity _____

Allergens: (Food, Tapes, Dyes, Other) _____

Allergy Band Applied ☐

MEDICATIONS: Medication Policy Explained ☐ Medications Brought In: To Pharmacy ☐ Sent Home ☐

Current Medications (including over the counter drugs):

MEDICATION	DOSE	FREQUENCY	LAST TAKEN		MEDICATION	DOSE	FREQUENCY	LAST TAKEN

USE OF: Tobacco ☐ How Much _____ How Long _____

Alcohol ☐ How Much _____ How Long _____

Uncontrolled Substances/Drugs ☐ Type _____ How Long _____

Reason for Hospitalization/Expected Treatment (patient perception) _____

Past Illness: Heart Disease ☐ Hypertension ☐ Kidney Disease ☐ Hepatitis ☐ Seizures ☐ Neuro Disease ☐ GI Disorder ☐ Lung Disease ☐

Infections ☐ Skin Disorder ☐ Emotional Disorder ☐ Arthritis ☐ Bleeding Disorder ☐ Diabetes ☐ Other ☐

Cancer ☐ Site _____ Injury ☐ _____

Past Surgeries _____

Past Hospitalizations _____

Family History _____

BLOOD: Has blood been donated for you to use during hospitalization? Yes ☐ No ☐

Previous Blood Products Transfusion/Reaction ☐ _____

ORGAN

DONATION: Are you an organ donor? Yes ☐ No ☐

SIGNATURE/TITLE_____ DATE_____ TIME_____

*Used with permission from Scottsdale Memorial Hospital, Scottsdale, Ariz.

UNIVERSAL SELF CARE NEEDS

RESPIRATION INCLUDING CIRCULATION

Chest Pain ☐ Describe _____

Pacemaker ☐ Palpitations ☐ Claudication ☐ Edema ☐ Dizziness ☐

Shortness of Breath ☐ Without Exercise ☐ With Exercise ☐ Cough ☐ Sputum ☐ Color _____

Other _____

NUTRITION/FLUID CHEMICAL BALANCE

Diet_____Dietary Habits_____

Fluid Intake: No Problems ☐ Excessive ☐ Deficient ☐ Force Fluids ☐ Restriction ☐ Explain_____

Weight: No Change ☐ Gain ☐ Loss ☐ Amount of Weight Change_____

Oral/Dental: No Problems ☐ Explain_____

GI: No Problems ☐ Nausea ☐ Vomiting ☐ Dysphagia ☐ Anorexia ☐ Explain_____

ELIMINATION

Bowel Pattern: Date of Last Stool_____Soft/Formed ☐ Diarrhea ☐ Constipation ☐ Incontinent ☐ Bloody ☐ Tarry ☐ Hemorrhoids ☐

Recent Change ☐ Describe_____

Bladder Pattern: No Problems ☐ Incontinence ☐ Urgency ☐ Frequency ☐ Nocturia ☐ Dysuria ☐ Odor ☐ Cloudy ☐ Retention ☐ Self Cath ☐

Recent Change ☐ Describe_____Ostomy ☐ Type_____

NORMALCY

Understands English: Yes ☐ No ☐ Able to: Read ☐ Write ☐ If no, identify_____

Memory Loss: No Problems ☐ Short Term ☐ Long Term ☐ Difficult Learning ☐

Hearing: Normal ☐ Impaired_____Vision: Normal ☐ Impaired_____

Cognition: Able to Follow Simple Commands ☐ Responds Appropriately to Questions ☐ Unable to Follow Commands ☐

REPRODUCTIVE

Female - Last menstrual period_____Last Pap test_____ Pregnant_____ Vaginal Discharge/Bleeding ☐

Male - Prostate Problems ☐ Hernias ☐ Describe_____

Completes BSE ☐ TSE ☐ Frequency _____

Patient Education Resource: Pamphlet ☐ CCTV ☐ Other ☐_____

PSYCHOSOCIAL/SPIRITUAL

How do you manage stress? _____ Religious Considerations _____

Special concerns regarding hospitalization: No ☐ Yes ☐ Explain_____

Experienced life changes in the past year? No ☐ Yes ☐ Explain _____

PROTECTION AND COMFORT

Discomfort/Pain: ☐ Describe _____

How do you manage pain? _____

Risk for Skin Impairment: Low ☐ Med ☐ High ☐ R/T: Age 65 yrs plus ☐ Altered Mentation ☐ Altered Nutritional Status ☐

Altered Mobility ☐ Decreased Activity ☐ Incontinence ☐ Other ☐_____

Risk for Fall R/T: Age 65 yrs plus ☐ Hx of Falling ☐ Significant Disease/Symptoms ☐ Altered Mobility ☐ Language or Communication Barriers ☐

Sensory/Perceptual Alterations ☐ Altered Mentation/Medication ☐

Other _____

SIGNATURE/TITLE_____DATE_____TIME_____

ACTIVITY AND REST

Energy Level: Tires Easily ☐ Average ☐ High Energy ☐   Needs Assistance: Cane ☐ Walker ☐ W/C ☐ Crutches ☐ Other_____

Independent all functions ☐ or specify code

CODES
0 = Independent   1 = Assistive Device
2 = Assistance from person
3 = Assistance from person and device
4 = Dependent/Unable

Eating/Drinking_____Bed Mobility_____Shopping_____Bathing_____Transferring_____Cooking_____

Dressing/Grooming_____Ambulating_____Home Maintenance_____Toileting_____Stair Climbing_____

Exercise Yes ☐ No ☐ Type _____   How often _____

Does anything limit your activity?_____

Usual hours of sleep?_____Sleep alterations ☐   Explain_____

DISCHARGE PLANNING ASSESSMENT

Others living at home with you/home living arrangements: _____

Support Systems (Close Friend/Family Member) with Phone Number _____

Who is able to help you with care at home? _____

Utilization of Community Resources: None ☐ Home Care ☐ Homemaker/Aide Service ☐ Meals on Wheels ☐ Church Group ☐

  Support Group ☐ Name _____

Services Pre-hospitalization: None ☐

Home Care ☐   If Yes, Agency _____

                    Last Visit Date _____

Meal Service ☐ Chore Service ☐ Other ☐ _____

Environmental: No Problems ☐

Architectural Barriers in Home: Yes ☐ No ☐ Bathroom easily accessable? Yes ☐ No ☐

Bed on First Level? Yes ☐ No ☐

Stairs in Home ☐ Stairs to Enter Home ☐ Specify _____

Transportation: No Problems ☐ Transport to Appointments ☐ Specify _____

Financial: No Problems ☐ Unable to Obtain Medications ☐ Assist with Insurance ☐

Other ☐ _____

Teaching Needs Prior to Discharge: Disease Process ☐ Medications ☐ ADL Training ☐ Treatments ☐ Equipment/Supplies ☐ Diabetes ☐

  Long Term Venous Cath/Dialysis Cath ☐ Diet ☐ Other ☐ _____

Barriers to Teaching: _____

DISCHARGE PLAN

Goal: Discharge: Home, Self-Care per Patient ☐ Home, Care Provided by Significant Other ☐ Support Needed by Home Care Agency ☐

Extended Care Facility ☐ Dependent on Response to Treatment ☐ Equipment ☐ Community Resources ☐ _____

Other _____

Referral Recommended: Soc Work ☐ HHC ☐ P.N. ☐ Medical Equip ☐ Cardiac Rehab ☐ Dietician ☐ Nurse Specialist ☐

Referral Ordered/List _____

GENERAL COMMENTS:

_____
_____
_____
_____
_____
_____
_____
_____
_____

Time Physical Assessment Completed _____ (see NCR)

SIGNATURE/TITLE_____DATE_____TIME_____

Example of a Nursing History Form Based on Sr. Callista Roy's Model.*

| Date | Time | Received From: ☐ ER ☐ _____ ☐ admitting ☐ doctor's office | VIA ☐ w/c ☐ ambulatory ☐ cart | Room | Family Physician | ☐ male ☐ female | Age |

| Temp. | | Pulse | ☐ Regular ☐ Irregular | ☐ Regular ☐ Irregular | Resp. | BP (LA) | BP (RA) | Height | Weight |

Informant: ☐ patient ☐ family member ☐ friend ☐ transfer form ☐ prior medical record / date: _____ ☐ interview per phone
☐ current ER record ☐ other _____

History and present status of chief complaint: _____
_____
_____
_____
_____
_____
_____

INTERDEPENDENCE – ROLE FUNCTION – SELF-CONCEPT

| Pain Present: ☐ no ☐ yes / location | Intensity Scale 1 (mild) – 10 (severe) | When did pain start? | How was pain managed at home? |

Allergies: (describe reaction) ☐ Medications ☐ food ☐ environment ☐ none   Allergy band on? ☐ yes ☐ N/A

PATIENT HISTORY:

No Yes
☐ ☐ Heart disease (MI, angina, CHF, arrhythmia, murmur, mitral valve prolapse, pacemaker)
☐ ☐ High Blood Pressure
☐ ☐ Stroke
☐ ☐ Respiratory (asthma, emphysema, bronchitis)
☐ ☐ Kidney (stones, infection, hemodialysis)
☐ ☐ Liver (hepatitis, mono, jaundice)
☐ ☐ Cancer
☐ ☐ Blood Disorder (bleeding, clots, anemia, phlebitis)

No Yes
☐ ☐ Blood Transfusion
☐ ☐ Diabetes
☐ ☐ Thyroid Disease
☐ ☐ Seizures/Fainting
☐ ☐ Muscle Disease
☐ ☐ Neck/Back Disorder, Arthritis
☐ ☐ Depression, Mental Illness
☐ ☐ Alcohol/Drug Abuse
☐ ☐ Communicable disease (TB, STD, ...)
☐ ☐ Other _____

Past Surgeries: ☐ none   Pt/Family Reactions to anesthesia: ☐ N/A ☐ no ☐ yes_____

Past Medical Hospitalizations: ☐ none   Recent xrays: ☐ no ☐ yes _____   Recent lab: ☐ no ☐ yes

FAMILY HEALTH HISTORY: (Check conditions that apply)   ☐ none
☐ cancer ☐ diabetes ☐ stroke ☐ high blood pressure ☐ heart disease ☐ muscle disease ☐ other _____

Medications: (prescription, O.T.C., recreational) Include dose and frequency.   Admission Nurse, note time last dose taken.
☐ None
_____
_____
_____

Are medications taken as prescribed: ☐ yes ☐ no ☐ N/A

Home Situation: (marital status, children, significant others, living environment – stairs, etc.)

NSG-001   **Admission Nursing Assessment** (page 1)   UVMC 3/88
                                                                                Rev. 3/92

* Used with permission from Upper Valley Medical Centers, Piqua, Oh.

Occupation:

Social History: (education, special learning needs, religion, hobbies)

Utililzation of community resources: ☐ no ☐ home care ☐ hospice ☐ Meals on Wheels ☐ church group ☐ support groups ☐ other_____

Personal Concerns: _____

Do you have any religious special requests? ☐ no ☐ yes_____

Emotional Status: ☐ calm ☐ anxious ☐ angry ☐ quiet ☐ talkative ☐ sad ☐ agitated ☐ other_____

Life changes in past 1-2 years? ☐ none ☐ change in health ☐ new baby ☐ marriage / divorce ☐ death someone close

☐ job / business related change ☐ other _____

Do you feel you deal successfully with stress? ☐ yes ☐ no ☐ depends on circumstance Describe:

NEUROLOGICAL

Mental Status: ☐ alert ☐ oriented ☐ disoriented ☐ restless ☐ drowsy ☐ unresponsive ☐ memory loss

☐ other _____

Speech: ☐ clear ☐ slurred ☐ garbled ☐ aphasic ☐ hoarse ☐ barriers/ foreign language_____

2	3	4	5	6	7	8	9	+ Reactive
								- Nonreactive
								± Sluggish

Right Eye:_____ -mm_____ Left Eye:_____ -mm_____

Ability to Move Extremities to Command
0 (no movement) 1 (weak) 2 (strong)

RA: LA: RL: LL:

SENSES

Vision Impairment: ☐ no ☐ yes ☐ glasses / contacts ☐ artificial eye ☐ cataracts ☐ glaucoma ☐ blind ☐ R ☐ L

Hearing Impairment: ☐ no ☐ yes partial deaf ☐ R ☐ L total deaf ☐ R ☐ L hearing aid ☐ R ☐ L

ACTIVITY / REST

Sleep: (Usual time of day and hours) _____

Sleep problems: ☐ none ☐ unrested after sleep ☐ insomnia ☐ nightmares ☐ other_____

SELF-CARE ABILITY (Check appropriate column)

ACTIVITY	0	1	2	3	4	5
Eating / Drinking						
Bathing						
Dressing / Grooming						
Toileting						
Bed mobility						
Transferring						
Ambulating						
Stair Climbing						
Shopping						
Cooking						
Home Maintenance						

0 - Independent
1 - Assistive Device
2 - Assistance from person
3 - Assistance from person & equipment
4 - Dependent/ unable
5 - Change in last week

FALL RISK EVALUATION

Age <3 or >75	10 points	
Confused and disoriented, hallucinating, senile	15 points	
History of falls	15 points	
Recent history of loss of consciousness, seizure disorder	15 points	
Unsteady on feet / amputation	10 points	
Poor eyesight	5 points	
Poor hearing	5 points	
Drug / alcohol problem, sedatives	5 points	
Postop condition / sedated	5 points	
Language barrier	5 points	
Attitude (resistant, belligerent, combative, fearful)	10 points	
Postural hypotension	5 points	
15 or more indicates risk Fall precautions started: ☐ yes ☐ no	TOTAL POINTS =	

Fall Band on ☐

Assistive Devices: ☐ none ☐ crutches ☐ bedside commode ☐ walker ☐ cane ☐ splint / brace ☐ wheelchair ☐ prosthesis

☐ other _____

Activity Tolerance: ☐ no problem ☐ weakness ☐ vertigo ☐ unsteady gait ☐ angina ☐ dyspnea ☐ dyspnea at rest

☐ other _____

Admission Nursing Assessment (page 2)

UPPER VALLEY MEDICAL CENTERS
PMMC STOUDER
ADMISSION NURSING ASSESSMENT

INSTRUCTIONS: Check all boxes that apply. For Surgical Admissions: complete white area at P.A.T. and grey area day of admission. *See Care Plan / 24 HR Nursing Assessment & Care Record. N/A-Not Applicable

OXYGENATION - SKIN INTEGRITY

Skin: ☐ Warm ☐ Hot ☐ Cool ☐ Dry ☐ Diaphoretic ☐ Clammy

Skin Color: ☐ Normal ☐ Pale ☐ Cyanotic ☐ Jaundiced ☐ Mottled ☐ Flushed

Edema: ☐ none ☐ yes / location: _____

Pedal Pulses: ☐ Present ☐ Abnormal / Explain: _____

Skin Lesions: (mark location of skin lesions by number on diagram)
☐ none ☐ scar (1) ☐ rash (2) ☐ wound or open area (3) ☐ bruise (4) ☐ incision (5) ☐ sutures / staples (6)
☐ abrasions (7) ☐ discolorations (8) ☐ other (9)
Describe: _____

Dressings: ☐ no ☐ yes / location: _____

Monitor pattern: ☐ N/A

Respirations: ☐ nonlabored ☐ labored ☐ rapid ☐ shallow

Heart sounds: ☐ audible ☐ abnormal

Cough: ☐ no ☐ yes ☐ non-productive ☐ productive / color: _____

Oxygen: ☐ no ☐ yes - method / amt.: _____

Tobacco Use: ☐ no ☐ yes / type: _____
_____ pkg./day x _____ years

Breath Sounds: ☐ clear ☐ abnormal / describe: _____

RISK PREDICTORS FOR SKIN BREAKDOWN

BRADEN SCALE

	1	2	3	4	
SENSORY PERCEPTION	1. COMPLETELY LIMITED	2. VERY LIMITED	3. SLIGHTLY LIMITED	4. NO IMPAIRMENT	
MOISTURE	1. CONSTANTLY MOIST	2. VERY MOIST	3. OCCASIONALLY MOIST	4. RARELY MOIST	
ACTIVITY	1. BEDFAST	2. CHAIRFAST	3. WALKS OCCASIONALLY	4. WALKS FREQUENTLY	
MOBILITY	1. COMPLETELY IMMOBILE	2. VERY LIMITED	3. SLIGHTLY LIMITED	4. NO LIMITATIONS	
NUTRITION	1. VERY POOR	2. PROBABLY INADEQUATE	3. ADEQUATE	4. EXCELLENT	
SHEAR & FRICTION	1. PROBLEM	2. POTENTIAL PROBLEM	3. NO APPARENT PROBLEM		

Score of 16 or less indicates that patient is a risk. Refer to SKIN CARE DECISION TREE. **TOTAL**

ELIMINATION

Abdomen: ☐ soft ☐ firm ☐ distended / girth _____ ☐ non-distended ☐ tender / location: _____

Bowel Sounds: ☐ present ☐ absent Last BM / color / character: _____

Bowel Pattern: ☐ diarrhea ☐ constipation ☐ blood in stool ☐ hemorrhoids
☐ no problem ☐ incontinence ☐ laxative / enema Use/List: _____

Bladder Pattern: ☐ burning ☐ nocturia (No. times/night) ☐ difficulty starting flow ☐ frequency
☐ no problem ☐ incontinence - ☐ total ☐ daytime ☐ night time ☐ occasional ☐ urgency ☐ hematuria

Drainage Tubes: ☐ none ☐ indwelling catheter (1) ☐ intermittant catheterization (2) _____ ☐ N/G (3) ☐ G-tube (4)
☐ chest tube (5) ☐ T-tube (6) ☐ penrose (7) ☐ ostomy (8) type: _____
☐ other (9) _____
Describe Drainage: _____

LYTES - NUTRITION

Current Diet/Restrictions: ☐ Regular Is diet followed: ☐ yes ☐ no Last fluid / food intake: _____ Appetite: ☐ good ☐ fair ☐ poor

Recent weight change last 6 months: ☐ no ☐ yes / describe: _____

Fluid Intake: ☐ restricted ☐ 0 - 5 glasses / day ☐ 5 - 10 glasses / day ☐ > 10 glasses / day

☐ Caffeine use: Amt. _____ ☐ Alcohol use: Type/Amt. _____

Eating disorders: ☐ none ☐ nausea ☐ emesis ☐ chewing / swallowing difficulty ☐ sore mouth ☐ taste alterations ☐ mouth ulcer
☐ indigestion ☐ ulcer ☐ mouth-white patches ☐ erythema ☐ other

Dentures: ☐ no ☐ yes / ☐ upper: ☐ full ☐ partial ☐ lower: ☐ full ☐ partial ☐ caps ☐ bridges ☐ loose teeth ☐ retainer ☐ crowns

IV: ☐ no ☐ yes – solution - rate - site - cath no. _____ ☐ IML ☐ vascular access device

Admission Nursing Assessment (page 3)

ADMISSION NURSING ASSESSMENT

ENDOCRINE

☐ N/A	Last Menstrual Period	Problems: ☐ none ☐ abnormal bleeding ☐ breast lump history ☐ vaginal drainage ☐ other ☐ breast feeding	Breast self-exam done: ☐ no ☐ yes Frequency:
	Pap smear requested during hospitalization: ☐ no ☐ yes* *See sticker on front of chart		Last Pap Exam:

☐ N/A Last Rectal Exam   Rectal exam requested during hospitalization: ☐ no ☐ yes*
*see sticker on front chart

Concerns about current or future effects of illness / surgery / treatment on:
☐ appearance ☐ male / female roles ☐ other _____

DISCHARGE PLANNING

What do you know about your present illness? _____

What information do you want or need about your illness? _____

How long do you expect to be in the hospital? _____

What concerns do you have about leaving the hospital? _____

What are your discharge plans? ☐ home ☐ home nurse ☐ nursing home ☐ other (specify)_____

Plans stated by ☐ pt. ☐ other _____

ANTICIPATED DISCHARGE NEEDS ASSESSMENT (Check appropriate discharge needs)

☐ Health Related Teaching	☐ Assistance with Daily Living ☐ eating ☐ drinking ☐ bathing ☐ dressing ☐ bed mobility ☐ transferring ☐ ambulating ☐ toileting ☐ stair climbing ☐ grooming	☐ Mental Health Evaluation Services	☐ Medical Supplies and Equipment(O_2 wound care, os-tomy, ambulation aids, hospital bed, etc.)
☐ Financial Assistance		☐ Assistance with Home Maintainance ☐ Shopping ☐ Meal Preparation ☐ Housekeeping ☐ Meals on Wheels	
☐ Transportation Assistance	☐ Inadequate Support Systems to Provide Care		

Referrals to: ☐ none ☐ dietician ☐ diabetes nurse ☐ infection control ☐ Enterostomal Nurse ☐ social service
☐ home health agency ☐ chaplain ☐ other_____

Person identified to help after discharge: _____

Discharge planning needs discussed with: ☐ pt. ☐ other / specify: _____

Emergency phone numbers: 1. _____ 2. _____

Additional Comments _____

☐ N/A   Durable Power of Attorney: ☐ yes   Living Will: ☐ yes   Physician Notified: ☐ yes

TEACHING

ADMISSION Day Teaching: Check boxes when instruction has been given to the patient/significant other

TO BE COMPLETED ON ALL PATIENTS:
☐ general description of unit
☐ nurse call control
☐ electric bed
☐ phone ☐ TV ☐ newspaper
☐ electrical equipment from home

☐ smoking policy
☐ visitor policy
☐ siderail - reason
☐ identification bracelet on
☐ Pt. Ed. Channel

TO BE COMPLETED ON PATIENTS AS APPLICABLE:
☐ pain medication request(s)
☐ activity orders - reason
☐ NPO/fluid restriction - reason
☐ IV fluids - reason
☐ monitor

☐ guard in attendance
☐ telemetry-discuss potential room change when monitor discontinued
☐ other_____

VALUABLES

VALUABLES: It is strongly recommended that valuables are left at home. If this is not possible, valuables may be deposited in the hospital safe. If additional items are brought into the hospital after admission or items are sent home please inform the nurse.

CODE: N=None   S=Safe   R=Kept in Room   H=Sent Home

	N	S	R	H		N	S	R	H		N	S	R	H	Other
billfold					glasses					jewelry					_____
money					contact lenses					bridges-upper/lower					_____
purse					hearing aid					dentures-upper/lower					_____
wig					prosthesis					religious items					_____
					retainer					medications from home					_____

☐ I agree that this is a statement of my belongings at the time of admission and I understand that the hospital will not be responsible for anything that I choose to keep at the hospital.   ☐ I understand the above instructions concerning orientation to the hospital

Patient/Relative Signature _____   Witness _____

DATE	TIME	P.A.T. NURSE'S SIGNATURE / ER	INT		INT	DATE	TIME
				Primary Survey R.N.: _____			
NOTE: When the assessment is not completed in full by one nurse, initials must accompany entries.				Additional R.N. Signatures: _____			
				☐ N/A Report given to: _____			

Admission Nursing Assessment (page 4)

Assessment Tools for the Family Client

Family Assessment Tool*

Family Demographic Information

Name (first) _____ (middle) _____ (last) _____

      (maiden name) _____

SS# _____ Address _____

_____

Telephone (home) (____) _____ (work) (____) _____

Contact of client (name) _____ (tele) (____) _____

DOB _____ Age _____ Race _____ Marital status _____

Military experience _____

Travel outside of U.S. _____

Occupation(s) (usual) _____ (current) _____

Average number of hours worked per day _____ Usual work days _____

Job satisfaction _____

Past occupations _____

If not currently employed, would you like to be? _____

Communication: English.   Understands _____ Speaks _____ Writes _____ Reads _____

Other language _____

Source of client payment for care _____

Means of transportation to health care facility _____

Information collected from (client) _____ (other source) _____

if other, degree of contact with client _____

*From Ross B and Cobb K: *Family nursing: a nursing process approach,* Menlo Park, Calif., 1990, Addison-Wesley. Used with permission.

Nurse's comments: _____

_____

_____

Date _____ Signature _____

Chief Complaint/Reason for Visit _____

_____

_____

Present Health of Family Members: _____

_____

_____

Past Health History of Family Members:

Vision _____

Hearing _____

Childhood diseases _____

Injuries _____

Surgeries _____

Hospitalization _____

Major illness _____

Allergies _____

Immunizations _____

Habits _____

    smoker _____ alcohol _____

    caffeine _____ hard drugs _____

Medications

    OTC _____

    Rx _____

Family History

Client and/or family member (clarify all "yes")

Disease	Yes	No	Comments
allergies	_____	_____	_____
tuberculosis	_____	_____	_____
hypertension	_____	_____	_____
heart disease	_____	_____	_____
diabetes	_____	_____	_____
cancer	_____	_____	_____
gallbladder	_____	_____	_____
kidney disease	_____	_____	_____
liver disease	_____	_____	_____
anemia	_____	_____	_____
thyroid	_____	_____	_____

Thrombosis _____ _____ _____

hyperlipidemia _____ _____ _____

uterine fibroids _____ _____ _____

STD _____ _____ _____

emotional illness _____ _____ _____

genetic disease _____ _____ _____

congenital _____ _____ _____

Obstetrical History _____

_____

Menstrual History _____

_____

Sexual History _____

_____

Interpersonal Relationships

Names and ages of family members _____

_____

Roles of members _____

_____

Previous marriage(s) _____

Housing _____

_____

Community _____

Past/Present stressors within family unit _____

_____

_____

_____

Nurse's Comments: _____

_____

Religious/Cultural Data

Country of birth _____ Spouse's country of birth _____

Customs, health belief, values of culture _____

_____

Folk medicine _____

Spiritual belief system _____

_____

Spiritual/cultural influence on health care decisions _____

_____

_____

Psychosocial Data

ADL:

exercise _____

leisure _____

nutrition _____

sleep _____

Income source _____

Educational level _____

Cognitive abilities _____

Developmental data _____

Response to illness _____

_____

_____

Response to care _____

_____

_____

Support system _____

_____

Nurse's comments _____

_____

_____

Date _____ Signature _____

Additional information/comments _____

_____

_____

_____

_____

_____

_____

An Assessment Guideline for Work with Families*

The assumption is made that each person and family is characterized by rhythmic developmental sequences which are constantly patterning/re-patterning in mutual simultaneous interaction with the environment. Because these dimensions are essentially boundaryless, there will appear to be some overlap

I. The Individual Sub-System Considerations
   A. Developmental
      1. Past developmental history of parents and children
         a. Parents' physical and emotional health at time of establishment of the family unit continuing into present time
         b. Developmental landmarks, i.e., age specific tasks, and physical growth for each person
         c. General psychosexual developmental considerations of members
         d. History of life traumas
         e. Present level of functioning of each member in regard to developmental tasks
   B. Biological
      1. General state of the physical health of each member
      2. Past and present difficulties and care
      3. Past and present physical level of functioning including motor skills, etc.
      4. Genetic factors affecting level of functioning
   C. Psychological
      1. General state of emotional health and psychological growth
      2. Past and present problems including care
      3. General level of functioning with regard to cognitive and affective elements
   D. Social
      1. Class and cultural factors—including types of support systems
      2. General social development of children and adults, i.e., school work and social realms
   E. The nurse as an individual (including development, values, biases, etc.)
II. Interactional Patterns
   A. Executive and sibling system relationships
      1. Clear versus breached generational levels (including inversions and exclusions)
      2. Negotiation patterns and levels
   B. Triadic and dyadic relationships
      1. Positive and negative vectors in relationships (e.g., scapegoating and favoritism)
      2. Cyclical nature of sequencing
   C. Communication patterns
      1. Clarity vs. distortions such as double messages
      2. Usual channels and modes
   D. Role relationships
      1. Role reciprocity and/or role confusion and inconsistency
      2. Complementarity and/or symmetrical patterns
      3. Ways in which intimacy is expressed
   E. Attachment patterns
      1. Commitment and detachment levels
      2. Individuation and enmeshment levels
      3. Mutuality and isolation levels
      4. Implicit and explicit expectations
III. Unique Characteristics of the Whole
   A. Family group psyche
      1. Problem-solving style; i.e., moving toward/against/away
      2. Capacity to validate reality
   B. Family mass
      1. Relative stability and/or disorganization
      2. Capacity for change, i.e., relative rigidity or flexibility

*From Whall AL: Nursing theory and the assessment of families, *J Psychiatr Nurs* 19:30-36, 1981. Reprinted with permission.

    C. Belief system
       1. Values, myths (including distortions such as sham and pseudomutuality)
       2. Rules regarding expression of beliefs
    D. Group dynamic characteristics
       1. Family power structure
       2. Leadership and problem-solving ability
       3. Cohesiveness and reference groups
       4. "Boundary" characteristics—who is allowed "in" and who is "out"
    E. Family developmental needs
       1. Maturational requirements
       2. Situational requirements
    F. Family typological actions
       1. Centripetal and/or centrifugal
       2. Open, random, or more rigid lifestyle
    G. Economic factors
       1. Distribution of income
       2. Income as related to needs
       3. Style of disbursement
IV. Environmental Interface Synchrony
    A. Developmental needs of family vs. community resources
    B. Family values as compared to community values and beliefs
    C. Requirements of community upon the family
    D. Effect of the family upon the community.

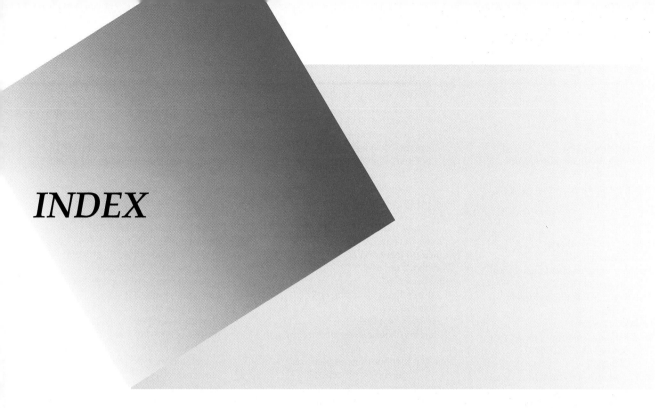

INDEX

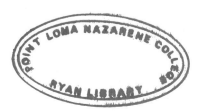